Research for Development

The series Research for Development serves as a vehicle for the presentation and dissemination of complex research and multidisciplinary projects. The published work is dedicated to fostering a high degree of innovation and to the sophisticated demonstration of new techniques or methods.

The aim of the Research for Development series is to promote well-balanced sustainable growth. This might take the form of measurable social and economic outcomes, in addition to environmental benefits, or improved efficiency in the use of resources; it might also involve an original mix of intervention schemes.

Research for Development focuses on the following topics and disciplines:

Urban regeneration and infrastructure, Info-mobility, transport, and logistics, Environment and the land, Cultural heritage and landscape, Energy, Innovation in processes and technologies, Applications of chemistry, materials, and nanotechnologies, Material science and biotechnology solutions, Physics results and related applications and aerospace, Ongoing training and continuing education.

Fondazione Politecnico di Milano collaborates as a special co-partner in this series by suggesting themes and evaluating proposals for new volumes. Research for Development addresses researchers, advanced graduate students, and policy and decision-makers around the world in government, industry, and civil society.

THE SERIES IS INDEXED IN SCOPUS

Andrea Bonarini · Serenella Besio

Robot Play for All

Developing Toys and Games for Disability

Fondazione Politecnico di Milano

Springer

Andrea Bonarini
Department of Electronics, Information and Bioengineering
Politecnico di Milano
Milan, Italy

Serenella Besio
Dipartimento di Scienze Umane e Sociali
Università degli studi di Bergamo
Bergamo, Italy

ISSN 2198-7300 ISSN 2198-7319 (electronic)
Research for Development
ISBN 978-3-031-05041-1 ISBN 978-3-031-05042-8 (eBook)
https://doi.org/10.1007/978-3-031-05042-8

This Springer imprint is published by the registered company Springer Nature Switzerland AG
The registered company address is: Gewerbestrasse 11, 6330 Cham, Switzerland

To all who love
and wish to play

Preface

This book is born to collect the experiences done in more than 10 years of development of robotic games for all, and to share them not only with the scientific community, but with all the people (caregivers, parents, makers, designers, players) that may be interested to explore this way of exploiting technology to improve the life of children with disabilities and people at large. The play experience is fundamental for everybody, and autonomous robots give the possibility to explore new ways to play where the device is no longer immaterial, but tri-dimensional enabling a relationship through the body, and no longer passive, but can actively participate in the play experience. This new dimension opens new ways of playing that rely on the real, physical world, and integrates the possibilities given by the new technologies, including Artificial Intelligence and Machine Learning.

A boost to the development of this experience has been given by the EU COST Action "LUDI: play for children with disabilities", where hundreds of people from tens of countries and different experiences and backgrounds met together to share knowledge and produce documents and books to support the development and the adoption of play as a mean to develop and integrate persons with disabilities. Some LUDI efforts were also dedicated to technology and robots and contributed to further develop the already ongoing activities in our universities.

This book is intended as a reference both to what has been done up to now in many contexts and countries, and to what could be done by exploiting the technology on the basis of a deeper knowledge of the users' needs. Together with a strong background on play, disability, and technology, many experiences are reported to make aware of issues and potential solutions, with the aim of giving all the stakeholders at least a good introduction to the many possibilities to develop robot-based play activities. What is presented here considers persons with disabilities, but it is valid for any situation where robots could be used to play, and it aims at supporting the development of inclusive play experiences that anybody can enjoy.

Milan, Italy
October 2022

Andrea Bonarini
Serenella Besio

Acknowledgements

We would like to acknowledge the contribution of the many students of Politecnico di Milano from Computer Engineering, Design, Bio-engineering, Mechanical Engineering, and Automation that have developed in the years many of the robots and play experiences we report in the book. Many others could not be included but contributed to the knowledge now shared within the Playbot4all[1] initiative at Politecnico di Milano.

We would also like to thank the many centres that accepted to test the developed prototypes and participate in the definition of specifications and in the evaluation of the prototypes, as well as their assistance that contributed to make the developers understand what they really needed and what they had liked to do.

The many figures that participated in the EU COST Action "LUDI: play for children with disability" generously shared their competencies and collaborated to frame a powerful set of practices that we wish will be spread as much as possible.

We would like to thank also colleagues and all the ones that contributed to the activities here reported, providing their invaluable support.

Last but not least, we would like to thank all the ones that supported us in the realization of this book with patience and competence.

[1] http://playbot4all.polimi.it.

Contents

Chapter 1
Introduction

Andrea Bonarini and Serenella Besio

Abstract What is the role of robots in defining playing activities, and in particular playing activities for all, where persons with different abilities can play and interact with each other thanks to the presence of a robot? Play is one of the basic activities people and most animals use to develop abilities and skills. The aim of this book is to frame the relevant aspects of playing with robots so as to provide foundations for a structured analysis of what has been so far presented in literature and experimented, and for an informed design of the huge amount of new playing experiences that could be implemented.

1.1 Background

What is the role of robots in defining playing activities, and in particular playing activities for all, where persons with different abilities can play and interact with each other thanks to the presence of a robot? Play is one of the basic activities people and most animals use to develop abilities and skills. In the last years, many robots are becoming affordable for the mass market, and they are beginning to become part of the set of devices present in many homes, schools, social, and care centres. From one side, toy companies have innovated their tradition and introduced animated, reacting toys on the mass market. On the other side, researchers, supported also by technological developments and the attitudes induced by the makers' movement, have brought robots also outside the production plants, into the society. As part of this global movement, robots started to introduce activities also involving persons with disabilities and the innovative possibility to interact with an artificial device, properly programmed.

Research on play in the last decades has developed constructs and approaches to frame the concept of play and drive the development of focused experiences and informed activities. This research has been developed mostly in areas related to Humanities, such as Psychology, Philosophy, Learning Sciences, and Sociology. From the technological standpoint, pushed by the success of videogames, research on games has involved Engineers, Computer Scientists, and Designers, who focused on the mechanics of games to obtain products that could have success on the market.

A. Bonarini and S. Besio, *Robot Play for All*, Research for Development,
https://doi.org/10.1007/978-3-031-05042-8_1

The two communities developed different approaches to study and develop play activities, with relatively few contact points.

In particular, within the technology-oriented community developing robots for persons with disabilities, there are tendencies to produce robotic games and playful activities, but there is often a lack of a methodological approach in the development and in the evaluation of the play experiences.

However, both areas—Humanities and Technology— share a common trend: instead of considering play as a scientific phenomenon "per se", they look at it as a particular, curious, and significant, activity within which other skills are expressed, manifested, and developed. Therefore, play is mainly treated as a useful context for carrying out research, development, education, and rehabilitation, through the identification and realization of objectives: for instance, cognitive growth, social learning, functional improvement, and emotional and psychological wellness.

For what concerns disability, this trend is mainly due to the fact that rehabilitation gains and functional advancements are permanently and predominantly addressed, mainly in the case of children. It is indispensable and desirable that societies focus on improving the functioning of individuals, through the progress of medicine, rehabilitation, and clinical disciplines in general including health technology, but it is equally necessary that a firm, convinced emphasis be placed on the role that societies play in defining the life conditions of persons with disabilities as well as in shaping their disability: this concerns not only macro-areas, such as policies, systems, and services but also meso- and micro-areas, such as the concrete contexts of life that are available, with their materials, technologies, people and relationships, knowledge, and attitudes.

Studying and developing new solutions to enable children with disabilities to play better, more satisfactorily, more autonomously, and more happily, is a goal that can be pursued and even achieved now, in a situated way, by adopting the right approach. This approach can only be multidisciplinary because children are extraordinary recipients of the facets that compose them, and of their life contexts; if we aim to propose and develop play experiences that could have a real meaning for them, and playful attractiveness, we need to put together just like the pieces of a puzzle knowledge coming from different disciplinary areas. On two conditions, however: that the common object of interest is the play itself, for the sake of play; and that the wishes and opinions of the children themselves are carefully and systematically taken into consideration: only players can tell how they would like to play, and even if the play works, if they like the play.

One of the first attempts to go towards this line has been the EU COST Action "LUDI: play for children with disabilities"[1] (2014–2018). Hundreds of researchers with all the involved backgrounds, from tens of countries, participated for 3 years in an intense exchange of knowledge that brought to the development of materials that can be considered as a checkpoint reference for this research field.

LUDI has gathered the R&D experiences existing in the playfield together with those coming from the clinical, educational, and technical fields, and, at the same

[1] http://www.ludi-network.eu.

time, it has strengthened among participants higher awareness about the importance of this topic. Three autonomous areas of research have been established, which refer to the main domains of the WHO ICF classification [764, 765]: disability (types of impairment, functional characteristics); play (definition, types and characteristics, evaluation, rights); environmental factors (not only technologies, relationships, play activities, and scenarios but also policies and rights); a fourth has been devoted to exploring and collecting the voice of children themselves. This highlighted how the possibilities and abilities to play are the results of a positive encounter between the functioning of the child's body and the opportunities offered for him/her to be active and to participate in social life, by virtue of the quality and effectiveness of contextual factors.

Due to the differences between the cultures and socio-political systems of the members of the network, it was needed to share a common working background, and the assumption of the ICF model in its systemic and ecological complexity has at the same time constituted a challenge and an achievement for the LUDI work.

The activities were coordinated by four working groups (WGs) from dedicated Task Forces; one of them—that gathered technicians, electronic and robotics engineers, designers, occupational therapists, toy experts, and psychologists—was devoted to the accessibility and usability of technologies and tools for play; it created a database of dedicated assistive technologies as well as a systematic review of existing guidelines in the field.

LUDI has produced seven books, a special issue in an international journal, and two training schools, where a training model, based on a multidisciplinary and participatory approach, has been first tested and then validated. During the schools, influenced also by the experience of "Hackability", a certain number of children presented their own "play dream" to a small multidisciplinary group of experts, that in some days presented a prototype of toy per each participant, ready to be tested.

LUDI aimed to produce an impact in both the scientific and social fields. Its multidisciplinarity has attracted the expertise and enthusiasm not only of researchers from many fields but also of politicians and business representatives. The convergence towards a single definition of play has highlighted the inaccuracy of previous constructs and proved useful for advancing research in the sector, increasing the comparability and transferability of the results.

The concept of "play for the sake of play" invited: (a) clinicians to abandon the primacy of rehabilitation objectives and to rediscover, behind the disability, the child with her rights; (b) robotic engineers and technicians, to rethink design from a playful rather than rehabilitative perspective and also to specialize it according to the various, different, types of play; (c) educators and professionals, to make a clear separation between playful and play-like activities in their work.

The adoption of the inclusive approach has highlighted: (a) the importance of playing with peers; (b) the rediscovery of the adult's role as mediator and scaffolder in the playful situation; (c) the importance of evaluating the usability of toys; (d) the search for new products capable of favouring it.

The critical analysis of existing knowledge in the technical field has led to widen the study also to (a) the accessibility of structures, contexts, and play tools; (b) the accessibility and usability of technologies and toys.

This book lies in the track traced by LUDI, putting together the experiences of two scholars coming from the two souls related to play: the Coordinator of LUDI, Serenella Besio, professor of Special Pedagogy at the University of Bergamo, Italy, and Andrea Bonarini, co-coordinator of the technology working group of LUDI, professor of Artificial Intelligence and of Robotics and Design, and Coordinator of the AI and Robotics Lab at Politecnico di Milano.

Although play is an activity that can be performed by anybody, and actually it is, this book focuses mostly on children, both because the largest part of research on play and robot play is oriented towards children, and because the experiences done in LUDI and before by the authors were mostly centred on children. However, many of the general considerations contained in this book are valid also for play activities oriented to the whole population, with and without disabilities.

1.2 Aims

This book aims, through the analysis of the many related aspects, to develop a framework to support the design of playful experiences with robots for all.

We would like to provide frameworks to access in a structured way the research done so far in the field, including contributions that concern different aspects, from the more physical and technological, to the more related to the design of playful activities and to disability. This is intended to become a reference for designers, researchers, and operators in clinical and educational fields to implement successful playing activities that could exploit the possibilities that a robot gives.

Examples of these robots are presented and analysed, coming both from market and research.

1.3 Structure

The book starts from the definition of "play", "toy", and "game", putting in evidence their values for everybody, and, in particular, for persons with disabilities. A strong background on the research about the play topic is provided in the first part, discussing the related issues and open problems. The relationship between play and disabilities and the role that play can have with persons with disabilities are also discussed considering different types of impairments and the relative issues. Characteristics of play activities and tools are matched with the role that play can have in the development of persons with disabilities, to provide a reference and a framework to analyse what has been done with robots in the field, and what it could be done considering the relevant aspects of play. The analysis carried out first makes evident the vastness of studies connected to the theme of play, with all its facets, and highlights the elements of uncertainty not yet resolved. Moreover, it declines the theme of play in relation to the most common types of disabilities, trying both to indicate the functional limitations that should be considered to design any activity or product in the field, and the possible directions to circumvent them or to facilitate their overcoming.

In the second part, the role of robots in playing activities is analysed, focusing on the many aspects that should be considered to design a playful robot, including, among others: shape, materials, interaction, abilities, and behaviours. The design of a robot should consider the playing activities where it is possible to exploit its unique characteristics, such as the possibility to act and react to signals, in order to offer interesting experiences. These play activities should be designed to engage the players even when they have special needs, which are considered when discussing how robots can be used for this task.

Then, having set a framework that includes all the aspects relevant for the design of playing activities, in Part III some robots present on the market and others developed in research labs (including the ones developed at Politecnico di Milano—AI and Robotics Lab in more than ten years) are analysed along the defined dimensions, to make evident what has been done till now, and what could be done in the next future. Selected examples are provided to show the variety of possibilities, while pointers to the rich literature may support the interested reader to go deeper into this "white rabbit hole". The introduction of robots in playful activities with persons with disabilities may also raise ethical, social, and psychological issues that are discussed in a dedicated chapter, together with possible measures to reduce their impact. From all this material, open issues, research directions, and possibilities for new developments are finally envisioned.

Although there is a strong orientation in considering robotic play activities accessible for persons with disabilities, the presented frameworks and solutions may be interesting for everybody; in most cases, the developed play activities have successfully involved both persons with and without disabilities, since play is for all, any age, any ability: everyone likes to play.

Part I
Inclusive Play

This part is dedicated to frame the concept of play in general and its relationship with disability. The point of view of different authors is provided, putting in evidence the different types of play, their role in developing abilities, and the possibilities that persons with disabilities may have to exploit inclusive play.

This part is aimed at building a background and a reference framework for the different aspects of play that will be used as a reference in the rest of the book, and that will play a relevant role for further developments. The huge research efforts spent on play, and on its relationship with disability, are often confined in the Humanities area, while their results and methodologies would be an important resource for the development of new approaches also based on new technologies.

Chapter 2
Play and Games

Serenella Besio

Abstract What is play? Philosophers, psychologists, sociologists, designers, and computer scientists have given definitions trying to capture the essence of this activity that has been recognized as an essential component of the development process of people (and animals). We present the different definitions and the different types of playful activities and games, as they have been classified, along different dimensions, in structured frameworks. We put in evidence the role of play in the people development process and the accessibility conditions of each type of play activity.

2.1 Introduction: Impregnability of Pay

Play is an endless and inexhaustible topic of study that has aroused interest in researchers since the past centuries, proposing interpretations that are never stable rather always evolving. It is in fact as broad, complex, elusive, impregnable, astonishing as concrete play activities are. In his fascinating picture of the topic, Eberle underlines that "play is a roomy subject, broad in human experience, rich and various over time and place" [228]:214. It is especially typical of childhood, but it appears at any age of the individual's life and of the human history, occurring in every geographical area and in every culture. It does not belong only to human beings, but also to animals.

However, play changes during the child's development, acquiring over time different forms that have been interpreted, by various authors, as "stages" or as "types". These typologies do not remain stainless stable, but rather intertwine the one with the other, become more complex, acquiring new meanings and requiring new competences. In this way, play develops, covers all ages, changes constantly but also always remain the same, as if it implied a deep core that never changes and makes it self-evident, different from any other human activity.

Play is intrinsically rich in contradictions and welcomes opposites: it can be free or fixed by shared rules, it can adopt an active or a passive form—the actor and the spectator. It can be solitary or social without losing fun; children who seemingly play alone are rather playing with an imaginary partner, while gamers may play together at a distance on the Internet without ever meeting in person. In addition, the same

A. Bonarini and S. Besio, *Robot Play for All*, Research for Development,
https://doi.org/10.1007/978-3-031-05042-8_2

actions are perceived as wearisome and unpleasant if performed out of obligation or duty, and as amusing or desirable if done for fun: should we conclude that play "can be a matter of degree, too?" [228]:215.

Play has also been defined as ambiguous [686], it hides its secrets to the most attentive observer and to the most sophisticated researcher. On the other hand, everybody feels expert in play, for having been a child and having played, and everybody knows the feelings it may produce: happiness, getting lost, suspension of reality. We all blissfully experienced its contradictions: rigid rules and uncontrolled fantasy, absolute concentration and total lightness, symmetry and order, rapidly turning into chaos and disorder [333].

Within these antinomies lies the human experience of play, a frustrating dichotomy that is always resolved through action. This duality is so deeply rooted in the phenomenon of play that Sutton-Smith [687] based his last "theory of play" on it, called "coevolutionary multiplex of functions". And this was 10 years after his famous analysis of the *Ambiguity of Play*, in which he described the "seven rhetorics" that led play scholars to create insuperable barriers.[1] "And since play could not be decoupled from its rhetorics, the subject itself remained deeply ambiguous" [228]:219. Although complex, play is always loaded of value, correlated to the spirit of the time, connected to the practices—educational, clinical—and to the contexts in which it is carried out. It "contains multiple patterns of meaning over time experienced differently by players participating in the same play episode and by any other person observing the play phenomena" [373]:400. This fluidity of interpretations is also reflected in language: in English, "the word appears as a transitive and intransitive verb, as a noun, and as an adjective. [It] describes actions, the lack of action, and attitudes. The definitions encompass both causes and effects. When coupled with other words, play conveys a surprising assortment of meanings" [228]:217.[2]

Play is also peculiar for being a unique, unrepeatable area of life that was clearly identified as a "frame" by Gregory Bateson [48]. "Play enactments can be said to happen within the play frame and the negotiations or disputes outside a frame; together, they form a complex, multi-layered whole" [373]:400. We immediately recognize the possibility to enter this frame, when the gleam in the gaze of a child invites us,[3] even without words, to play. "Then, in a moment, the adult feels like a child again, and those sensations come back alive, real, unchanged over time. In some happy cases, that gleam in the eyes of those who accept or launch a playful provocation can also be encountered in an elderly person, reviving the liveliness of childhood time" [68].

---

[1] They are progress, fate, power, identity, imaginary, self, frivolity [686].

[2] "To play on words is to manipulate them, to play off is to react to, to play with is to join or to manipulate, to play out is to follow through. To play up is to step up to the plate with teeth gritted. To play down is to minimize. To play 'possum' is to disguise yourself. To play it cool is to chill out" (Murray, Bradley, Craigie, Onions, (eds.) Oxford English Dictionary, 1970, 972–77).

[3] This very distinctive gleam is a real signal, spread among humans but culturally sensitive, to invite starting a play session. It is totally akin to the "play bow" of dogs, wolves, and other canids and to the "play face" of primates [141].

Tackling the issue of play is neither easy nor trivial; it demands structural and scientific choices and requires caution and depth. In what follows a short overview of play is proposed, according to the various disciplines dealing with it, collected into four sections on play: its nature, its functions, its characteristics, its definitions. In facing this challenge, this work will be inspired by Sutton-Smith who "encouraged researchers to retain the spirit of play in the study of it, enjoy the process, and stay always creatively open to its mysteries and ambiguities" [373]:401.

2.2 The Nature of Play

In spite of the studies developed over the centuries, the numerous interpretations proposed, and the natural evolution of the play itself as an activity, yet "its nature and function remain contested" [652]:1. Contemporary studies of play are mainly located in the literature of the 70s and the 80s of the last century; in recent years, a renewed interest has arisen on the area, with greater awareness on its complexity; to reach a comprehensive understanding of it, knowledge from different disciplines must be connected and intermingled: evolutionary biology, neuroscience, philosophical and psycho-educational sciences, anthropology, sociology, cultural, and media studies [652] but also, mainly today, technology, and robotics.

2.2.1 Anthropology: Times and Geographies

The origin of play is lost in the mists of time. It seems to belong to the human species since the very beginning. We can consider the primitives' paintings in the caves as a first expression of playfulness, as well as their use of propitiatory masks highlighted in the rock engravings (dating up to 30,000 years ago).

The oldest known toy—a parallelepiped in clay with round recesses—was found in Bulgaria, dating back to the 5th millennium BC [68]. Egyptians made dolls from cloth or majolica, as well as wooden or stone toys, while Romans made sweets in the form of letters and invented games involving imitation and comparison. Toys were usually buried in children's graves among the Sumerians, the Egyptians, the Greeks, and the Romans [23, 481]).

Literature in the fields of education, pedagogy, and anthropology is rich in publications concerning toys, which have characterized the various periods of human life and help to outline a picture of the society and culture of their time. *Toys as culture* is one of the most authoritative books by Brian Sutton-Smith [685], in this line of research. Studies also exist about cultural documents that testify the life of childhood over the centuries, through the representation of their toys. Paintings, such as the renown *Children's Games* of Pieter Bruegel the Elder (1560) and other ones of the same era, have been analysed and discussed [555]:281 to draw clues about everyday life, dominant ideas of childhood, community, time.[4]

Like everything related to play, the world of toys is constantly changing; today, the technological products and games represent a salient element, and they demand a socio-anthropological change in the sector, because they may imply consequences in various aspects of play, not only in the infant area.

This universality of play over time might be only apparent, however fascinating; in fact, it mainly refers to studies addressed to the Western society. For example, play in foraging societies—populations "managing to maintain the oldest way of living on Earth despite constant pressures [...] to give up their autonomy" [107]:302, interesting for their similarity to first human communities—offers the opportunity to study "how play may underpin the social development of the [typical] unique set of cultural traits" (ibidem). Children's play of these populations shows the same characteristics of "civilized" ones: it is based on imitation "of the values, ideas, practices, and material culture they see around them in their culture" [107]:316, it assumes the forms of work-pretence play, adopts ritual forms, and includes creative elements. Differently from other children, these ones are much more autonomous in their play, their games are mostly non-competitive, they trust themselves and their group; perhaps, predictably, their exploration mainly concerns nature and is less pre-prepared by humans. Moreover, the idea proposed by Gray [299] that these societies are "suffused with play", with children free to play all day—thus potentially resulting in suppressing dominance and enacting a great degree of social cooperation and sharing—is not supported by Boyette, who did not find in his observations such a liberty to play nor a diffused social sense of playfulness. He warns against the "romantic" idea that "play leads to egalitarianism. Play among foragers [...] also facilitates learning subsistence skills, ethnobotanical knowledge, how to share, and so on. Additionally, play in other societies contribute to learning inequality and competition" [107]:315. And he concludes: "Play universally serves, as it does in other species, as a psychological state that opens body and mind to learning behaviours and cognitive orientations that are of use in the environment in which a child lives" [107]:316.

Analogous conclusions have been drawn by authors working on the play present in indigenous communities: since play activities "mirror and reinterpret the surrounding culture" [295]:367, they also include changes due to the contact with the more "civilized" community. Anyway, some authors [565] suggest that direct contact with nature might be responsible of their deep respect for the environment, but give them also the capacity to "face the challenges and risks offered by the physical environment in their free and unsupervised daily play activities" [295]:367.

An original point of view on the influence exerted by the surrounding culture and values on play development and its concrete realization is provided by a study on Confucian territories [378]. The traditional Confucian values (benevolence, righteous-

[4] To testify the historical-cultural importance of keeping trace of the artefacts and forms of play, numerous museums of toys exist in Europe and in the rest of the world, addressed to various categories and to different purposes.

ness, courteousness, wisdom, filial piety, self-restraint), addressed to instil harmony and collaboration in reciprocal relationships, gave high importance to children's education and academic success, and depreciated the value of play, considered a waste of time compared to the hard work of learning. For this reason, "in traditional Confucian societies [children] were typically less involved in free, independent or exploratory play. [...] They were implicitly expected to be ideal and play harmoniously with others" [378]:349.

With recent globalization, teachers became interested in the Western idea of play as a learning experience, while overall values shifted towards independence, parallel status, insubordination. Families consider now play as a reward, and at the same time many play objects, environments and styles of the Western societies are introduced in these countries.[5] In addition, some play, especially media and technological play, are "now being used as an agentic venue for children to go beyond the 'Confucian shadow'" [641]:353. Paradoxically, the authors note, today in these cultures "children have become more immersed in structured and subject-specific education play, with much less free time to be involved in outdoor, collaborative and group play" [641]:354 that, even if adult controlled, was anyway proposed in more traditional times.

2.2.2 *From Ethology to Neuroscience*

The awareness that not only humans, but other animal species are able to play is considered a proof in favour of the hypothesis that play is—at least partially—an innate competence.[6] Play probably originated in the first mammals, at least 70 million years ago [146]. Today researchers agree that it probably belongs not only to mammals, but also to all vertebrate classes as well to some social insects, such as wasps [206]. Pointedly Burghardt [140, 141] has done prominent research and established important milestones in the field, such as the proposal of a definition of play,[7] as well as the discussion about "the evolutionary, developmental, functional, causal and experiential aspects of play [that may] differ considerably" [143]:10. After examination of the three major theories of the nineteenth century about the

[5] Singer et al. [641] conducted a study involving 2.400 children from North and South America, Africa, Europe, and Asia in which they demonstrated that the major free time activity for children was watching television.

[6] "Because other mammals play, it is exceedingly unlikely that this talent arose spontaneously in our own species as a feature of our exclusive property right. Instead play is widely shared and adaptive and, in fact, has enhanced the survival of our graduating class—mammals—over the very long haul. Jaak Panksepp, the founder of the discipline of affective neuroscience, and his colleagues discovered that frisky rats laugh while they wrestle (much as we humans do) and will wither socially if deprived of play. We last shared a common ancestor with them nearly seventy-five million years ago. The antiquity of play only deepens the sense of play as both fundamental and necessary" [228]:227. The author's reference here is at: Panksepp, J. (2004). *Affective Neuroscience: The Foundations of Human and Animal Emotions, Oxford University Press.*

[7] See Sect. 2.5.

origins of play, he created an innovative synthesis capable of providing a convincing interpretative outline of the evolution of play.

The first is Spencer's surplus energy theory [656], according to which the parental care of "advanced" mammals towards youth is the causal origin of play, because it gives them "the metabolic energetic reserves enabling them to blow off excess energy through apparently useless behaviour" [143]:14. Groos [303] elaborated on this idea within its instinct practice theory, by proposing that "carefree youth allowed animals to perfect the skills they would later need for survival in a relatively safe context" (ibidem). The third one, the recapitulation theory,[8] was proposed by Hall (1904), arguing that play, especially in humans, could be explained as a recapitulation of behaviour from ancestral stages that reproduce the development of the species itself [337]:367.

All these theories have been criticized, dismissed, and also pilloried; surprisingly, Burghardt, adopting "an ecumenical approach to the work of these thoughtful pioneers [...], combined their insights into a broad-scale theoretical approach, [the] surplus resource theory", which includes "diverse behavioural repertoire and parental care": behavioural and cognitive repertoire in some vertebrates, especially mammals, may result "from a re-organization of the ontogeny of some response systems", and play may be evolved "in response to the motivational and stimulus needs of the young animals" [143].

Three processes of play have been then identified by Burghardt: the primary process play, which is not done for any adaptive scope (i.e., provoked simply "by the need or drive to be active" or by "lowered thresholds to stimuli", etc.); the secondary process play that "serves to maintain functions, such as physical fitness or sensory and motor abilities"; the tertiary process play that "truly increases an animal's competence in various domains (foraging, defensive social among others) and may even produce evolutionary and culturally important novel and innovative behaviour" [143]:15. Both the secondary and the tertiary processes can derive from the primary one, and all three belong to the repertoire of many animals, humans included. An additional and fascinating aspect of these ethological studies is the role of the process of domestication both in facilitating play and in influencing the onset of different play variants and trajectories. Burghardt et al. [142] have demonstrated differences in the ontogeny of the object play among breeds. Furthermore, humans and animals may also play together; perhaps domestication of some animals—e.g., dogs from wolves, and other species—may have played "a crucial role in human evolution" [652]:2.

Developing on these themes, Gray [300] first observes that animals at play may exhibit core elements of morality; this mainly happens in social play—i.e., among primates, dogs, etc.—where "players must control their actions to avoid hurting or frightening one other" [300]:96 and this, in turn, may enable them coexist and cooperate.

---

[8] Inspired by Haeckel (1874), according to whom ontogeny recapitulates phylogeny. This is mainly applicable to the human foetus development which shows, even in short phases, traits of other species that can be considered as ancestors.

Research on the social play of animals—mainly, rats—is today very promising for it gives the opportunity to improve knowledge on its relation with the development of brain and behaviour. Contemporary neuroscientists are interested in finding the "deep-brain mechanisms that make play possible" [337]:364. Siviy [644] and other authors demonstrated that prefrontal cortex, responsible for executive functions, is engaged in the fighting play of rats; in turn, other studies [537] confirmed that play fighting experience in the juvenile period of these animals modifies the development of these parts of the cortex, also provoking "improvements in executive functions skills and associated social competence" [143]:24.

Trezza et al. [710] propose an overview of the "neurotransmitter systems that modulate social play behaviour in rats", the most studied species in the field. In particular, after analysis of a wealth of studies, they could conclude that: opioid neurotransmission is related to "pleasurable properties", cannabinoids and noradrenaline likely influence both emotional and cognitive aspects; dopamine is implicated in motivation (ibidem). This puts into evidence that specific cerebral localizations are involved in managing play activities: localized sites, such as the nucleus accumbens and the basolateral amygdala, as well as distributed networks of prefrontal and subcortical brain structures. The authors conclude: "our understanding of how social play behaviour comes about in the brain has substantially increased in the last decade [...] but much more detailed information will be necessary to fully understand the brain mechanisms of play" [710]:40; particularly, a huge work should be done to interpret the way the different neurotransmitter systems interact in managing the play activity as well as the way the subcomponents of social play are modulated by the neural mechanisms.

The sensorimotor play—also called practice play—whose importance has always been valued by preeminent scholars,[9] today receives particular attention for its connections with the study of the child's brain development: "the early manifestations of infant play typically involve [...] the visual, sensory, and motor areas of the brain [that] are actively developing during the first year of life and [make] connections to the emotional brain centres" [61]:125.

Exactly during this phase of the child's life, it becomes possible to acknowledge that brain maturation and play development show many similar peculiar characteristics. They both involve phase shifts (with "periods of disequilibrium and recursive elements"), "move toward order, with emerging patterns of attractor states", show "sensitive dependence on initial conditions because small inputs [....] may cause disparate results", show "interdependence because all levels are interrelated [and have] both stable and dynamic alternating periods". Thus, both of them "can be characterized as [...] non-linear dynamic" systems [61]:135.[10]

---

[9] Among the others: Jean Piaget, Jerome Bruner, Eleanor Gibson, and Esther Thelen.

[10] Since sensorimotor play experience seems to be crucial, the debate on the influence of technological toys on the brain maturation as well as on play processes is open today [61], see also Sect. 2.8.

2.2.3 *Classic Theories: Philosophical and Pedagogical Conceptions*[11]

Even accepting the use of the word "classic" to define the prominent theories of their own era, yet it is difficult to choose the scholars for this very short review, whose scope is mainly to highlight, after the rise of scientific interest on the subject, the intervention of new meanings and interpretations. It is worth remembering that the conceptions briefly here reported always arise within well-defined socio-cultural and historical-geographical areas. They are closely related to the contexts where they were born and in turn contributed to their development. Since the play these authors are considering is predominantly the infantile one, every assertion always builds on contemporary ideas of childhood and of community life.

Since the ancient Greece, play has been recognized as a peculiar activity of the human being, at any age. According to Plato (428-348 BC), children between 3- and 6-y-old should spend most of their time—in a place consecrated to the gods—in free play activities, socialize with their peers, learn the social norms and rules, between fantasy and discipline. The great philosopher shows a very modern attitude, where mutual relationships of play participants naturally allow for moral growth. Aristotle (384-322 BC) distinguished play from work, because it lacks necessity, and, like virtue and happiness, is rather characterized by freedom and self-sufficiency.

Basically, however, in ancient times, play was mainly represented by the development of gymnastic and sport skills to prepare for war. In the Middle Age, in the area we call today Western countries, under the prevailing religious influence, play was considered as a possible source of moral promiscuity, and some games dangerous for moral development: thus, it was kept under control, but it was also deemed necessary to give vent to the energies—as Fénelon (1651-1715) asserts—to let the children's "great heat" escape. For him, as a French Catholic archbishop, play could be functional to the needs of education, making study more pleasurable, but it might also make children overly excited, becoming a source of sinful thoughts.

Conversely, Locke's (1632-1704) idea of play can be considered a precursor of modern pedagogy, as an empiricist and a forerunner of Enlightenment; according to him, toys must not be purchased, but made by the children themselves.[12] Study should be just as fun as play, and if a child wants to continue to play, he/she is not yet ready to study; the efforts made by children while playing give a pedagogical advantage to the teachers, which is worth exploiting in the most effective way.

The era of Enlightenment represents the great turning point in the European history regarding education, because pedagogy puts the focus on creating responsible citizens and disseminating social values and the educational process must move within this framework. The educational utility of play is clear at this point: the German pedagogist Basedow (1724-1790) proposed that practical teaching is appropriate to

[11] This paragraph is partially inspired to Besio [67].

[12] "Little stones, a pack of cards, a mother's keys, and other similar items that they can't hurt themselves with are fun for children just as much as those things that are bought at such a dear price in stores and that go bad or break in a very short time" (Locke, 1918, orig. ed. 1693).

education for all, regardless of class and religion, while pleasant teaching adheres to the needs of students; he was the first to link play with educational activity, where fun was an integral part of the educational project through play.

The German poet and philosopher Schiller (1759-1805), perfect representative of Romanticism, stressed the dual nature of human beings, made of a sensuous and a formal drive, both inescapable to form a whole being. Since the two poles are conflicting, it is exactly the ludic impulse that can mediate between them: "when people play, they control their baser emotions by placing these within framework of rationally considered rules and restraints" [337]:363. Through play, people exploit their full capacities for living in the world: "Man plays only when he is in the full sense of the word a man and he is only wholly a man when he is playing" (Schiller, cited ibidem). But when can this happen? Only when people feel satisfied with themselves and their lives; superabundance is needed for play being in act: like animals, "creatures play when they feel themselves in full possession of their powers" [337]:363.

Perhaps the German pedagogist Fröbel (1782–1852) has been influenced by Schiller, but only thanks to him play acquires its full educational value: he is convinced that play stimulates the imagination and allows the child to relate with him/herself and with the world. To carry out these functions, play cannot be solitary, but should occur within a group, and must allow children to practice skills and roles as adults. Fröbel invented the mechanism of "gifts" offered to children to favour their overall growth, in body and mind [568]. He encouraged also children to engage in self-directed manipulations of the material world, so that they can join scientific knowledge with an aesthetic experience [335]. Movement and play must be developed together and gradually at different ages; moreover, play can support teaching both physical strength and moral and spiritual determination that are intertwined.

Fröbel's educational project is based on some fundamental features that are still quite interesting: (a) play is a planned part of the school day; the adult must not act in an authoritative manner; (b) the use of structured educational materials that carry out the explicit function of teachings; (c) play must be correlated to the environment in which it happens and be open to contact with nature; (d) the creative and cognitive aspects present in play must be safeguarded and nurtured at the same time; (e) the link between play and life is explicit; the recreational behaviour can become a social behaviour. Fröbel opened the first kindergarten in the history, in 1837, incorporating play—that he considered the highest phase of child development—into early childhood school programmes. The progressive school educator of the first quarter of the twentieth century then built upon Fröbel's emphasis on the importance of play.

Between the nineteenth and the first decades of the twentieth century, big changes in society and culture took place: on one hand, the industrialized world was beginning to take its contemporary form, on the other hand, the social sciences arose and then consolidated, conceived as scientifically grounded, "for understanding human behaviour and experience" [337]:363. In society at large, "ideals of personal development, self-realization [...] become commonplace and influence many fields of study, including play" and "this view [...] remains a dominant theme in contemporary play studies" (ibidem).

A world apart, one might say, is represented by Maria Montessori (1870–1952), whose life widely leans on the twentieth century. Her world-famous "method" encourages children to "play" "with elements that have implications for adult life, such as toy hammers, dishes, and ovens. According to her, children desire self-guided activity with culturally valued items instead of fantasy-based role play" [335]:193; they also "enjoy the social validation that comes from sharing their activities with peers" (ibidem). Her entire educational system is based on the seriousness of adult work. The play impulse in children is really a work impulse; its two main characteristics—the tendency to be active and the tendency to be experimental—can be assets of education.

For the US pedagogist and philosopher Dewey (1859–1952), the relationship with materials is of great importance: materials are seen as real tools, if the situation is governed by playful spirit, which commits children to the inherent value of what they are doing and excites their creativity. The value of play is greatly emphasized, as something that builds the person, through experiences but also by habits of self-directed enquiry. Doing is also the key concept proposed by Winnicott (1896-1971) who postulated an indeterminate place between an "inside" of the child and an "outside": "to control what is outside, one has to do things, not simply to think or to wish, and doing things takes time. Playing is doing" [755]:41. The symbolic makes it possible to separate these two worlds—for example thank to "special objects" called "transitional objects"—and to create a third one, called by Winnicott "play space" and "illusion space", a space of the experience created by the child, as a product of his/her mental activity and of his/her action on reality.

Eugen Fink (1905–1975) seems to anticipate a contemporary idea of play as total abandonment to a dense reality, a sort of happy nothing made of concentration and oddness: "Play resembles an oasis of happiness that we happen upon in the desert of our Tantalus-like seeking and pursuit of happiness. We are abducted by play. By playing we are released a bit from the mechanism of life—as if we were transported to another celestial body, where life appears easier, more ethereal, happier" [253].

"In common [the two last] educational theorists emphasize the value of play—or at least the playful spirit—as something that builds the person, not only through the development of experience-based skills and knowledge but also by habits of self-directed inquiry" [335].

2.2.4 *Three Pillars of Psychology*

Psychology is still today the discipline that more than all the others has deepened the theme of play, making it one of its central objects of study. Play has been considered, according to the various authors, an activity able to promote individual progress, to focus self-exploration, to connect intimately to imagination [337]:368. These themes, anyway, should contrast with tradition, where play is considered "a vehicle for frivolity, that it engages fate, it explores power relations, and [...] it articulates community identity" (ibidem). In both cases, it might be asserted that play is "a distinctive pathway for building identity, capability, and experience" [335].

For the purposes of this work, at least three major pillars in different areas of psychology need to be cited. As (and perhaps even more so) in the case of the other fields of play study, this presentation cannot exhaust the harvest of existing reflections and research but constitute only a light indispensable substrate.

According to Freud (1856–1939), play responds and is led by the principle of pleasure, which first appears in the children's ludic activities. As known, according to him only some elements of psychic functioning are conscious; awareness works also at deeper levels, that may come suddenly to consciousness. Play gives the opportunity to "imagine alternative patterns for thought, feeling and behaviour" [337]:369 and also to explore these alternatives.

Since "every child at play [...] creates a world of his own [...] rearranges the things of his world and orders it in a new way that pleases to him better" [271]:45, play is an exercise of pleasure and fulfilment of wishes: and the principal wish is to be and to act like an adult [478]. Instead of being mere fantasy or daydreaming, play "protects the player from the usual repercussions of the words, gestures and other behaviours" [337]:369. Later, in his work *Beyond the Pleasure Principle* (1928/1967), after observation of a young child's game with a reel, Freud sustained that play might let the child dominate an unpleasant emotion, replacing it with a pleasant one, provoked by the control on the psyche's urges and the regulation of all the elements of the situation. The therapeutic development of these assertions, from the work of Anna Freud on, is well known in the field.

Subsequent scholars in the psychodynamic field identified the symbolic act and the use of symbolic objects that arise in play as the prominent elements for the child's psycho-emotional development; pointedly, Erikson interprets play as an "attempt to synchronize the bodily and the social processes with the Self" (1966, cit. in [337]:369). Since then, the separation/identification process starts and proceeds. Related feelings and emotions help the child to adapt to reality and deal with the problems that he/she encounters in real life: "This is an experience that allows the child to check his/her phantasmal events and vicissitudes, on a manipulated and controlled reality, in an illusory dimension (and real together), which favours both an examination of reality and the exercise of concrete skills with a focus on adaptation" [262].

Play is central to Piaget's (1896–1980) thinking. More systematically and significantly than other authors, he highlighted the relationships between play and the child's cognitive development (1945). The learning process is due to an interaction between "the biologically (and psychologically) developing child and the challenges presented by the physical (and ultimately symbolically configured) environment" [337]:370. Humans learn what the real world consists of and how it functions through experience, in an active manner, acting on it, provoking changes, making predictions about the consequences of their actions and verifying them. The interaction takes two forms: personal adjustment—or accommodation—to environmental changes through the adoption of behavioural techniques and practice/implementation—assimilation—of these techniques on the environment.

Play is "pure extreme or pure assimilation, when behavioural techniques are repeated 'pure for functional pleasure"' (ibidem).[13]

These schemata become more and more complex as the child grows, to include "control of object and symbolic manipulation [until] play involves the manipulation of ideas" (ivi:371). Balancing between these two poles produces adaptation, the most important process governing human development within the environment.

Starting from these assumptions, the author emphasizes, in particular, how play favours and supports symbolic mental activity and asserts that it carries out two basic functions: on one hand, it consolidates the capabilities the subjects already possess and, on the other hand, it strengthens their possibilities to act effectively on reality [66]. According to Piaget, play develops along stages that are age-related; each stage develops and grows in complexity, then exhausts its developmental function for the individual and is replaced by the following one, which in turn maintains with the previous one direct and recognizable relationships. These stages are presented as "invariant [....] qualitatively different [and] typically cumulative, in that later ones build off earlier levels. Furthermore, later stages are thought to be more complex, rationally controlled and abstract" [333]:16. Play develops and proceeds from one stage to the other one, mainly due to intellectual development, to which it is closely combined, since its inception.

It was the Russian psychologist Vygotskij (1896–1934) who, before and more than others (1933/1981), highlighted the social nature of children's play and, at the same time, its role in fostering their social development. "His approach focused much more clearly on action-in-the-world or interaction than on the playful expression of pre-formed ideas and wishes". Rejecting both Piaget's intellectual and Freud's feeling-based play, he argued that "play is a blending of thought, feeling, and action" [337]:371. Children are immersed in the world around them, including objects, adults, peers, and they acknowledge its influence on themselves. Social environments produce challenges that urge them to respond and consequently change; peers have a fundamental role in this process, because they can act more effectively, thus becoming another occasion of change; and the roles of challenger or questioner may be inverted. "The result is a setting marked by imaginative inter-subjectivity, where each person (ideally) takes seriously the invitation of the others" [337]:372.

Then, play is both a product and a producer of social activity, it provides children with the opportunity of subordinating their behaviours to rules and only later develops voluntary behavioural self-control as an internal function. This process of interiorization is stimulated by self-reflection, comparison with others, clarification, and explanation. Despite its eminently social nature, play has other important functions: reduction of tension and fatigue, opportunity to act and experiment the ability to control emotions, actualization of dreams and wishes, development of learning and cognitive skills. Rules and constraints become very important: the pleasure associated with play is exactly due to the restrictions voluntarily imposed on the ludic activity.

---

[13] This assertion has been contrasted by other scholars, for whom accommodation is equally important in the play behaviour [683].

The role played by the social context and the relationships within allow Vygotskij to lay the foundations for the most compelling concept of his theoretical framework: "Play is a source of development and creates the Zone of Proximal Development (ZPD)" (Vygotskij, 1934/1962), which is the "distance between the level of independent performance and the level of assisted performance" [95]:206. In other words, play is the leading activity for children in preschool and kindergarten age. Within the ZPD, the entire child's development takes place, and in this sense, it is possible to state that it is play that creates development [67].

2.2.5 Cultural Studies

As an inherent component of human life, play has been explored in depth also by scholars coming from many other branches (sociology, anthropology, history, etc.). Their contributions, rather being collateral, have been instead significant to understand the intermingled relationships between play, societies, and cultures: the existing representations of the theme have been enriched and the novel interpretations have in turn inspired the nearby sectors, including the educational and technical ones that this volume intends to explore. For this reason, in what follows some short lines are spent on this area.

Huizinga (1872–1945) describes play first as a "well-defined quality of action", "a special form of activity" [356]:4 marked by five defining traits[14]; as such, it takes the form of the driving force of all human activities, a sort of primordial "big bang" from which civilization itself comes from: "culture is played from the very beginning" [356]:47. Play characterizes the *Homo Ludens* as a cultural animal and is a creator of culture [67]. It occupies a sort of blank space between instinct and will [228]; mainly in its social form, it is "the vehicle by which people publicly display their character, capabilities, and status, not only as individuals but as communities. [...] Play is an important agency of social and cultural change" [335]:194.

Caillois (1913–1978) was both an admirer and a critic of Huizinga's work. Particularly, in *Man, Play and Games*, he sustained that "the more rule-bound or game-based forms of play (*ludus*) should be distinguished from play's more spontaneous, free-flowing forms (*paidia*)" [337]:378.[15] Then he developed a thesis about the evolutionary nature of play, from a propitiating and sacred form of the origins—including a desire of discovering abandonment and even death—to today's social game-like form, addressed to organization and rationality. The very function of play is to regulate uncontrolled desires and impulses—deriving from *agon*—to put their significance into perspective, thus tempering and making coherent a person's experience [334].

[14] See Sect. 2.4.

[15] He then identified four main types of play that are very famous in related literature and considered important for their inspiring power in scholars: *agon* (social contest), *alea* (exploration of chance), *mimicry* (imaginative disguise and role performance), *ilinx* (turbulence or vertigo); furtherly, he "layed out these types, ranging between *ludus* (rule-bound, game-based) and *paidia* (free-flowing) on a continuum" [337]:378.

Nevertheless, controlled play is no longer play, it loses its nature of attractive and joyful fun. Freedom in play is spontaneity, immediacy, carefreeness: "a basic freedom is central to play in order to stimulate distraction and fantasy" [149]:27. "Free play is a luxury activity and it belongs to free men. Hungry people don't play" (ibidem:14).

The cultural context has been again called into question, as a frame of roles and behaviours, by the anthropologist Bateson (1904–1980): what the child learns from play is not how to behave according to certain rules or roles, rather that there are types of roles and categories of rules [67]. The author (1956) identified and highlighted the experience of "being within playing", calling it a frame: "It is a mode of organization of behaviour—one way of fitting pieces of activity together" [483]:92. The essence of play is in its being a meta-communication; the message "this is play" serves as a filter to start a new situation: a dimension different from reality, governed by specific rules, shared by players. This frame adopts a "deuteron-type" logic, which includes contexts, relationships, and their modes of functioning; players share a paradoxical ludic feature: they agree on what is "true" and what is "make believe", maintaining this framework throughout the course of the play activity [102], they defend it against intruders, and if someone violates a rule, he/she is ruled out. "To stop that play, another meta-communication should happen—'I won't play anymore'—that dissolves the frame" [67]:16.

2.3 Functions of Play

Why do animals and people play? To which needs does this activity respond? Which adaptive functions does it support, being so deeply rooted—in time and in space—stable but also changing, instinctive but also sensitive to learning?

Scholars of the field have always put similar questions about, if any, the meaning and purpose of this activity in the life of the individuals and of the species, and numerous, different, answers have been produced during time.

In what follows, a list of the most significant hypotheses on the functions of play that got credit in the field is presented. For each function, the following aspects are indicated: the type, the main way the function of play acts in the considered field (evolutionary, developmental, cultural), one representative researcher who proposed it, with only one related reference.[16]

As a background for this review, it is worth reminding that, according to the play theorist Sutton-Smith, play should be considered as a "coevolutionary multiplex of functions" [687]:111, due to its multiple characteristics, across a variety of relevant functional domains that are "genetic, affective, performative, experiential, and culturally relative" (ibidem:116). Moreover, today it is still considered questionable if play really has—or should have—demonstrable functions or scopes: for this reason, the proposed summary list has the only goal to try to organize, under this respect, the

[16] It should be noted also that in the part of the list devoted to the evolutionary studies, some related advantages are marked with an asterisk, to emphasize that statement is scientifically controversial.

most remarkable works in the existing wide literature on the theme. It does neither aim to be exhaustive, definitive, or to impose hierarchies of validity and importance among the cited authors indicated. Being play—as said—an impregnable field of studies, the works included in the list belong to different cultural traditions [593] and consequently they refer to different scientific methodologies, from the experimental to the speculative one.

The selection criteria here adopted concern the solidity, in their own area, of the studies cited, as well as the degree of interest they arouse in relation to the topic covered by this volume. Possible functions of play, in fact, might prove very useful when planning research in the field, since the expected related advantages might suggest ideas on the criteria to be adopted for demonstrating the effectiveness of a play activity and of a tool use. As it will be discussed,[17] measuring changes or results obtained by the implementation of ludic activities and the adoption of play instruments is neither trivial or reliable.

Evolutionary Functions in Animal Species

- Practice motor skills
  - Acquire basic motor skills (running, jumping, climbing, etc.) [63].
  - Enhance motor ability, provide the needed experience to develop the nervous system [145].
  - Prepare to adopt protection behaviours, thus avoiding predators [291].
  - Acquire precopulatory behaviours [538].
  - Gain high dominance state in adulthood [92].
- Enforce resilience
  - Develop the physical and emotional abilities to face possible survival challenges [240].
- Introduce innovation
  - Generate, just for fun, novel behaviours that turn out to be useful ("play is the mother of invention") [13, 300].
- Propose cooperation in social play
  - Exhibit core elements of "morality" [55, 56].
  - Enable animal to form social bonds, thus cooperating during adulthood [190].
  - Establish new relationships, thus facilitating entering a hierarchical society [178].

[17] See Sect. 2.10.1.

- Train for the unexpected
  - Train to deal with the emotional feeling of being surprised or disoriented or disabled [664].
  - Train to struggle and escape from thrilling and dangerous situations deliberately created [536].
- Generate novel behaviours
  - Provide an ability necessary to survival [483].
  - Provide a flexible substrate to the individual's cognitive system [483].
- Cope with stress
  - Vent the intrinsic surplus energy [303].
  - Reduce aggression, thus ameliorating social tension [628].
- Dimension (duration) of play
  - More time devoted to play increase individual fitness, thus favouring survival [153, 240].

Evolutionary Functions in Individuals

- Offer preparatory practice
  - Train activities that ensure preservation of the organism (Kant).
  - Train functional and useful abilities [181].
  - Maintain useful habits that otherwise would disappear [162].
- Provoke adaptation
  - Test skills useful for environmental adaptation. Exercise skills preparatory to adult roles in life [303].
  - Explore new situations in new environments [441].
  - Look for optimal solutions to environmental challenges [441].
  - Exploit people's full capacities for living in the world [656].
  - Essential to adequate human development in Western societies [653].
- Introduce creativity
  - Express the innate creative attitude of human beings, further developing into work [274].
  - Occasionally create novelty that can prove useful to face a new contingency in "reality", thus resulting in adaptation [482].
  - Reinforce animal and human variability, thus nullifying the rigidity that sets in after successful adaption [686].

  - Novel behaviours in playing with objects spread among peers and become dominant ("seeding hypothesis of play"); novelty attracts peers' attention. The behavioural flexibility in play with objects may be an evolutionary driver [627].
  - Support cognitive abilities and competences through assimilation, play creates opportunities to experience and act on the environment and as the child grows, it offers increasing complex cognitive challenges and conflicts. By developing through stages, it provokes and contemporarily accompanies the initiation of higher cognitive functions (practice play/sensorimotor functions; symbolic play/language; play with rules/operative thinking and reasoning). Play is the spring of the child's cognitive development [548].
  - As the causal agent of ZPD—through social interaction—play is also the main drive for cognitive development. The mature make-believe play originates abstract thinking, symbolic representation and imagination [737].

- Support social abilities and competences

  - In free play, children learn social norms and rules (Plato).
  - Through the relation with the social contexts (peers and adults), play creates and develops the ZPD. Social contexts with variability in play competence establish a correlation between play, self-regulation, and following direction [305, 737].
  - Mastery social interactions [231].

- Support psycho-emotional abilities

  - Recreation (Aristotle).
  - Let the children's "great heat" escape (Fénelon).
  - Deal with surprise and fear. Vent the intrinsic surplus energy [303].
  - Express dynamic feelings—fear, anger, desire, love, ambition, conflict, rivalry—in a magnificent way. Give the child the opportunity to deal with these feelings in fantasy [270].
  - Produce "functional pleasure" [548].
  - Through emotion control, delay the achievement of immediate pleasure, giving rise to imagination in play. Reduce tension and fatigue [737].
  - Symbolic acts and objects—e.g., a blanket—as substitutes of reality, give rise to the separation/identification process [755].
  - Play contents assume a prominent role in representing feelings and emotions, dealing with problems and focus on adaptation [262].
  - Master fear, both physically and psychologically [607].

Functions in Culture

- Drive new cultural meanings

  - Mark the development of societies towards more complex and advanced ones that shift interaction from selfish, sensory, and destructive engagements in those

that are more sublimated and aesthetic. Prepare participants to ponder and actuate the ideal [656].
- Create the human culture, through attributing meanings, commenting, making it possible to develop art, science, history, and humour. Preserve the play spirit itself [356].
- Express total and joyful freedom in the *paidia*—primitive—form. Regulate unplayful and uncontrolled impulses by tempering them and making coherent a person's experience [149].
- Ignite knowledge about the different frameworks or contexts of behaviour and the possible roles and styles in relationships [48].
- Manifest self-representation; allow the experience of "otherness". Give rise to freedom of decision, which, however in the same time, is threatened and irrevocably limited; play becomes the player's lord, every play is a "being played" [276].

Functions in Specific Social and Health Conditions of Individuals

- Face situations of political violence (war, terrorism)
  - "Bolstering resilience in the face of adversity, coping during a traumatic event, processing such events in their aftermath" [187].
  - May have adaptational significance to support the emergence of positive affect in children, with respect to the adults' high levels of anxiety (Bonanno et al., 2011).
  - Create a coherent trauma narrative in play is associated with better coping with the events and with post-traumatic growth [186].
  - Share subjective private experience with others thus taking advantage of the positive value of social engagement against the development of psychopathology [314].
- Cope effectively with various medical procedures and hospital visits
  - Offer activities that children relish outside (normative play). Explore basic equipment and supplies (medical play),promote emotional expression, enhance development and well-being (therapeutic play) [154].

2.4 Characteristics of Play

Another traditional way adopted by scholars to discuss, interpret, and describe the multifaceted and impenetrable topic of play has been listing its essential traits or characteristics. Considered as a whole, each of these—numerous—lists might be considered as a tentative epistemology of play: as if the authors, overwhelmed by the complexity and difficulty of the task, abandon the objective of giving a complete and organic structure to their work, and devote themselves to identify details, peculiar characteristics of their object of study.[18] In what follows, three of these lists will be presented, for their peculiarity in the play studies' landscape.[19]

2.4.1 LUDI—Characteristics of Play

The first two lists that are presented have been developed by the LUDI Action [72], devoted, respectively, to play characteristics and play fundamentals, where distinctive traits of play, common to all the identified play types[20] able to design its special peculiarity, have been grouped: the characteristics refer to qualities, intrinsic attributes, while the fundamentals related more to the concrete activity of playing. Both were derived from an accurate analysis of the literature carried out as part of the research process. For each typology, the researchers' proposals are presented.

- Feeling of freedom
  Play associates to freedom, immediateness, spontaneity. It is the first trait marked by Caillois: "Controlled play is no longer play", it loses its attractiveness and joyful fun. "[It] is central to stimulate distraction and fantasy [...] and is indispensable [...] to the most organized forms of play" [149]:27. Freedom has also overlooked implications, such as licentiousness in play gestures, words, jokes. According to Sutton-Smith: "For the children who take part to the jokery, there need be no limit to the shocks they can include in this kind of unorthodox play" [687]:91.
- Concentration, intensity
  Freedom is never associated with laziness, rather with concentration, intensity, density [253]. Tension [356] means to be totally absorbed, is the desire to achieve, to be successful. Being fully involved and feeling within a special condition of life are two co-existing attitudes [66]. "In this intensity, this power of maddening, lies the very essence, the primordial quality of play" [356]:3.

[18] A detailed and sound review of studies describing play by collecting its main traits has been included in some works of Henricks [332]:2015.

[19] For the sake of completeness, the characteristics identified by some of the authors included in the previous paragraphs are shown in what follows. For Huizinga, the five main traits of play are: its voluntary nature, its difference from ordinary or "real" life, its qualities of seclusion and limitation, its combination of order and disorder, and its connection to secrecy. According to Bateson [48], play has five main characteristics: unfinalization, creativity, not literalness, flexibility, and pleasure. Caillois singles out six traits of play: it is free, separate, uncertain, unproductive, governed by rules, and marked by make-believe. "He criticized Huizinga for emphasizing the idea of secrecy", by arguing that "play works to the detriment of the secret and mysterious" [336]:117. Sutton-Smith also produces his list of characteristics: chanciness, fluidity, ambiguity, particularity, diversity of perspective (ibidem).

[20] More details on the types of play within the LUDI Action will be discussed in Chapter 3.

- Pleasure, fun
  "Nature gave us play, with its tension, its mirth, and its fun" [356]:3. But Vygotskij [737] contrasts this interpretation by putting instead the bond, the limit, at the basis of the pleasure inherent to play. According to Freud, human play is led by the principle of pleasure. The pleasure produced by play does not run out spontaneously in the excitement of the moment, rather it leaves traces on the individual's feelings in relation to life itself: "[play's positive pleasure] makes it possible to live more fully in the world, no matter how boring or painful or even dangerous ordinary reality might seem" [687]:95.
- Serious mode
  "The pleasure of play is not always manifested in delight or glee or laughter. Play can be a very serious business but still within play the act of doing is clearly rewarding in the sense that it incites its own repetition" [483]:91. The play in which the child is intensively involved is always seriously challenging him/her. In fiction or in playful concentration, several 'make believe' acts are accomplished "seriously", but the realism of such acts must never let the two contexts overlap.
- Curiosity, surprise
  Although play makes positive use of repetition and schemes, its preferential sign is discontinuity. It pursues and uses flexibility, constantly seeking changes in forms or in contents. Often it comes out from the unexpected, from surprise [228]. Teasing, particularly studied by Sutton-Smith, is related to the feeling of surprise or even shock; in some cultures, it seems relevant in the play relationships between the child and the adult, becoming a means of social learning.
- Intrinsic motivation
  Intrinsic motivation is the main drive of play, not only or not so much to achieve a result, rather to keep alive the play process itself. Any type of play provides the pleasurable feeling of "being in" play, rather than to achieve a result. "Winning a game or achieving a result is important insofar as they are symbols of the dynamics and the challenge that were involved in their attainment" [483]:93. Play and games are intrinsically motivated, do not tend to satisfy primary physical needs, and does not depend on external rules or social obligations [102].
- Challenge
  Play is a challenging process and from the player—child or adult—demands commitment and seriousness (a careless player is reprimanded by his or her companions and is asked to "play for real"). Challenge has a special role in soliciting specific feelings in the player and provoking in turn new tension, demanding additional concentration. It might be in act both in solitary and collective play, in this second case, issues concerning collaboration and competition are unavoidably introduced.

LUDI—Fundamentals of Play

- The concept of frame
  Play is a special context in life, a frame [48] that one can get in, get out, that can be suspended for a while, in which behaviours, meanings, rules, and roles are different from reality (are in-lusio, according to Huizinga [356]). Players create,

recognize, and agree on this play frame, that is, at the same time, invisible and concrete and that they inhabit and defend both from intruders and sceptics.

- The need of doing
  Play is related to the human fundamental need to be active, to interact with the world around. "To control what is outside, one has to do things, not simply to think or to wish, and doing things takes time. Playing is doing" [755]:41. The process of doing seems to be interesting per se, and more important than its results. Children themselves impose limitations and constraints to their activity, thus obtaining both the goals of being reassured by repetition and feeling challenged by novelty.
- The role of imagination and fantasy
  Play is also the main door for entering "another reality" [235]:221-222, for evoking situations, combining representations, developing thought; it is the door to the profusion of symbols, language, metaphors, creativity, and imagination. According to Vygotskij, "play is a transitional stage in the development of imagination, [...] a specific human form of conscious activity. Like all functions of consciousness, it originally arises from action" [737]:8.
- The importance of the rules
  Rules in play are not limited to games; they are rather intrinsic to all the kinds of play at any developmental age, first created by children themselves and later socially agreed-upon. According to Vygotskij, "the essential attribute in play is a rule that has become a desire" and Bondioli underlines that children take pleasure in "self-submitting to the rule of giving up spontaneous and impulsive actions" [102]. In some cases, rules can put the players into trouble: getting out of it is the gist of play. It is worth noting that one of the basic lines of demarcation in the interpretation of play between the two giants of the field, Piaget and Vygotskij, is located precisely on this topic.
- The social aspects of play
  Play is social in two main senses: because children learn to play in dual relationships or in groups, and because most of the types and modes of play require social contexts. Play relationships with peers are irreplaceable in childhood to learn by imitation, to face different opinions, to acknowledge the need for mediation, to develop skills of cooperation, and to overcome conflicts. Adult and parental influence is vital for the child to start and learn how to play: at the beginning, they can be protagonist models, and then—by gradually fading their interaction—they can become prompters, scaffolders, companions, and spectators.
- The play development in childhood
  Play develops and changes along childhood; it becomes more complex, it changes its features and its focus, by addressing different tools and/or ways to interpret the reality and the human beings. Research identified different types of play and showed that a given type of play prevails in certain developmental phases, then it merges with others, and it may disappear but also re-emerge in different forms, in different times of life.

2.4.2 Henricks: Qualities of Play

The list of qualities proposed by Henricks (started with the work dated 2006 [332] and then refined in 2015 [336]) is presented, for it authoritatively echoes the tradition of the sector, whereas inserting an innovative and contemporary viewpoint. His "distinguishing qualities of play" have been classified with respect to the six different perspectives that he singled out for describing play; they also have been contrasted with three other special human behaviours that are not play: work, ritual, and communitas.[21]. Eberle sustains that Henricks' attributes of play appear very useful as possible criteria and "once having so identified these criteria, apply them as standards" [228]:215. For each perspective, the related qualities are detailed.

- Play as Action
  - Transformation: When people play, they try to impose their will on external circumstances [...] they try to render otherness according to their own orientation, strategies, or schemes do this in order to test, expand, and solidify their own power. Even if they change the world very modestly, they feel confirmed by this assertive mood.
  - Consummation: It denotes the sense of commitment to happenings in the present; play is process-oriented, it gives attention *to means rather to ends*. Since often it requires speed, it is emotionally charged and expressive. This quality includes also the concepts of *intrinsic motivation, non-instrumental expenditure, waste*, and it is also related to the self-imposed boundaries to play, thus including *seclusion, limitation, secrecy, and make-believe*.
- Play as Interaction
  - Contestiveness: Play is an assertive, *contestive* stance towards the world. This competition is often to obtain something but the interaction occurs with materials and symbolic elements. Players want and need difficulties and *obstacles*, they select forms of play that have "too"—heavy, difficult, high, rough—characteristics.
  - Unpredictability: Players prefer objects which are able to respond directly instead of merely resisting or that are able to confound by their failure to response as expected. Play needs an optimal level of unpredictability that challenges the players' declared goals. It is *tense, uncertain, unexpected*. Creatures want to inhabit contexts that make real the prospects of dissatisfaction. Only then do accomplishments give them pleasure.

---

[21] The list has been elaborated from the contents of Henrick's book *Play and the Human Condition* [336]. Many sentences are taken from the text; the parts in italics refer to characteristics and qualities singled out by other scholars that inspired Henricks' work and have been grouped in his classification.

- Play as Activity
  - Self-regulation: In play, rules arise as agreements of the participants (it is *free*, it is *voluntary*). Play celebrates creativity and *improvisational potential*, it pursues challenge and novelty (it is *order and disorder, equilibrial and disequilibrial*). While players invent restrictions, they are fascinated by inventing predicaments and new ways to respond to them.
  - Being episodic: Play events are *episodes* repeated and returned (*recursive*), but never the same. Play activities often feature repetitions of narrowly defined actions; often play is time spent performing small behaviours again and again. But it is players who determine what these behaviours are, what rules apply and how those rules are to be enforced, etc.
- Play as Disposition
  - Curiosity: It is a prelude to actual play experiences; people want to put their capabilities into action, watching is not enough. They want to put their hands on the playing materials, because they don't know how this process will go: and it is precisely because they want to be involved (*continuation desire, optimism*).
- Play as Experience
  - Anticipation: People play because they desire to know what it will feel like to be the executors of a newly constructed moment [see also Curiosity, above].
  - Feelings of the present: An alternation of fun (excitement, exploration, disorders) (*flow, engagement, total absorption, diminished consciousness of self, entraining*) and exhilaration (pleasurable restoration, order) (strategic disengagement).
  - Feelings of remembrance: Feeling of gratification, that is, the sense of being pleasurably spent, including elements of self-congratulation. Frustration, anxiety, boredom, failure, and fatigue can also be present: smaller doses enhance keep the play going, too many of them may cause its end.
- Play as Context
  - Ascending meaning: It focuses on how people construct the character of situations; play is a rebellion against the forms and forces of the world; they try to manage behaviour their way. Psychologically emboldened, they willfully destabilize bodies, environments, societies, and culture. This process may be envisioned as an upward movement.

2.4.3 Eberle: Elements of Play

The last group of characteristics reported in what follows concern the very innovative list of six basic elements advanced by Eberle [228], who, totally changing perspective, invites to consider play not as a "thing", rather as a "series of connected events [such as] other processes that unfold and move along at varying rates" (ibidem:220). In this sense, the author compares play to known processes in other fields of study—neuroscience, cellular biology, meteorology, software engineering, etc.—that "out of their own resources and over time gather shape and structure spontaneously"; these phenomena are called "emergence", that is, "the arising of novel and coherent structures, patterns, and properties, during the process of self-organization in complex systems"[22] (ibidem).

Play is one of those processes, which start their growth from simple rules and then acquire a complex form. Eberle's proposal concerning the play elements is thus interesting not merely for its components—emotional and personal rewards for participants—rather for the relationships established between them, as well as for the complex design of the structural system, which offers both a description and a hypothesis of play development through these elements.

He envisages play as "an emergent, spiralling process, much like a vortex, that participants enter and then find themselves being carried forward within" [338]:37. The non-linear process proceeds from the first to the sixth element that represent "different patterns of awareness that combine and deepen as one moves through the event" (ibidem). These elements should be read "as conveniences, as manners of speaking, and above all, as moving images more akin to concepts in aesthetics and philosophy" [228]:222. The elements, represented as wheels, in their rotation picture an imaginary line swirling from each of the elements as a scale that slides into its opposite, that is, the non-play (respectively, anticipation/obsession; surprise/shock, terror; pleasure/excess; understanding/indifference; strength/heedlessness; poise/abstraction). In addition, each "element takes on explanatory power as it subdivides into eight "expressions"[23] synonyms of varying potency" (ibidem).

Within each play event, but also along the play development in childhood, the transition from one element to another occurs when each level has reached its maximum level. "Wheels spin within wheels in this diagram that appears more as a field of possibility and less as a linear certainty" (ibidem:230). The diagram lets also describe changes of play according with time, place, and culture; it registers changes of people, due to their maturation and increased experience: "Remove an individual disk from the spiral, and you have an individual moment of play. Set it running forward, and you have a picture of play over time" (ibidem).

- Anticipation

  Play begins in imaginative, predictive, and pleasurable tension. Preparation to play is to begin to play: there is an instant or an interval that separates what had not been from what soon will be play (when the neighbourhood kids knock at the door,

[22] The definition, cited by Eberle, belongs to the management theorist Jeffrey Goldstein, and is contained in the article *Emergence as a Construct: History and Issues*, "Emergence", 1999, 1:49.

[23] Eberle envisaged also, for each element, a corresponding counterpart of "not play". For further details concerning both this aspect and the eight "expressions" please refer to the aforementioned author's work.

the dealer shuffles and cuts a deck of cards, the referee's whistle blows, the school bell rings recess, etc.). In the interval of a game waiting for—or thinking to—the opponent's next move improves a lot one's own concentration and performance. Play begins with a disposition to play: this state of readiness, whether mild, or intense, already feels rewarding as it makes way for play.

- Surprise
  Surprise occurs when the novelty breaks into habit: usually, this provokes hilarity; but laughter and surprise can arise also when the event is expected, such as in the case of the repetition of a game of peekaboo: and this represents the only apparent paradox of the relationship between anticipation and surprise. Since memory and prediction share a neural substrate, players in a state of anticipation may be "remembering" a future pleasure. Surprise is a reward, if the players are prepared to appreciate it: for example, they keep play challenging by choosing up equal sides, by negotiating rules that handicap the strongest or most skilled players or positions, and by introducing technologies that allow peak performances.
- Pleasure
  It is the keystone of play, both as a defining trait and an incentive to play some more; it drives play. Players experience pleasure in intensifying shades of satisfaction, buoyancy, gratification, joy, happiness, delight, glee, and fun. Play would not be playful if it were not fun. But pleasure is mostly momentary and exactly for this reason it applies more easily to play as a process rather than a static thing. It is strictly connected to all the other elements: anticipation entails and promises pleasure; discovery and surprise bring to pleasure; understanding points to insight and sensitivity as rewards of play; considering strength as creativity, the power of this sort of pleasure is clear; and the full experience of poise produces pleasurable feelings.
- Understanding
  This element delivers emotional and intellectual abilities. The needed mutuality and sensitivity stir from the first mutual exchanges in life, in the attunement between mother and infant (that contains the first three elements) and proceed through the development of a "theory of mind". Then, group play soon sharpens appreciation of the utility of fairness, without which children will suffer. Full growth of mutual understanding cannot be achieved without play and other kinds of human contact. Understanding of both empathy and knowledge also feeds back into play. At the same time, tolerance, mutuality, and sensitivity flow from play, and they also instruct play, making it richer, more complex, and once again, more pleasurable.
- Strength
  Strength of mind and body flows from understanding that trains physical and mental abilities. The ideas of bulging muscles and blinding speed remind to the strength of the circus strongman or of the super hero of a comic book. But players garner also strength in the form of mastery and control: one must be flexible enough to be resilient, ingenious enough to avoid the rough spots, and lively enough to bend without breaking. By playing, people enlarge their abilities, augment their sense of fairness, thus steeling against fear and pain. They become able to face

fantasy monsters and to play down such physical discomforts as breathlessness, weariness, dizziness, side stitches, and muscle strain. Play strengthens social skills too: it creates new friendships, rearranges the old ones, and train to read others' intentions. A stronger self makes the individual more attractive as playmate and partner. Wit, ingenuity, creativity, drive, and passion are all expressions of strength.

- Poise
  Play reserves poise as a reward for the luckiest players who experience increasing dimensions of dignity, grace, composure, ease, wit, fulfilment, and spontaneity. These expressions of poise are social, plainly, but they extend to the physical, too. Play pleasurably enhances proprioception—the awareness of our bodies in space, the dynamic sense of the relation of its parts—but the sense of balance decreases over time. Play trains the body, feeds the mind, shores up the feelings, and tutors good social judgement, making people better rounded and more attractive. Benefits of poise are acknowledged in physical, intellectual, emotional, and social ways.

2.5 Definitions of Play

Rivers of ink have been spilled to find a universally accepted definition of play, especially in different cultural environments,[24] but, since it began to be studied and analysed in an effort to recognize and understand it, play escaped any definition that tried to fix it, define it, and encode it. In contrast to this wealth of reflections, however, there is astonishing evidence: in fact, the scholars have not found, over time, an agreement on a single definition of the phenomenon. And if this finding can, on the one hand, freshen the enthusiasm of those who exalt the elusiveness and the mystery of play, on the other, as Burghardt [141] has effectively argued, it challenges the scientific validity of different play studies. Without a shared definition it is not possible to compare results, to test hypothesis, to identify research lines or assess the progress in the knowledge on play [68]. In what follows, only a few proposals will be presented: apart from the first, which is a tribute to the scholar who has dealt with this problem more than others, the other three are of specific interest for the purposes of this volume.

[24] Again, for the sake of completeness, the definitions of play of some of the main cited authors are reported in what follows. For Huizinga, play is a particular pattern shared across human cultures that precedes their development; it is a free activity standing quite consciously outside "ordinary" life as being "not serious", but at the same time absorbing the player intensely and utterly. It is an activity connected with no material interest, and no profit can be gained by it. It proceeds within its own proper boundaries of time and space according to fixed rules and in an orderly manner [356]:13. Bateson identifies the essence of play in its being a metalanguage: since it is something that "is not what it seems", for a playful activity to be truly such every player must be able to affirm: "This is a game", that is, there must be the awareness that the action is fictitious and that it "meta-communicates" this fiction. Caillois defines play mainly through its characteristics, but he also asserts that it is "an occasion of pure waste: waste of time, energy, ingenuity, skill, and often of money" and he adds: "as for the professionals [...] it is clear that they are workers and not players" [149]:5.

2.5.1 *Sutton-Smith's Definition*

Sutton-Smith (1924-2015) tried all his life to find a satisfactory definition of play, but he continually recognized the difficulty of the task due to the impregnability of the theme and in the last years he seemed to abandon the intention. For him, in fact, the issue is afflicted by many problems, such as "vagueness and imprecision, [...] confusion that spring from the specialized languages and approaches [...] the competing ideological and ethical assumptions about play" [228]:218.[25] Nevertheless, two years after the proposal of "rhetorics", he thought it was possible to glimpse a plausible solution in the drift and imprecision itself and he proposed the following definition:

> "Play, as a unique form of adaptive variability, instigates an imagined but equilibrial reality within which disequilibrial exigencies can be paradoxically simulated and give rise to the pleasurable effects of excitement and optimism. The genres of such play are humour, skill, pretense, fantasy, risk, contest, and celebrations, all of which are selective simulations of paradoxical variability" [687]:253.

As Eberle comments, "the definition is circular, incomplete, and difficult to unpack" [228]:219. Such a definition ends by encouraging scholars to isolate in their ivory towers, avoiding confrontation with colleagues and it threatens to become a disquisition of enlarged proportions, e.g., about the "genres" of play to include or to skip.

2.5.2 *The LUDI Action Choice: Garvey's Definition*

For its purposes of studying, renovating, and increasing the play of children with disabilities, the Action LUDI had to share a definition of its main topic, among scholars belonging to various disciplines very distant from each other. After careful literature analysis, LUDI adopted Garvey's proposal:

> "Play is a range of voluntary, intrinsically motivated activities associated with recreational pleasure and enjoyment" [279]:4.

The definition is at the same time wide and flexible and offered interesting and promising features for the Action itself: it includes all the possible types of ludic

[25] Trying to capture its multifaceted essence, Sutton-Smith proposed in 1997 [686] to subdivide play into seven "rhetorics" deriving from different kinds of culture, and above all by the fact that play demonstrates to fail "to outgrow disciplines, their discourses and current climates of opinion" (ibidem). See also Sect. 2.5.1.

activities[26] and considers three significant dimensions that are typical of the infant play: it is pleasurable (recreational pleasure and enjoyment), autotelic (voluntary), intrinsically motivated [134].

Being LUDI a research project clearly addressed to action and intervention in many fields of childhood (social, educational, juridical, rehabilitative, etc.), its members were mainly concentrated on concrete play activities: for this reason, in order to apply the chosen definition in the most coherent way, it was necessary to make a precise distinction between play activities and play-like activities,[27] thus emphasizing the needed focus on the concept of "play for the sake of play".

2.5.3 Burghardt's Definition

In order to properly develop his studies, the ethologist Burghardt [141], in a text that is now unavoidable in the field, sets himself the goal of reaching an exhaustive and shareable definition of play, to make the related research area more scientifically sound.

He proposes five criteria for identifying it in animals. Playful behaviour in his opinion (ivi:70-82): (1) "it is not fully functional in the form or the context in which it is expressed", that is, it does not have a purpose immediately related to it; (2) "it is spontaneous, voluntary, intentional, pleasurable, rewarding, reinforcing, or autotelic (done 'for its own sake')"; (3)"it differs from other ethnotypic behaviours structurally or temporally in at least one of the following aspects: it is incomplete (generally through neglected or dropped final elements), exaggerated, awkward, or precocious; or, it involves behaviour patterns with modified forms, sequences, or targeting"; (4) "it performs repeatedly, in a similar but not rigidly stereotyped, form, during at least a portion of the animal's ontogeny"; (5) "it initiated when an animal is adequately fed, healthy, free from stress (e.g., predator threat, harsh microclimate, social instability) or from intense competitive systems (e.g., feeding, mating, predator avoidance); in other words, the animal is in a 'relaxed field'".

Burghardt's proposal of systematization has the express purpose of initiating new studies in the sector, which can be set up according to a classic scientific approach. In fact, Burghardt argues that "all five criteria must be met in at least one respect before the play label can be confidently attached to any specific instance of behaviour" (ivi:79). Studied in this way, "it should be possible to cut through some of the confusion as to what play means in a phyletic perspective" (ivi:82) and also to classify it, verify its characteristics, perhaps also applying quantitative measures, evaluate its modifiability and the tools and methods for eliciting it.

---

[26] The types of play will be treated in detail in Sect. 2.6.

[27] This distinction will be reconsidered more in detail in Sect. 2.10.2.

Within the described framework, Burghardt proposes the following definition:

"Play is repeated, incompletely functional behaviour differing from more serious versions structurally, contextually, or ontogenetically, and initiated voluntary when the animal is in a relaxed or low-stress setting" (ivi: 82).

Assuming the necessary differences in language and context of application, Burghardt's characteristics of play are also typical of human playful behaviour. To what extent, under what conditions, could they be considered exhaustive in the representation of the human play? Can we adapt Burghardt's definition of animal play to the human play?

What seems promising in this hypothesis is the evolution of play from the instinctual naturalness to more flexible and complex types, connected to the onset of the relationship with other individuals; two lines of future research can be envisaged. The first: to identify traces of continuity between species: in other words, the elements of similarity and overlap that make animals' play—especially primates—similar to human play. The second: to find more precisely the discontinuity between them; where is it located? Is the symbolic function the main responsible for it? These two lines of reflection might produce important advances on the role of both the emergence of the symbol and the socio-relational component—more refined and complex in humans—in the development of play [68].

2.5.4 Eberle's Definition

According to Eberle, "play unfolds as a series of fortunate events driven by emotional experiences" [228]:231. The framework proposed by this author, based on six elements[28] connected to each other thanks to the developmental process of play, graphically represented by revolving and rotating wheels, can contain most of the play characteristics described in literature, and include any type of play. Anyway, play should be defined in order to distinguish it from similar developmental and multifaceted behaviours: "we need to extract a working definition for play that accounts for play as an event that unfolds spontaneously (but not randomly), that notices the volition of the participants (but still accounts for both rule making and rule breaking), and that recognizes its benefits (while acknowledging the risks)" (ibidem:229).

Other occurrences should be respected by this awaited definition: (a) any individual belongs to his/her own social and psychological networks and has a history of his/her own; (b) play belongs to the individual's intentions and viewpoints, it cannot be "pulled away from where and when and with whom it takes place" (ibidem).

The author proposes to imagine play "both rotating and revolving like a Tilt-a-Whirl thrill ride [...], an emergent self-feeding process where causes and effects are

[28] See Sect. 2.4.3.

linked"; its elements are strictly intermingled: anticipation "leads to surprise that gives rise to pleasure which enlarges understanding, which in turn builds strength [...] which contributes to the poise that again enables our anticipation" (ibidem). "It is as if a play event sits on a platform, where each element spins on its own axis as the whole corkscrews through time" (ibidem). As a conclusion of this complex, articulated description of play as a collection of interrelated elements in one or more recursive cycles, Eberle proposes (ibidem) his definition of play[29]:

> "Play is an ancient, voluntary, 'emergent' process driven by pleasure that yet strengthens our muscles, instructs our social skills, tempers and deepens our positive emotions, and enables a state of balance that leaves us poised to play some more".

2.6 Types of Play

Scholars have always recognized that play and games can take many different forms, however not infinite in number. Not only do these forms persist with the passage of generations—despite the obvious cultural and environmental changes—but they also occur, with due differences, in geographically and anthropologically distant populations.

In many cases, the same previously mentioned researchers have advanced proposals for plausible classifications of types of play. Regardless of their belonging to broader explanatory schemes of play, some types—despite widely shared—have been questioned.

For example, the predominant way to study play with objects does not persuade Pellegrini, who deems that scholars are too focused solely on a generic functional use of them. The author proposes a classification of object uses—exploration, construction, tool use, and tool making–each of which has "different developmental histories and different implications for using objects to solve problems" [535]:178, thus different connections with the child's development. He also underlines that "the importance of social interaction around object uses in early cognitive development [...] has been ignored" (p. 165); although object play can be solitary, Pellegrini stresses its role in social learning: "interactions with objects take place in social contexts and [...] children spend considerable time observing others using objects" [535, 706]. In one of his studies [535], he sustained that novel uses of objects "attract the attention of peers and may spread through the population, depending on their usefulness" [534]:176: he labelled the capacity of these novel behaviours to out-compete alternatives as the "seeding hypothesis" of play.

A type of play that is not that much represented in current literature is play fighting that can be considered the Cinderella role in the field of types of play:

[29] The definition has been refined in collaboration with Stuart-Brown.

better known as rough play, it is defined as a "verbally and physically cooperative play behaviour involving at least two children, where all participants enjoyably and voluntarily engage in reciprocal role-playing that includes aggressive make-believe themes, actions, and words; yet lacks intent to harm either emotionally or physically" [323]:108. Its numerous forms (rough-and-tumble, risky play, superhero play, etc.) are often viewed with a certain suspicion by adults, due to a "general lack of understanding of their playful nature and the misconception that all rough play includes intent to harm" [324]:200. On the contrary, many convergent research studies exist, supported also by authoritative educational initiatives, that emphasize positive aspects of such type of play "for learning and skill development" [652]:3; professionals in the field should be accordingly educated on how it can be best supported.

A frequently observed feature is that the development of play in the single individual presents recognizable and typical characteristics in different phases of life, frequently interpreted as evolutionary forms of the same phenomenon. These evolving types of play have been deeply studied in relation to the overall, social, and cognitive, development of the child. In these works, due to its easy observation and its universality, the development of play has often taken a central role and has been interpreted as a driving force.

2.6.1 Piaget and Vygotskij: Child Development Through Play Development[30]

This area of study has represented one of the main research interests of the two giants in developmental psychology and pedagogy, Jean Piaget and Lev Vygotskij. The differences that separate the two researchers precisely regarding the types of play, from one hand help to understand their respective conceptions of play, and from the other hand urge the contemporary play researcher to pay acute attention to detail, while being fully aware of the complexity and richness of the implicit underlying issues.

The importance of symbolic in play for Piaget [548] is well known: the phenomenon of symbolism manifests in the child's life "as soon as [he/she] leaves the sensorimotor level to the representational thought" [549]:679 and it is an inevitable result of the action of distortion, an attribute of assimilation. Unlike the previous stage—called practice play by the author—symbolic play gradually disengages from frequent repetition, and behaviours can be merely evocated, thus opening to the combination of representations in a form that anticipates thought. However, practice play and symbolic play are strictly related: "symbolic play is to practice play how the representative intelligence is to sensorimotor intelligence. This matching at two different levels should be added to another at the same level: symbolic play is to representative intelligence how practice play is to sensorimotor intelligence" [549]:690.

[30] This paragraph is mainly inspired by Besio [67].

The schemes drawn from real life are first applied to inadequate objects and later evoked, up to the consciousness of "pretend"; from pretend play, a free combination of symbols, human creativity, metaphorical transformation of reality will arise.

Nevertheless, neither pretend or symbolic play are based on rules, because the rule is grafted on social skills—such as bargaining and mediation—which occur only when the phase of egocentrism has been surpassed.[31] A rule, for Piaget, can exist on an individual basis—thus, it can be changed at will—and has an objectual content, or on a social basis, resulting from an agreement between the players, who find a compromise between different wills and intentions. Both types of rules are based on conventionality; thus, they are not compatible with pretend play, which has only a subjective nature. Consistently, the author singles out rule-based play as a standalone play stage, the third and last one in his hierarchy.

Vygotskij [737, 738] prefers to avoid using the concept of "symbol" in play, because too connected to the cognitive aspects of growth, and rather to use the concept of imagination: play is a "transitional stage" in the development of imagination. In this way, Vygotskij totally reverses a previously common belief that imagination precedes play: "Imagination is a new formation that is not present in the consciousness of the very young child, is totally absent in animals, and represents a specific human form of conscious activity. Like all functions of consciousness, it originally arises from action" but the process advances during human development: "we can say that imagination in adolescents and schoolchildren is play without action" [737]:8. In addition, according to him, play "is not the predominant form of activity [of the child], but is, in a certain sense, the leading source of development in preschool years" [737]:6.

He stresses mainly the value of the dramatic or make-believe play typical of preschoolers and children of primary school age. Thus, he does not include movement, object manipulation, or explorations in the concept of play. "Make-believe play has three components, as children: (1) create an imaginary situation; (2) take on and act out roles; (3) follow a set of rules determined by specific roles" [96]:438. These three components have an important role in the formation of the child's mind, in the development of abstract thinking and of conscious and voluntary behaviours.

A profound basic line of demarcation in the interpretation of play between the two authors concerns the rules in play. Vygotskij's position is completely antithetical to Piaget's: play "is not completely spontaneous but is instead contingent on players abiding by asset of rules" (ibidem); this rule is already intrinsic to pretend play, the first Vygotskijan type. It has an important psycho-developmental function, but also a critical and direct influence on the effectiveness and success of the ludic activity. In fact, it obliges the child to control his/her immediate impulses, even by acting against them: in competition games, the player must submit to data constraints, in pretend play "the action is subject to the meaning, while, in real life, the action wins out over meaning" [737]:552. Thus, Vygotskij can state that, in play, freedom is only

[31] This is the first phase of Piaget's stage-based theory of cognitive development; from the egocentric stage, the child gradually comes to recognize that other people (and minds) have separate perspectives on objects, events, relationships.

illusory: "While playing, children are free, they determine their actions starting from their self, but [...] their actions are subject to a well-defined meaning, and they act according to the meanings of things" (ibidem). "Play is always a blending of thought, feelings and action: action leads the player to realize new, unanticipated thoughts and feelings" [338]:371.[32] For Vygotskij, "the essential attribute in play is a rule that has become a desire" [278]:580. As a powerful indicator of a child's development, play cannot be neutral with respect to the interpretations of the ways in which it carries out its role.

The positions of Piaget and Vygotskij represent two significant lines of study that produced important followers and advancements. On the one hand, the Piagetian idea proposes a hierarchical alternation between the stages of play. Play is interpreted through an epistemology that provides "invariant and qualitative different stages of development; such stages are typically cumulative, in that later ones build off earlier levels. Furthermore, later stages are thought to be more complex, rationally controlled and abstract. Indeed, human development itself is sometimes equated to the creation and maintenance of personal schemas that feature increasing degrees of integration and control" [333]:16. Moreover, play develops and proceeds from stage to stage, substantially thanks to intellectual development, with which it is considered closely related, since its inception.[33]

On the other hand, the approach inspired by cultural psychology and then by constructivism, while identifying an evolution—not rigidly hierarchical—in characteristics, types, and degrees of complexity of children's play, stresses the value of inter-individual variability, avoids the correlation between every type of play and a predefined chronological age of the child and does not support the idea of a linear progression between stages [596]. Moreover, this approach points out the influence of many concomitant factors, and not only of the cognitive ones: desires, volitions, emotions, experiences, and social contexts of life.

This position is deeply inspired by Vygotskij, whose core idea is that "the history of human development is a complex interplay between the processes of natural development that are determined biologically and the processes of cultural development brought about by the interaction of the growing individual with other people" [95]:204. The high mental functions, in his view, first appear and are built within the social relations which the child is immersed in, and secondly, they become psychological and biological functions of the individual. To put it directly in his own

[32] This statement fully reveals the Marxist matrix of the author's thought, in contrast to Freud's position, entirely feeling- and emotion-based.

[33] The practice play of infancy becomes "more sophisticated as the child's ability to act intelligently develops. When children's sensory-motor schemes become sufficiently coordinated to construct the concept of object permanence, the ability to represent absent realities becomes possible" [12]:235. During growth, "intellectual development from early to late childhood includes an increasing ability to mentally coordinate concepts that are needed to adapt to the natural, physical and social worlds. These changes influence children's symbolic play. As children come to understand the importance of reciprocity in relationships (especially as experienced in peer relationships), they develop a deeper understanding of the necessity to conform to social rules and conventions, including following the rules in games" (ibidem).

words: "Every function in the cultural development of the child appears on the stage twice [...]: first, as social, then as psychological [...]. This pertains equally to voluntary attention, to logical memory, to the formation of concepts and to the development of will" [738]:136. It is exactly in the social contexts that Vygotskij lay the foundations of the Zone of Proximal Development (ZPD), where the child's development takes place. Being play the most important activity within ZPD, the author can assert that play creates child's development.[34]

2.6.2 The Concept of Mature Play and Its Levels

Elkonin [231] elaborated Vygotskij's concept of play as a leading activity "to specify the types of interactions between the child and the social environment, that lead to achievement of the developmental accomplishment in one period of life and that will prepare him for the next period" [96]:441.

Together with his students, he was able to demonstrate that play creates a Zone of Proximal Development (ZPD)[35] where children can function "a head taller than themselves", as Vygotskij stated. Through a series of experiments they compared children's performance on various tasks in play and play situations: the gap between play and non-play performance was high in children who "were assumed to be at the peak of mature play", it did not exist for children who "have not yet developed advanced forms of play [and] for [the older ones] who no longer needed the support of play to support their behaviours" [96]:442. These results confirm Vygotskij's hypothesis that "play is the source of development" but they demonstrate also that new child's behaviours "become apparent in play far earlier than they do in other activities" [737]:16.

To the purpose of finding if a certain level of play should be reached in order to be beneficial, Elkonin proposed the idea of mature play, the "unique form of children's activity" [231]:19, the real source of development in childhood, with the intent of distinguishing it from other forms of playful activities adopted by children.

Mature play has three characteristics, along the three types of make-believe play envisaged by Vygotskij (imaginary situation, roles, and rules)[36]: (a) the child's ability to use objects as substitutes that are very poorly resembling to those they symbolize: they only should perform the same function; as play develops, these objects can become unnecessary and be substituted by gestures; (b) "the child's ability to take on and sustain a specific role by consistently engaging in pretend actions, speech and interactions that fit this particular character"; as play develops, these roles become richer and relationships between them more complex; (c) "a high quality of play scenarios, that integrate many themes and span the time of several days or weeks";

[34] See Sect. 2.2.5.

[35] See Sect. 2.2.5.

[36] The main source of the description of the mature play and its level is the already cited article of Bodrova et al. [96].

the more mature the play, the more articulated the play planning (ivi:443). Elkonin identified four levels of mature play, along these three types. They are described in more detail here below. Level 4 should be considered the full expression of the mature play. There is a relationship between the child's age and the level of play, but not all the children reach the highest level of mature play at the end of their kindergarten.

Elkonin: Mature Play

- Level 1. The main contents of play are actions with objects directed at the play partner (e.g., the actions of a mother feeding children); actions are stereotypical, repetitive, apparently without no order, the script is limited to the core content, without action preceding or following it. If a child produces acts that are inconsistent with the script, nobody objects. The roles exist, but are determined by the situation, not the reverse. Children do not name the roles they play, nor the roles their peers are playing.
- Level 2. Actions with objects are similar to the previous level, but the sequence of actions must be accurate and respect the structure of the real life. If a child produces a mistake in sequence, the other players do not accept it, even if they do not explain what was done wrong. Children name the roles they are playing; the actions related to the role are more clearly dominated.
- Level 3. The focus of the play is the role, and the actions related to it. Some interactions occur demonstrating that the awareness about the reciprocal roles of players is increased (e.g., a player-student asks a player-teacher to give her a coloured pencil). The roles are distinct and clearly attributed and children label them before the beginning of play. The role guides the players' behaviours, as well as the logic of the actions, which become more varied and complex. Speech becomes part of play, adopting specific intonation, vocabulary, and styles, in accordance with the role and the scenario, even if some occurrences of non-play speech may intervene. If a child leaves the assigned role, the other players object: and usually the child explains his/her mistake and tries to fix it.
- Level 4. The main content is here performing actions adequately related to the relationships between the existing roles in the scenario. The roles are well defined, and the child maintains his/her role throughout the entire play session. "The 'role-related speech' is consistent with the role played by the child who uses it, as well as with the role of the child to whom this speech is addressed" (ivi:444). The sequence of actions fully complies with what happens in real life, with a great variety and accuracy of execution. The rules of real life are used as reference for the play rules; actions addressed to different players are coherent with the interlocutor's role. When children object because of a mistake or a rule break, they also can explain the reason for their complaint.

2.6.3 The LUDI Action: Types of Play

The study of the evolutionary nature of play and the analysis of its effective development through subsequent stages—as well as its correlation with the overall child development—have always attracted scholars in the field.

The three typologies proposed by Piaget led the way to many other proposals, in form of classifications, that are not related to the process evolutionary nature. The flourishing of these proposals[37] hints at a latent dissatisfaction on the completeness of the existing classifications; the scientific debate stressed above all the obsolescence of the radical ruptures between play stages, because they seem rather to intermingle, each feeding the other, to re-emerge later in time and in different forms.

Yet, researchers, professional operators, and experts in general need to know and distinguish them on a common basis. In fact, the identification of different types of play, their emergence in different periods of the individual's development, together with their growing complexities and intertwining over time are matters of specific interest for those wishing to explore play as a specific topic of interest. Particularly, such awareness gives the opportunity to study more in-depth—and to knowingly intervene on—play activities, for what concerns the type and the complexity of play, but also the equipment of settings, the adoption of tools and mediators, the kind of relationships.

To accomplish this practical scope, LUDI developed its own classification of types of play, after deep analysis on the field literature. This model makes it possible to respect and safeguard the following five elements of evidence concerning the evolutionary mode of the included types of play and their relationships: (a) in case of regular conditions of child development, and of environmental or socio-cultural contexts, each type has a peculiar onset in a precise developmental age; (b) there is a characteristic progression between the types of play, during development; (c) environmental contexts, human relationships, and technological innovations may give rise to new types of play, which are made by an amalgam between those already known, with varying degrees of involvement of their characteristics, or different skill requirements; (d) the types of play can coexist in different phases of life; (e) each type of play can re-emerge, be reactivated, reveal itself anew, in different developmental stages, remodelled and re-contextualized or simply reproduced by pure ludic spirit [68].

Play requires, claims, and builds up different competences and abilities during development; it manifests immediately, co-evolves with the child, benefits from new skills becoming more and more complex, offering increasingly higher challenges, and stimulating the construction of new—cognitive and social—skills.

Within this model, each type of play, instead of being rigidly separated from the others, involves the competences of the previous one without exhausting them,

[37] Johnson and Dong [373]:401 cite the most recent proposals as follows: Pellegrini and Smith [535] suggest locomotor play, social play, parallel play, object play, language play, and pretend play; Fjortoft [255] uses functional play, constructive play, and symbolic play; Whitebread [750] offers five types: physical, play with objects, symbolic, pretence/socio-dramatic, and games with rules.

Table 2.1 LUDI classification of play [134]

Dimension	Type of play
Cognitive	Practice
	Symbolic
	Constructive
	Play with rules
Social	Solitary
	Parallel
	Associative
	Cooperative

because it re-elaborates and readjusts them at a new level. At that point, these competences are no longer the same; they are contaminated, more complex, and new. A graphical representation of this proposed model would probably not be a continuum of a unidirectional timeline, rather a spiral line, showing the different periods of onset, the progression of each type, their possible coexistence in time, but also the possible contamination between them and even the somewhat reworked reactivation of some of them, in other life periods. Thus, abandoning the hypothesis of adopting a model built on rigidly separated stages, the LUDI model is based on two dimensions, for each of which four main types of play have been singled out (Table 2.1).

While the types of the cognitive dimension have been mainly inspired by the corresponding proposals of Piaget [548] and Parten [528], those related to the social dimension have been derived by Smilansky's studies [650].[38] Each type of play appears at a certain point of the child's life, usually according to the order shown in the table, in the form of an embryonic new group of behaviours, and it becomes more and more complex during time. Furthermore, soon each type of play intertwines with the other ones, which already belong to the child's repertoire, provoking changes in them; vice versa, in some cases, very basic patterns of primitive types of play appear again to support more advanced play activities.

But this blending occurs notwithstanding the dimension the types of play belong: Pellegrini's studies[39] have demonstrated, for example, how direct and deep is the interdependence between the object play and the social context where it comes off; in addition, each play activity can be carried out both in a solitary and in a cooperative form: and this may happen at different ages (since being able to play cooperatively is to be acquired during development), or simply because of contingent situations (no peers are available to play in that moment). Then there is another way in which the cognitive and social dimensions of play meet and overlap: Goffman point out that before starting to play, people "acknowledge that the situation will be of a certain

[38] However, there is a strong accordance between this categorization and that contained in the ICF-CY [765], which will be discussed in Chapter 3.

[39] See Sect. 2.6.

type" [290][40]; even if this statement is more suited to the case of games, in general, it has background implications for the creation and success of play situations and particularly in the educational field.

In the following, the LUDI proposal of types of play according to the two dimensions is shortly presented in more detail, making also reference to the most recent advancements in the related research. For each item, the first paragraph reports the definition contained in the text by Bulgarelli and Bianquin [134], while the second holds additional clarifications for the purposes of this volume as well as references to further research specifically dedicated to the topic. In [134], detailed information is available on the methodology adopted for the construction of the model as well as on the identified bibliographic references.

LUDI Types of Play: Cognitive Dimension

- *Practice play.* This type of play refers to two main aspects: (1) simple body actions or experimentation of body (movements with hands, arms, legs, head and face, vocalizations, etc.); (2) visual and tactile experimentation of objects (children can explore objects with their senses, can manipulate them, practice and use the objects as they are meant to). Moreover, children explore causes and effects (i.e., drop an object and listen to the sound it produces). Typically, in this type of play, movements and experimentations are repeated several times. This type of play is typical in the first and second year of life. Recently revalued for being a precursor to other levels of social, emotional, and cognitive development [217] thanks to new studies in neuroscience. Koziol et al. [403] state that "higher-level executive functioning skills are based on these early sensorimotor experiences". Bergen [61] offers a detailed description of the development of sensorimotor play (sic) of the child, who gradually decentralizes from his/her own body to the objects, whereas his/her actions on them become more effective and goal-oriented. Sensorimotor development is socially initiated and supported by parents and peers. From an epistemological perspective, enactivism [130], perceptual theory [60, 285], and dynamic systems' theory [697] are engaged in this area.
- *Symbolic play.* This type of play implies giving new signification to objects, persons, actions, or events: thus, children symbolically use objects as they were something else, produce pretend play, and make-believe activities. There are several levels of symbolic play with growing complexity: (a) simulation of actions by the child; in this stage, only the body is involved; (b) simulation with objects; (c) simulation with substitution, in which the objects become other than what they are; (d) use of absent objects. Role-playing or socio-dramatic play is another type of symbolic play, where children act out roles in life scenes; they assign

[40] He identifies seven traits of play in this regard: (a) blocking of the ordinary functions and consequences of activity; (b) exaggeration of some behaviours; (c) interruptions of behaviour sequences; (d) repetitiveness of these behaviours; (e) event's relative freedom or "voluntarism"; (f) practice of role-switching, mainly by alternating dominance and subordination positions; (g) separation from external needs [338]:375–376.

roles to others and plan scenes. It involves narrative competence. The simplest expressions of this type of play typically emerge at the end of the second year of life. Nicolopoulou [503] offers an exhaustive description of the development of pretend and social pretend play, from the object substitution to the role-play and socio-dramatic play. He then confirms the universality of this type of play, while recognizing its sensitivity to the influence of cultural and socio-economic factors. While first proving an exploration of pretend play viewed as central in the development of cognitive and social development [430], a subsequent critical review of existing research in the field [432] raised a lively discussion about the role of pretend play, about its usefulness or necessity to promote child development. To Harris [321], it is critical for imagination development whereas role-play helps to promote social understanding and theory of mind, thus enhancing mental understanding. According to Weisberg and Gopnick [745], pretend play prepares children to counterfactual and hypothetical reasoning required for interacting in the real world.

- *Constructive play.*
  This play consists in gathering, combining, arranging, and fitting more elements to form a whole and achieve a specific goal. It usually involves blocks and interlocking building materials (i.e., building a tower of small cubes). In this type of play, the child combines sensorimotor/practice repetitive play with symbolic representation of ideas: children engage in self-regulated creation or construction of a product or a problem solution. It appears in the second year of life. Constructive play acquired the dignity of a devoted type from Smilansky on 1968 [650], creeping in between practice and symbolic play: in fact, it requires both complex and refined psychomotor skills and abilities to hypothesize work plans and monitor their implementation. The dispute is still open about whether or not it is a type of play. A possible alternative category might be "using and making tools" [315], but literature is scarce [534]. This would involve learning to use a tool according to cultural conventions as well as using an object to solve a problem for which it has not been designed (a more divergent and complex action). Tool use increases in preschool children, while making tools develops through middle childhood. The supportive role of adults in letting this interest grow is crucial [706].
- *Play with rules.* This play consists of games with a specific code and rules accepted and followed by the players. It is usually combined with the other three types. It appears in preschool time, from the third year of life.
  According to many authors, all playing involves rules, while others prefer to limit them to a specific type[715]. Winther-Lindqvist proposes this definition: "Games are competitive with a particular goal in deciding between a winner/loser (individual or team) which is determined through enacting and performing particular roles/tasks within the constraints of explicit rules" [756]:224. Playing games gives the opportunity to explore existential themes, such as agency in a group, identity as a player, relationships with others, and it offers the occasion to experience socio-emotional responses to victory, defeat, and frustration. Rules can be external to the game or internal, and in this case they can be invented along the way; their restrictive and transformative function is needed for the game to take the particular

form it has. Anyway, children play their games in their natural settings, they tend both to apply and negotiate rules, as well as to discuss about their application, correctness, and usefulness. This is the most interesting reason for they are also socially generative.

LUDI Types of Play: Social Dimension

- *Solitary play*. Occupying oneself in purposeful, sustained engagement in activities with objects, toys, materials, or games. The child plays alone and independently even if surrounded by other children.
- *Parallel play*. Engaging in purposeful, sustained activities with objects, toys, materials, or games in the presence of other persons also engaged in play, but not joining in their activities. The child plays independently at the same activity, at the same time, and at the same place.
- *Associative play*. The child is still focused on a separate activity, but there is a considerable amount of sharing, lending, taking turns, and attending to the activities of one's peers.
- *Cooperative play*. Joining others in sustained engagement in activities with objects, toys, materials, or games with a shared goal or purpose. Children can organize their play and/or activity cooperatively with a common goal and are able to differentiate and assign roles.

2.7 A World Apart? Games

Regardless of the various classifications, the different forms of play overlap, then blend, and separate again; nevertheless, by middle childhood tend to mutate into rule-governed, game-like activities [652]:2. "Games are a structured and competitive form of play. Key components of games are rules, which should be understood, freely accepted and followed by the players. Most games involve more than one player, thereby encouraging development of social relationships" [574]:68. "Rules are not just for organizing games and making them fair, they keep games interesting and keep games going. But rules will vary widely in their stringency too" [228]:215.

As already seen in this work, some authors consider that rules are involved in any type of play, while others state that they are specific of a particular type: Winther-Lindqvist proposes an intermediate position: "rules are involved in all playing [but] they are unequally dominant in different forms of playing" [756]:222. As said, games are strictly related to socialization and social development: they offer the opportunity to exercise and experiment social rules and roles, they give rise to communities, that may involve both children and adults; sometimes games acquire a different nature when they merge with sport or profitable initiatives but even so they maintain something in common with the game from which they derive—for example, the emotions as well as the involvement of players and spectators.

Rules of the games represent the right constraints that make the game possible with its form; they regulate the relationships among the players as well as the context where they deploy. But rule making implies rule breaking too: their existence does not guarantee that the players adhere to them. In addition, "games generally involve mental or physical stimulation, and often both. In many situations, a game is supported by objects, instrumental to the game, such as cards, a rope, a ball or a computer.

The gaming situation can also be abstract, as in word games" [574]:68. Games can be invented, but most of them are "culturally recognized and well-known activities like soccer, chess, tennis, and the like" (ibidem). They are also associated with "a dispositional stance toward the indeterminate" [456]:208.

Feelings and emotion towards fate are always implicated when being a game player, but they are counterbalanced by skill and mastery, in a continuous tension, until victory or defeat. The experience of taking part to a game may be different according to the player's attitude to win, or simply to join. According to Winther-Lindqvist, "gaming is a distinct play form because performance is more about this committed engagement to mastering the tasks within the rules (and possibly winning) than it is exploring imagined scenarios" [756]:225.

During the 60s and the 70s research in the social and anthropological fields studied in-depth children's games in the streets and playgrounds, revealing that they play with their social status and interpersonal influence (ibidem; [622]) within the game and with their ability to negotiate and mastery rules, despite their ambiguity, thus developing skills in socio-cultural practices [354]. To better understand children's games and gain new knowledge on the meaning of gaming among children in their own contexts, Hughes (1991) proposed three different forms of rules that should always be considered when making research in this area: the explicit rules of the game that define the identity of the game, the rules of the social context, and higher order gaming rules: rules for rules. These last two "reflect the institutional setting or context for the game and the particular relationships among the players" [756]:229: the rules for the rules are responsible of when and how the various existing rules should be respected, and why, in some concrete situations.

2.8 Short Reflections on Play and Technology

It is not possible discussing the theme of play today without at least mentioning the impressing dissemination of available resources and technological tools, most of which addressed to play and games; because of their preponderance in the everyday world, it is impossible that their use does not imply changes in play modes and ideas in the next future.

Bergen [61] reflects on the possible consequences that the use of technological devices from very early childhood can have on their development, including neurological ones. It has now been demonstrated, in fact, that play activities have direct influence on the brain maturation, and therefore it can be hypothesized that a particular activity, such as that suggested and supported by technology-augmented toys, can induce modifications that must be considered. Most of these devices are used for a long duration of time, and they do not require a wide variety or complexity of sensorimotor actions, mainly pointing and pressing. If the time spent by children in contact with these tools substitutes the time spent in other kinds of sensorimotor activities, many developmental consequences might be expected from this loss.

Also, the interaction these devices require is elementary, since children are expected only to react to simple stimuli (although captivating), instead of acting in different ways on various objects that have a wide variety of affordance qualities. "Thus, such play materials may involve a narrower set of physical, cognitive, and social-emotional experiences" [61]:137. For these reasons, it is possible that "this type of play material may differently affect brain development, sensorimotor play, and the types of social and cognitive schema that are strengthened in such play.

At present, the long-term effects of such play on children's socio-cultural competence and enactive cognition is unknown" but if it is correct, as some researchers have stated that "the final pattern of life-long connectivity is established during the first few post-natal years, through activity-dependent mechanisms" [11]:1, "then the effect of these newer technological devices on infant sensorimotor play must be examined" (ibidem).

The digital world, nevertheless, must be observed also from additional perspectives. Scott [624], for example, critically analyses the modern digital technologies as a salient aspect of the socio-cultural environment that have great influence on children's play and interpret this phenomenon within the cultural and media studies tradition. Roskos observes that play is pervading everyday life, exploiting together online and offline digital and nondigital ludic opportunities. The "child's digital habitus—their internalized digital culture—affords them new ways of seeing, acting, and playing in the world", and it is the new scenario that "forces us all to look anew at what play is and what it can do" [595]:538.

Promising emergent lines of research are ongoing in these fields. Digitization has also spread to the education and school sectors, and many tools that are available today to support learning at all academic levels are based on playful environments, exploiting the attractive and motivating qualities that play can offer. These are play-like activities, which make learning more captivating, and prove useful mainly in exercise and repetition. At the same time, further novelty comes from technological design.

Lund [447], who proposed the name "playware" for technological systems that support physical play is convinced of the power of play, considered as a free activity based on mere pleasure. He therefore includes in playware the use of intelligent technologies to develop recreational activities called games, and also "intelligent hardware and software, oriented both to the production of games and of fun playful experiences" [446]:6. Playware must be adaptive and anticipatory, modular, programmable, and self-configurable; moreover, it can be personalized. Play is the essential objective of the developed tools and is presented as the sole criterion for measuring their effectiveness. Since the outcomes of the application of the playware are often assessed in the health area, in this case play represent a background for the activity, a way to entice the user to action and to make the task acceptable and desirable [71].

Also robots are technological tools that could be used for playing physical games; they are concrete and three dimensional, therefore they can be explored with all the senses of the body and guarantee a physical contact—aspects that are by no means negligible as regards the relationship with the human interlocutor and the play opportunities they suggest. Robotic systems, sometimes sophisticated, can be used to support object manipulation by children, especially motor impaired ones [233]. Furthermore, with respect to the common playware, they are mobile devices, able to propose and react, so opening a still different way of playing. Robots are the topic of this book, and they will widely treated in Part II and Part III.

2.9 Contexts and Mediators of Play

In this section, we will present those elements that are enabling the play activities: context and mediators.

2.9.1 Environments

The main attitudes to adopt, in planning and building life and play environments, should be flexibility and open-mindedness, so that these sites, indoor or outdoor, natural or artificial, restored and accommodated or brand new, may guarantee everyone's inclusion, regardless of their individual characteristics, and are capable of supporting the processes of social participation.

Environments are the "containers" of play and games: that is, spaces where play occurs and develops, spaces that suggest and give rise to playing. Play environments and materials have changed during time "due to changes in attitudes about children" [682]:667 who have been more and more proposed built places for playing rather than outdoor and natural ones [177].[41] These spaces built by the adults for the children have also represented the separation between the childhood and adulthood; anyway, "although play designers may envision a way of interacting with a

[41] "Outdoor play is today a critical part of play development [since] for many years the amount of time spent outdoors for children has been declining" [682]:673. Despite the demonstration of the well-being caused by living outdoor spaces [442], on the one hand there seems to be an acute resistance on the part of parents, who have an unrealistic perception of the risks associated with outdoor activities [681], and on the other it seems that the predominance of sedentary activities related to the use of digital media take children away from these experiences. Both nature and forest playgrounds encourage risky play; their play value is enhanced by "multifunctional materials like sand and water [as well as] the complexity of the landscape". Moreover, "open-endedness allows the child to decide which type of play activity she wishes to pursue" [682]:675.

play space, children rarely confine themselves by choice to those predetermined ideas" [682]:668.

If it is true that any child finds his/her own way to play in any space, in any situation, with any type of objects, it is also true that fascinating, mysterious, open, flexible spaces, nice and well-formed, may suggest new ways of playing, foster relationships, thoughts and ideas, create a productive and fruitful integrating background [777] where exploration, examination, attempts, trials, imitation can be implemented, roles can be acted, and rules can find their sense. Even the most solitary player plays within a context, whatever it is, and we may argue that colours, lights, sounds, objects, aesthetics characteristics in that environment, or feelings and emotions perceived there, in some ways have inspired that play activity.

Moreover, probably that player has at least a companion, or can find it, and the ludic exchange can soon start, through imitation—near or at a distance—dialogue, arrangements, negotiation of roles, and decision about rules. Probably that player has his/her own personal history about play: playful attitudes, support by the adults, school educational styles, and play occasions in life.

In short, environments—natural sites or architectural structures—are never neutral, distant, and meaningless. They are perceived and lived in many different ways that always correspond to the idea of use they offer, or, in the case of educational contexts, to the intentionality of use that underlies them. They may provoke feelings and moods, support attention or distraction, inspire sociability, favour or prevent relationships.

Home is the first place where individuals find the right answers to their own daily needs; it is to be considered "a place rather than a building: a place for safety and belonging, and most significantly a core setting for developing primary relationships" [562, 620]. Safety and reliability are two unavoidable characteristics of any house where children live and, consequently, play; anyway, to give children the opportunity to feel free to play, spaces should be properly organized, so that they can independently plan and carry out their activities but also involve adults and peers, possibly also "trespassing" their own area of the home. It should also not be forgotten that children, especially in their home, love to share everyone's space, even that of their parents, and play with normal household items—with kitchen and do-it-yourself equipment, with flowers and lights and carpets...

Therefore, above all, the parents' ideas about the importance of play in childhood are at stake, since they guide the organization of times and spaces, prohibitions and permits, which make them available to be involved in playing, and to be part of it.

The issue of usability[42] of this type of environment is not so much a matter of real physical spaces—many houses are small or untidy, but full of widespread playfulness—but of cultural and socio-psychological attitudes (ideas of development, parent-child relationship, acknowledgement of the child's needs, time availability, etc.).

[42] Usability should be considered the "extent to which a product can be used by specified users to achieve specified goals with effectiveness, efficiency and satisfaction in a specified context of use" (ISO 9241-11:1998, 3.1). In this case, the term is applied, by extension, to environments.

The introduction of play spaces within education institutions has been considered controversial: on the one hand, purists have sustained that when play is organized and controlled by adults is no longer play [407] or that play has nothing to do with curriculum development [680], on the other, the possibilists have considered that any environment devoted to children is a place where play can be practiced. Indeed, following the ideas of distinguishing educators such as Dewey and Pratt, they interpreted this option as a fruitful occasion: such an environment, in fact, may support play through socialization, and play has a decisive role in child development [275].

Among the spaces where play can be practiced, stands for originality the notable "Reggio Emilia approach",[43] for which the design and aesthetics of the physical environment are of utmost importance. As Malaguzzi said: "Our objective, which we will always pursue, [was] to create an amiable environment where children, families, and teachers feel at ease" (Malaguzzi in [229]: 41, [457]). Within this approach "the physical environment receives much attention and supports exchange and relationships through physical qualities of transparency, reflectiveness, openness, harmony, softness and light. A classroom atmosphere of playfulness and joy pervades" [230]:9. A friendly, warm space, capable of involving and encouraging the participation of all, including political administrators; a space that does not reject anyone because it is designed for the needs of people with very different characteristics, and which at the same time is projected to guarantee everyone's right to access the services offered.

This kind of environment should "allow for maximum movement, interdependence, and interaction. [It] must be set up to interface the cognitive realm with the realm of relationship and affect. Thus, there should also be connection between [...] thought and action, and between individual and interpersonal autonomies" [229]:41–44. Areas should be assured to those who would like to stay and play alone, as well as to those who would exchange ideas and share activities with peers. Thanks to a strict collaboration between architects, designers, and educational professionals, a detailed framework of inspiring concepts for designing such environments, where children can play, develop, learn, and share precious time together, has been developed [167]; among the numerous characteristics and qualities described, the most directly related to play are presented in what follows.

- *Overall softness*. Space should be "livable and serene [and] functional while remaining aware that different dimensions and relationships can coexist and that the people involved can communicate and work together" [229]:323.
- *A relational space* that makes it possible to share creative ideas and strategies, to explore and exchange among adults and with the children.

[43] The long history of the "Reggio Emilia Approach" (Reggio Emilia is a town in central Italy; the work group is also known as Reggio Children) starts in the second half of the nineteenth century and unfolds over the years with a series of significant stages. This path has led it today to be recognized in the world for its originality and effectiveness [343] and to come into contact with 145 countries and territories in the world. Loris Malaguzzi has been the initiator and the real protagonist of this movement of thought and action. https://www.reggiochildren.it/en/reggio-emilia-approach/.

- *Continuity with surroundings environments and social connections.* "The relationship among people can be extended as a dialogue with the world of objects. [...] Furthermore, relationship creates continuity with all that is within the space of the school and with what is outside" (ivi:323).
- *Multiple sensorial experiences.* "An environment that invites sensory experience by creating a variety of features, stimulating perceptions, and helping children become aware of them can support meaningful sensorial experiences" (ibidem).
- *Colour.* "It is necessary to use a chromatic range with many shades and to offer children a subtler colour scheme with many colours" (ivi:324).
- *Light.* "Lighting should offer an environment illuminated from a variety of sources: incandescent, fluorescent, vapor, halogen, etc., in order to make optimal use of the full range of possibilities. Light should be able to create shadows [and] should provide concentrated as well as diffuse light and different colour 'temperatures': warm white, cool white, rose white" (ibidem).
- *Materials.* "The materials used should be rich and varied. They should create a multisensory setting with surfaces which are smooth and rough, wet and dry, opaque, bright, translucent, and transparent. They should have different features which change over a period of time (wood, stone, flowers, fabrics) or remain unchanged (glass, steel)" (ibidem).
- *Flexibility and adaptation.* Such a space should be adaptable and flexible so that it "can either signal to adults the need to modify it, or [it] can directly proceed to modify the space as they use it" (ibidem). This gives the possibility to play in a solitary or parallel way or with others.

Guidelines such as those offered by the "Reggio Children" team may support in specifying usability aspects of ludic environments, but for these environments are really fully inclusive—that means to let everyone be successful in achieving his/her daily and desired activities and participate with the others on an equal basis—they should be also accessible.[44]

"Physical accessibility to sites/locations for play remains [...] a logical precursor to play itself. If the physical environment is not accessible" for all, some persons will be excluded from that environment, and this "exclusion [has, in turn, the consequence] to reinforce negative attitudinal barriers towards" diversity in general, and particularly disability [44]:20.

Within the wider perspective of Universal Design,[45] interventions on environments, products, and services should "ensure that anyone, including future genera-

[44] According to ISO (Guide 71:2014), accessibility should be interpreted as the "the extent to which products, systems, services, environments and facilities can be used by people from a population with the widest range of characteristics and capabilities to achieve a specified goal in a specified context of use". https://www.iso.org/standard/57385.html.

[45] Universal Design [668] is a popular design approach and it should be interpreted as the "design of products, environments, programmes and services to be usable by all people, to the greatest extent possible, without the need for adaptation or specialized design". The construct shall not exclude assistive devices for particular groups or persons with disabilities where this is needed. It is sometimes substituted, without changing meaning, with terms such as universal design, accessible design, design for all, barrier-free design, inclusive design and transgenerational. (ISO, Guide 71:2014).

tions, regardless of age, gender, capacities or cultural background, can participate in social, economic, cultural and leisure activities with equal opportunities".[46] These statements and the related awaited political measures concern also a special kind of environments devoted to leisure time in infancy and not only [651].

Accessibility of playground accessibility and of the related equipment has become a hot topic in the scientific literature of the sector, and it has been deeply analysed within the research studies conducted by LUDI [44, 234, 620]. However, for these spaces can exploit all their potential play value in providing fun and social sharing, the playground should respond also to the right usability criteria: for example, according to the preferences of the child, it should be wide enough, offer safety hazards, variety of stimulation, etc. [450]. While "accessible environments are usually guided by minimum standards set out in legislation in each country [....] usability means that [...] the play opportunities" offered are really available for everyone: "good playground design for accessibility and usability considers varied needs of the broadest range of users possible" [450]:105.

2.9.2 *Mediators: Toys*

In his analysis of the role of repetition in play, Walter Benjamin, a profound and passionate scholar of this theme, showed his antinomic view to Freud's, for whom children use to repeat "everything that has made a great impression on them in real life, and in doing so [...] they make themselves master of the situation" [558]:726. Benjamin was instead convinced that "there is a tendency to [...] view the realm of children's toys as distinct, as belonging to a 'fantasy realm' or 'fairy-tale land' of 'pure childhood'" (ivi:729).

The difference between the two positions is placed precisely on the directionality of the action made by the child: in fact, it is not the imaginative content of a child's toys that determines playing, rather the fact that the "child wants to pull something, and so he becomes a horse, he wants to play with sand, and so he turns into a baker; he wants to hide, and so he turns into a robber or a policeman" [558]:730.[47]

Benjamin's intuition is still today very engaging and problematizing.[48] The child can be viewed as the starter of the play process, seeking something that may respond to his/her need to know and explore. Obviously, as Pellegrini has pointed out,[49] the imitation of "the others" (adults and peers) has a not secondary role in the initiation of this process, especially when the activities carried out by the others seem to produce

[46] Design for All Foundation. http://designforall.org/.

[47] Reference by the author: Walter Benjamin, *Selected Writings*, 4 vols., ed. Marcus Bullock, Howard Eiland, and Michael W. Jennings (Cambridge, MA: Harvard UP, 1996–2003) vol. 2, 120.

[48] In fact, the devaluation of imagination as a source of play (that is, in contrast with the Vygotskijan perspective) does not seem convincing as a description of the child's playful activity. However, the avowal of the power of the physical action on things and in the surrounding space, even in the case of the symbolic play phase, seems intriguing.

[49] See Sect. 2.6.

useful results (whatever that means) or arouse new curiosity. This is equivalent to saying that the context around the child has a crucial role in instilling curiosity, thus highlighting the circular pattern between individual and environment.

Exactly like scientists, very young children, during sensorimotor play, "experiment with what objects can do and learn what the affordances of the objects enable them to do" [61]:129 [293]. By applying the gestures and the movements they are able to do at any given age, "they enjoy manipulative materials such as clay, water, paint; begin to use simple puzzles; and build with blocks", while when around the age 2 they can feel more active and brave, and start climbing, riding, jumping, and using objects that can be pulled and pushed. Or, when motor coordination is refined, they enjoy "poking fingers into holes, picking up small objects, and using toys activated by buttons or knobs [but also] make marks [with] crayons, pencils, and chalk" (ibidem). This list of the child's skills that evolve in accordance with the shift of interest to ever-different objects and toys seems to justify Benjamin's hypothesis.

So, if objects and toys do not contain in themselves a "fantasy realm", they anyway have specific characteristics that offer children many useful perceptual information on how they can be used: "the stimulus features of the environment, labelled 'affordances' [...] enable experiencing direct perceptual knowledge and thus action related to that knowledge" [61]:134, [285]; thanks to affordances, perception can be inferred "through the spontaneous exploratory activity and play", that is, directly from the environment. According to Gibson, the perceptual development then contributes to higher order thinking, as well as to social understanding. Working out Gibson's theoretical proposal, Carr "noted that affordances of objects have three characteristics relevant for understanding the types of playful actions young children use when they interact with toys and other objects: (1) transparency, i.e., the object signals which actions can be used; (2) challenge, i.e., different objects have many or few actions that can be used; and (3) accessibility, i.e., objects differ in how easily various actions can be used" [60]:132, [162].

Toys are not essential for play: it is common observation that players are able to "bend" the available objects around them to satisfy their wishes and needs. Or they can build the toys they need, and—as already noted by Pellegrini[50]—this activity can be embedded in playing. Yet, toys exist since the dawn of time: a delicate gift by adults to children that has been also interpreted as a form of inheritance and cultural transmission,[51] however often simply done unknowingly, simply out of habit and tradition.

Toys and games, which belong everywhere to the concrete world of childhood, are the essential mediators between a child, his/her own Self, the others—children or adults—and the outer world. As mediators "between the physical reality and its symbolic representation, toys also empower a child to express his/her feelings, worries or concerns" [574]:67: they respond to the needs and the preferences of the children, give them occasion and support while acting on reality and on the

---

[50] See Sect. 2.6.

[51] The reference is here to Groos [303] and to the debate that followed, at a distance and at different times, on this topic, which involved the reflections of Benjamin and Freud [558].

others according to their plans or desires. Since the actions are different according to the various types of play, different types of toys have been invented and created throughout history to support them, thus making play a more sophisticated, inventive, engaging, and challenging activity.

In recent years, the relationship with the toy has become more complex due to the introduction, thanks to electronics, of "sensors that can perceive actions, so that the toy can autonomously react with varying degrees of complexity while maintaining its characteristics" [574]:68. In this case, the toy is no more a passive play partner, but "also as an agent that can decide to do what it 'wants'. These toys may provide other play challenges, where the player has to understand how the toy is behaving and adapt his/her activity to that of the toy" (ibidem).

This new presence on the toy market contributes to increase complexity into the controversial issue of the types of play. In fact, numerous lists of categories of play have been developed by toy companies, which often follow odd criteria and contribute to adding confusion in the field; these lists usually suit the needs of the various developmental stages of the child, but also include groupings that are mainly useful from a commercial point of view.

The toy industry, in particular, for what concerns electronic and digital games, is now relatively thriving. Thanks also to the effective advertising it relies on, at least in the north-western countries it is widespread enough to guide the preferences of children and families and ends up affecting the choices and the styles adopted in free time.

Despite the large audience it reaches, the issue of accessibility, which also in this case is decisive, remains a significant thorn in the side: in general, toy companies continue to develop products from the perspective of an average, skilled user, performing for his/her chronological age, belonging to a cultural background which is also average and predictable.

The issue of accessibility, on the contrary, is decisive for play activities open to all the possible differences existing in the human population, thus contributing, in a rapidly changing world, to guaranteeing the accomplishment of a generalized principle of social participation and inclusion.

Jansens and Bonarini deeply analysed the existing literature on usability and accessibility of toys and technologies for play, with special attention to the population of children with disabilities.[52] Their scoping review intended to collect guidelines and tools existing in the field, their "possible use possible use for different stakeholders involved in play for children with disabilities [as well as] their strengths and weaknesses" [367]:83. After careful review, they were able to select 10 guidelines (out of 54 products initially identified and collected within the on-purpose database), only 5 of which had a specific focus on play. The obtained results highlight the lack of tools for usability and accessibility measurement, the sole inclusion of digital games and apps within the considered areas of play (while robots, on the contrary, were

[52] The two studies were produced within the cohort of publications developed by the Action LUDI. As in the case of the other LUDI products, this means that many researchers of the Action collaborated to the final result.

absent), no consideration of the particular population of children. Their conclusions sound synthetic but insightful: "further research in this field is required to support designers and engineers in making inclusive toys and technologies as well as to support parents and professionals in applying these toys and technologies to strengthen transparent professional reasoning and, if possible, evidence-based practice. There is still work to be done by researchers, innovation managers and policy makers to support play processes in children with disabilities, to cooperate and to exchange expertise" [367]:100.

Then, the two authors took the challenge included in these conclusions, by developing guidelines for taking into consideration "usability and accessibility of toys and technologies for play for children with disabilities" [368]:106. The guidelines are addressed to various populations—parents and caregivers, professionals, makers, designers, and researchers—to the purpose of giving them "reflections and decision-making processes for choosing, adapting, designing or studying a toy or technology"; the theoretical aspects of this work are then supported by five different tools devoted, respectively, to the groups mentioned above.

As for play environments, also in the case of toys the issue of accessibility should develop in accordance with that of usability. Ray-Kaeser et al. first recommend that toys should respond to safety standards and "include specific quality requirements [that children value a lot], such as durability, comprehensibility, proper functioning as well as the potential for interaction and popularity" [573]:72 and secondly they propose a selection of the Universal Design principles that are related to play and games, inspired to the three general principles—multiple means of representation, multiple means of use and multiple means of play. Finally, they offer a sort of guideline in form of questions, to support people in selecting toys and games with the highest probability of success, based on the premise that "the best toy is the one that matches the child's characteristics (skills and abilities, personal preferences) and the play characteristics (level of challenge, demands and requirements of the activity)" (ivi:74). As a consequence, questions are addressed "to consider the features of the toy or game, the child's abilities, needs and preferences, the activity promoted by the toy or game and the expected play context" (ibidem).

Also the TUET (Toys and games Usability Evaluation Tool[53]) [192] was developed in the context of the activities promoted by the LUDI Action and particularly in the area of usability of toys and games. As sustained by the three authors, it is a "method of analysis to evaluate play materials by considering the physical characteristics that are appropriate for children with hearing, visual, or upper-limb motor impairments" and it is intended for a wide audience of users, among which the toy companies, professionals in the fields of education and rehabilitation, toy librarians, and parents. Its use will support all these people to "design, select and adapt toys and games to the needs of all children".

Translated into four additional languages besides English, it represents the current arrival of the work carried out for the last decades by two significant institutions on

[53] http://www.tuet.eu.

the European territory (AIJU in Spain[54] and FM2J in France[55]) in the study of the usability and accessibility of play and toys, and in the application of this knowledge in favour of children with different skills and their life contexts, as well as, more generally, in favour of a more inclusive society.

2.9.3 Mediators: Play Companions

The fact that play has a prevailing social nature, even when it takes place in solitary mode, is now widely shared and that imitation, at a distance and apparently unintentional or expressly proposed by the interlocutor, is one of the main evolutionary engines of the complexity of play, is equally well known. Finally, the fact that play, like any emergent process, starts from an "innate predisposition" and grows towards more complex manifestations and structures, thanks to a blending process of relationships and actions active in the contexts of life, is one of the most promising hypotheses existing today in the study field of play.

Particularly, "Vygotskij conceptualized play as the creation of an imaginary situation, where players change the meaning of objects and actions to give them a new sense. [...] It is argued here that [the growing] repertoires of signs, and the meaning systems attributed to them, are highly culturally situated" [256]:420. Over time, the theoretical framework proposed by Vygotskij, which values the constructive contamination between the individuals and their living environments as a distinctive mark of their own growth and points out play as the engine for development, has proved to be productive of significant research and has obtained numerous experimental confirmations, which also resulted in the creation of effective intervention tools.

On this background, over the years, there has been a continuous growth of research that has tried to identify, clarify, and enhance the role of the child's social contexts, to make them become more aware and therefore more effective, in the construction of his/her harmonious social and cognitive development. As a consequence, these studies have analysed the typology and quality of these social contexts, since they inevitably call into question the theoretical conceptions of child and childhood, of relationship between peers and between adult and child, as well as, of course, of play. In what follows, adopting the perspective of social constructivism, a brief collection of these studies is presented to highlight the role of play companions—including both adults and peers—in co-constructing play skills and supporting play development.

Adults

Two interesting studies, a laboratory one by Lillard [431] and a naturalistic one by Ugaste [722], found that mothers are actively engaged in teaching play to their children.

---

[54] AIJU, Technological Institute for Children's Products and Leisure, Ibi, Alicante, España. http://www.aiju.es.

[55] FM2J, Centre national de Formation aux Métiers du Jeu et du Jouet. Caluire-et-Cuire, Lyon, France. http://www.fm2j.com.

Lillard showed that US mothers of 18-month-old children use to teach pretence by adopting specific body attitudes that signal children they are pretending: exaggerated actions, number of words doubled, augmented use of the pronoun "we", louder speech, long smiles, and longer periods of gaze exchange. All these behaviours, according to the author, "are akin to social referencing", and children during these exchanges "correspondingly displayed smiling back and performing pretence more often" [256]:421.

Ugaste noted that most of the joint play activities between mothers and their 5/6-year-old children in Estonia were related to academic skills; anyway, they "involved humour and magic [were] described as fun" while using toys was considered boring "unless they afforded the possibility to add something to them and change their function". In addition, "when children played with their mothers, the play lasted longer, and the level of the play was much more complex, with more play scripts, than when children played alone" (ibidem).

Other studies [281] suggest that the role of the adult is fundamental for the development of play. Nevertheless, this type of studies risks containing—or give rise to—bias in cross-cultural comparison, due to the different values attributed to play and childhood (and consequently to the role of the adult in children's play) in different areas, also in relation to underlying socio-environmental factors. Literature shows a variability in beliefs and practices [466] in this area. For example, families of Yucatec Mayan children do not actively participate to their play activities [280]; Caribbean parents do not include play among the needed pre-schooling activities [594]; some communities use to value work over play [170]. As noted by Göncü et al., the problem with these studies is that the concept itself of play should be reframed, to better understand the effective participation or indifference towards it: "play is only a partially understood activity, the meaning of which varies as a result of the perspective from which it is examined" [292]:155, for example, teasing in some communities "is a form of symbolic representation and [...] this and other forms of representation should be carefully considered when undertaking research into play across cultures" (ivi:175). The risk to impose a monocultural conception of play in study design is today widely discussed [219]: Lillard et al. [430], for example, claim for "a universal model of play to support children's development" [256]:423. For sure, knowing the meaning assigned by families and communities to the issues of play, its value, and the parents' role are unavoidable to gain new insights for reliable research in the field.

Hedegaard and Fleer [329] set up a 12-month naturalistic study in Australia—a land where cultures meet and coexist without substantially overlapping or intertwining—that put clearly into evidence that, while play was evidently used in family "for scholastic achievement [...] in the traditional sense of numeracy and literacy" [256]:430, the most inventive aspects of play were displaced to the joyful parent-child relationship, mainly in "the semiotic activity of creating a collective imaginary situation. [For example,] the adults regularly engaged their children in the process of changing the meaning of objects and actions to give them a new sense. [Additionally,] learning academic content was primarily embedded in family play, and concepts were amplified by adults to help children pay attention to them" (ibidem). Moreover, the study reached another inspiring result: "the adults and siblings appeared to be in tune with each other's development when in play". Adults gave more time and space for participation to the younger, or accelerated in favour of the older ones. Thus, the adults' careful behaviour "contributed to the maintenance and development of the collective play" [256]:432. The authors first conclude about the need to rethink pretend play, and the related social practice; then, they also observed interesting aspects concerned with games with rules that were "collectively introduced, supported, and narrated. [More precisely], the adults either were embedded in the play as players or were near the children's play [in both cases having the opportunity] to expand the play through their direct or indirect roles inside the play. What was different from previous research was that the adults genuinely played with their children, rather than pretending to be a player or a novice" [256]:433. Despite having a long duration and being conducted in depth, this study's conclusions are limited because it concerns only one family, but it is suggestive enough to understand that ideas and practices of play within the family are tuned with the cultural ideas of the wider society, thus playing a supporting role for aligning children with the community values.

Numerous play scholars, within the socio-constructivist approach, have for some years now taken radical positions regarding the role that the adult plays in the development of the child's play. According to them, without the supporting—or, better, scaffolding[56]—role of the adult, play does not exploit its full potential and the whole child development is affected, in particular, for what concerns self-regulation skills [87]. They also argue that—especially in the educational field [736]—the crucial role of play for learning is now increasingly overlooked, and that adults are losing their ability to interact playfully with children.

Moreover, according to many authors, make-believe play today is not only different from the past, but it has declined in both quality and quantity [372, 384]. A wealth of research, accompanied by tools and methods, has been carried out in this area. The precursor of these applicative studies is Elkonin, for whom make-believe play—the type of play he is most interested in—does not develop spontaneously, rather it is "an outgrowth of specific interactions young children have with their older peers and adults" [96]:447. For play "to become a truly 'leading activity' that drives child development forward,[57] children need to engage in specific interactions with adults who would lead children in their leading activity" (ibidem). Therefore, in case these interactions are absent or low quality, children do not reach the expected level of "mature play", getting stuck in immature levels of play.

[56] Scaffolding [129, 763], from a metaphorical point of view, can be imagined as the concrete "platform" that allows bridging the gap from a lower (or supported) to a higher (or autonomous) degree of competence. It is defined as a process by which a partner more skilled at a task changes the degree and quality of support provided to a less skilled partner, so that the partner can become more experienced. This process can make use of: (a) a gradual feedback system (explicit or implicit); (b) a mechanism for fading the precedents; (c) specific skill training programmes; (d) transfer activities, created ad hoc, of the skills and knowledge acquired [69].

[57] For more details about Elkonin's theoretical proposal, see also Sect. 2.6.2.

Possible further causes of this situation can be sought in some pejorative cultural changes: the fact that toys today appear more and more realistic—frustrating imagination—that adults tend to directly establish restricted forms of leisure and recreation as well as to impose limits and constraints, especially in relation to the perceived risk that the time dedicated to free play even in educational contexts is much shorter than in the past and that the opportunities for sharing activities between older and younger children have been reduced in the school, thus impoverishing the opportunities to develop new skills for imitation, mutual discovery, exchange, and dialogue.

For all these reasons, some researchers became convinced that "to achieve rapid progress in the quality of play, play scaffolding [...] needs to be designed to strategically target its most critical components" [96]:448. To this purpose, Bodrova and Leong [94] published their work *Tools of the Mind*, defined as "a Vygotskijan-based early childhood curriculum". Its use has demonstrated "to increase children's levels of self-regulation/executive function and to improve their academic performance in preschool and kindergarten" [42, 88, 96, 218]. It proposes a method to conduct make-believe activities able to support preschool children in reaching the phase of "mature play", through playful learning mixed with planning activities. It is based on four areas of increasing difficulty: (a) Scaffolding the Use of Toys and Props in a Symbolic Way; (b) Scaffolding the Development of Consistent and Extended Play Scenarios; (c) Scaffolding the Development and Maintenance of Play Roles and Rules; and (d) Planning for Play [96]. Very interestingly, the authors open the door to an extremely promising new harvest of research, reminding that the concept of "mature play" is still to be explored in depth in the case of other types of play—e.g., "building with blocks, movement games, and board games and computer games"[58]—that are sensitive to different chronological and developmental phases of children: for each of them the right "scaffolding areas" are still to be discovered, analysed, and experimented within further evolutive processes. Bodrova and Leong's proposal offers a further element of originality in that the materials developed do not concentrate only on the observation of the child but include also the scaffolding activity carried out by the teacher: then, two "categories" of subjects represent the focuses of their intervention. This clearly highlights the intention to look at the process as a system, in its aspects of relationality and circularity, thus ensuring evidence to the complexity of the process itself, as well as to the related methodology.

This methodological choice has been confirmed by the works of Hakkarainen and Bredikyte, who consider crucial the role of the adult as a mediator in play, but maintain the impossibility to study this theme within "a classical experimental design, because an adult is a distorting variable between cause and effect" [312]:458; they rather propose to adopt "a cultural-historical paradigm [where] causality can be called 'systemic, psychological, circular, or mutual'" (ivi:459).

Within the LUDI Action awareness on the importance of the role of the adult as a mediator of play was widely shared, as well as the need to increase the adults'

[58] With respect to the LUDI play types (see Sect. 2.6.3), these categories should be, respectively, translated into: constructive play, practice play, play with rules.

competence in promoting—and taking part to—the play activity. Bianquin [78] advanced also a structured proposal on the different facets that the adult's role might take. First there is the role of "builder of rights" (ivi:52). Information and awareness about the importance of play for the child development should be properly spread among parents, professionals, educators, and policy-makers. Since play is a right, appropriate time, space and relationships must be granted, as well as respect for the child's preferences, needs, and attitudes. The second is "promoter of inclusion". Play cannot segregate nor be segregated. It claims for participation, on equal basis, for sharing fun, desires, and plans without any constraint but the rules of the play itself: "providing inclusive opportunities", organizing inclusive and accessible environments, planning play activities able to grant everyone's participation in any occasion offered within the community life, are full responsibility of the adult. Promoting inclusion may also mean being able to offer children modelling inclusive behaviours, so that they can have a useful and good source for imitation, thus learning decentration, kindness, and collaboration. The third role presented—"scaffolder"—has been already discussed here; the author chose to distinguish three different sub-types, and areas of application: (a) observer, that requires a detailed and deep knowledge of the child to understand his/her real play wishes and needs, without running into prejudicial or hasty evaluations that would lead to ineffective play proposals; (b) activator, that should "identify the best promising conditions from which play can spring, exist and evolve" and then implement them; (c) partner, that gives the opportunity to play together with the child, following and supporting his/her directions and desires, without introducing additional and external goals (ivi: pp. 53–54).

Peers

Peers are partners of play, too, and according to some theoretical models they are an essential and indispensable component of it. They may be even more effective than adults, in provoking change in their companions, because they can take the role of "challenger or questioner: the result is a setting marked by imaginative intersubjectivity, where each person (ideally) takes seriously the invitations of the other" [338]:372. Nevertheless, there is no in-depth literature on this specific topic. Studies in clinical psychology focus on the development of relationships between peers, including play as one of the possible occurrences [328].

The best known and most widely used study in this regard, that of Parten, dates back to 1932; it proposes a systematization of the child social development through play development, by identifying a progression in infant behaviours, which would develop from the single individual to the dyad and subsequently to the larger group of peers. This model appears unsatisfactory today; first of all, in Sutton-Smith's longitudinal study [684] Parten's progression wasn't respected; then, further awareness raised on the complexity of the play phenomenon, as well as on its many facets. For example, some research today highlights the importance of the group in developing the pretend play phase [329], while some argue that collaborative behaviours can be highlighted in earlier stages [439].

A tool still in use in the sector, which gives some additional indications, is the *Peer Play Scale*, developed by Howes in 1980. The scale is intended to explore and show "a continuum toward more mature development" [351]:371. It introduces two conceptual notions—complexity in the use of an object or activity and complexity of social exchanges—to analyse them both in separate and comparative mode. The first three levels "are similar in object use (parallel) but represent increasingly mature forms of social exchanges (from lack of awareness to mutual recognition and finally interaction). Levels 4 and 5 are similar in advanced object use (reciprocal and complementarity) and dissimilar in social exchanges" (ibidem). According to this model, peer interaction in play can be described from simple undifferentiated responses (children look at each other but do not interact in other modes), through differentiated but not yet integrated ones (children socially engage without using object complementary, or the reverse), to organized and integrated responses in both the social and inanimate domains (children engage in social exchanges and also in complementary play activities).

Although Howes's study significantly refines the analysis of the social development of child play in its early stages, it is undoubtedly possible to point out the absence of more sophisticated and in-depth research relating to later evolutions. In fact, if cooperation among peers is an important final goal, it would be useful to be able to recognize in this social behaviour more details, facets, and evolutionary elements over time.

Currently, the role of peers in playing seems to receive more attention in the field of socio-cultural studies, where play is studied as one of the expressions of the communities' life and relationships among peers while playing are a not infrequently a focus of research (e.g., [295, 378]).

2.9.4 *"Le cadre ludique"*

Contexts and mediators of play have been described in detail in this paragraph: they are co-protagonists, together with the children, of the play activities, therefore responsible for the success of what happens inside them: that you have fun, that you make friends, that you start inventing, and that you feel active and participating.

Yet, to do this, it is necessary that each element is consistent with the others and that the whole situation they produce really works: many balances must be considered and maintained, but novelties must also be able to be accepted, and the occasions of disturbance or boredom must be eliminated.

In 2016 Périno presented her model, called *cadre ludique*—play setting or play frame—which can be a very useful methodological tool for intervention but also for reflection.

It is mainly conceived for educational or leisure time settings, but most of the proposed suggestions are perfectly suited to familiar and occasional spaces; the presence of the adult is always foreseen. The author proposes a definition of this construct as follows: "an attempt for play to exist in respect of its constitutional antinomies, behind which they can fit: to be alone and in relation, to be oneself and another, to know and not to know, to foresee the unforeseeable, to be a child and a player, a parent and a professional, to feel free and be subject to the rules..." [541]:102. It consists of six elements: (a) a devoted space that serves as a "container" to those who play and might justify the possible presence of adults; (b) separate play areas, differentiated and organized according to players' particular interests at different ages; (c) objects chosen and made available by adults; (d) presence of adults, who may be accompanying persons or various types of professionals; (e) a rule for using that special places, with references to the play duration; and (f) possibly, a relationship of belonging. If the players are young or very young, the elements may become more precise as well as the shared rules. The *cadre ludique* has five functions [541]:

(a) It is a frame of reference for the play situation: it gives play the right to exist as an educational activity per se; it attributes to play its own space and the right needed time; it guarantees a frame of reference different from the familiar ones; it assures inclusive play for everybody and it can be implemented everywhere.
(b) It provides a solution to the paradox of the player autonomy-security: it concretely and carefully considers the issues related both to the physical and to the affective and mental security, and these protective activities are always oriented to guarantee the exploitation of the individual's autonomy.
(c) It provides support for socialization through the organization of spaces according to the presumed skills of the players, which makes it possible to bring them together according to their close interests and more or less similar play needs; it gives rise to interactions between children thanks to complementary roles, while for older players, the setting provides elements of "relational comfort": the distribution of players in the space, according to common needs and similar skills, limits turbulence and conflicts.
(d) It gives meaning to the presence of the adults: they can be invited to immerse themselves in play areas, or to stay away, or to simply be there, without exercising the power that is naturally devolved to them; it gives adults a clear visibility, since they can exercise their roles, in a way that reminds to the "right distance", both physical and psychological, but, facing the children's freedom, they may also feel free from the usual authority, and more available for new types of interactions.
(e) It defines a context for observation or research activities; this special space in fact can facilitate the entry into play of children, free them from perceived limitations, or, on the contrary, it can reveal some difficulties. This particular function of the playful setting may then become the ideal space to deepen the individual's or the group's needs, as well as to study the play itself as a scientific and pedagogical theme.

In her work, the author presents and discusses the model in detail by including the basic principles that guide the play activity within the setting—as described in its components—together with suggestions for the concrete organization of the space, accompanied by directions for the arrangement of contexts that best favour the different types of play.

2.10 Research in Play

Play is an impregnable construct, is an ambiguous [686] and vague concept, it cannot count on a shared and unique definition, it cannot count on stable categorizations of typologies and characteristics, and it is not even known what is—if any—its function in the life of human beings. All human beings play and in this they are similar to many animal species, primarily mammals [141]; they have been playing since the dawn of time, and they play at any age, particularly in childhood, in every context, in every condition of physical, psychological, and economic well-being.

And yet, it is not easy to trace the similarities between the various manifestations of play, which are sensitive to the variety of species, time, age, place, and culture. Highlighting its recursive and elusive characteristic, play is an expression of culture—it is itself the origin of culture [356]—but its quality and its representations depend on the cultural interpretations given to it. "The above and other ways of thinking about play are typically very much ahead of our ability to render play empirically manageable" [373]:401.

Placed on this background, play does not seem a researchable phenomenon (Schlosberg, 1947). And yet, it does not seem correct to say that it is "scientifically useless" [373]:399. In the final part of their chapter, after appropriate analysis and discussion, the authors themselves conclude that "play is not scientifically nonsensical" [373]:410.

It's evident and sometimes overwhelming presence in ethology research, in the studies on the development and behaviour of human beings at all ages, in all conditions and environments, on the functioning of the communities in various geographical areas, its use or intentional exploitation in institutional activities—above all in scholastic and psycho-educational fields—its social diffusion at every level (from the infant's toy to the videogame, from the social media to advertisement), its flow into artistic expressions, but also everyone's belief that the sensations caused by play are unique and inimitable: all this demonstrates its unavoidable usefulness, perhaps even its necessity.

Two Questions

A culture that neglects a phenomenon of this magnitude would be short-sighted or guilty. And, in fact, culture and science have never neglected it: but how did they act so far? And then, to develop solid research in this sector, how to carry out reliable studies that may be subject to processes of comparison, falsification, repetition, generalization?

The first question could find some answers in the contents of the previous paragraphs. There have been valid attempts at systematization and in-depth analysis of the existing literature, and in recent decades many critical reviews have tried to give a logical, or historical, or disciplinary articulation to this harvest of works (e.g., [228, 333, 686]; with reference to LUDI, see also [72]). The fact that, however, the analysed studies belong to distant cultural traditions (for example, philosophical, pedagogical, anthropological-cultural, psychological, technological, etc.) makes their exegetical analysis even more difficult.

The masterful success is now represented by the fundamental book of Burghardt [141], which has marked the way to give a definitive turning point to the scientific field on play. Some of the studies considered in this chapter, for example, in the anthropological and socio-cultural areas, demonstrate to adopt a clear methodological approach and were able to reach reliable results, for example, through naturalistic studies and case studies (e.g., [295, 312, 378]).

Research has also advanced in the psychological field based on a solid methodological structure (e.g., [96, 534], among others), and precisely for this reason they also led to the development of tools usable in educational practice, or in research itself, thus available for further field validation.

Instead, it frequently happens that the play construct is used in a generic way without resorting to precise definitions or clear references relating to its description, evaluation, and possible measure. By way of example, the results of a survey are shortly reported that have been conducted on the final proceedings of the six most important international robotics conferences over 10 years (2009-2019); the survey intended to obtain information on works that included the words disability and play/game. Out of 112 studies found relating to play, 22 were devoted also to disability; a further analysis confirmed that these works concerned the topic "play/game and disability". Of these, only two reported a definition of play, while in the others the term was used in an unscientific way (for example, without specifying the type, without adopting any criteria for measurement or evaluation, with no reference to studies in the field of play/game); in some cases, the words play and game were used as synonyms, betraying the indefiniteness of the adopted construct. In addition, play was never the objective of the research or project presented, but rather a means to achieve external goals, which were placed in the health and/or rehabilitation area [71].

To answer to the second question posed above—*how to develop solid research in the field?*—the work of Johnson and Dong proves very useful. The authors recognize the complexity of the task of studying play—"the enormity of outlining the conceptual challenge in studying play" [373]:399. Nonetheless, they give a presentation of standard quantitative and qualitative methods used in researching play, with specific reference and examples to the issue of play. The document is important for researchers who want to start field and experimental activities in this area, and reading is recommended. They conclude that "still, a gulf exists between play in research and in conception. Conceptual evidence about play is abundant, growing, and worthwhile, but it must be joined with new empirical work targeting what we are learning from our constructions" (ivi:410).

They also suggest new possible and promising trends in research, such as (a) choosing a research paradigm "player led" rather than "researcher led", so as to involve more directly the protagonists in the process; (b) preferring mixed methods of research; (c) adopting innovative techniques more related to reflexive strategy to better know and understand players' views and experiences of play. "By including the player's perspective some depth is gained" (ivi:411).

Finally, since research on play includes very often practitioners in the field—teachers, educators, parents, various types of professionals—Sigel's proposal [638] of adopting a "'proximity index' in reference to the nearness or remoteness between researchers' and practitioners' views" [373]:411 seems particularly stimulating. "An effort must be made by those doing new research with player-led procedures to understand what kinds of play occur; what play looks like, feels like, and how it is experienced by players; and how play is understood by players and practitioners. This seems now to be a needed complement to efforts by traditional quantitative, qualitative, and mixed-methods researchers" (ibidem).

2.10.1 Tools for Play Assessment[59]

As deeply discussed here, play is the most important activity in childhood, and as such it can be observed and evaluated per se or being completely intermingled with all the other developmental areas, it can be used as a means for evaluating other evolutionary aspects of the child. Therefore, traditionally play assessment is divided into two areas: play assessment and play-based assessment.

A very detailed and comprehensive review of existing tools in both areas has been done within the Action LUDI, in which one book has been devoted to *Evaluation of children's play* [75]. Every tool proposed for play assessment is strictly related to the definition of play it encompasses and, of course, to the dimensions of play it intends to evaluate.

Tools do exist for measuring the development of play within certain types or the progress from one type to the subsequent one—and the list of types of course is coherent with the related definition of play—or the relationships with peers, with adults, and with the different contexts.

Play can be analysed in naturalistic environments, but also—in this case requiring more carefulness—within adult-initiated play. Outcomes of the application of these tools are improvements in settings where children live or spend their time, investigation on individuals, or collective progress in play.

Ray-Kaeser et al. [573] include, in this group, some assessment tools that analyse play as a general behaviour:

- The Assessment of Ludic Behaviour [248][60](see Sect. 2.10.2), addressed "to document and describe the qualitative aspects of a child's free play behaviour, play interests, ludic abilities, ludic attitude and communication in play, concepts derived from the Ludic Model" [573]:21 of the same author.
- The Test of Pretend Play—TOPP [422].

---

[59] This paragraph has been widely inspired by Ray-Kaeser et al. [573].

[60] The authors include here also the ToP and the TOES that are mentioned below.

- The Child Initiated Pretend Play Assessment—ChIPPA [666].
- The Peer Play Scale—PPS [351].
- The Revised Knox Preschool Play Scale—RKPPS [398] provides information on the child's developmental maturity in relation to play; it includes four dimensions for assessment (space management, material management, pretence-symbolic, participation) and it provides a play and as a profile of the child's play abilities in the four dimensions.

These tests are more precisely oriented and are addressed to deepen some forms of play, on the basis of a previously existing framework of interpretation. Play-based assessment tools are intended to measure some developmental skills in the child (e.g., motor, communication, thinking, etc.) that can be detected through play observation. The related measures for each skill have been settled by experts in the specific area of child development. They can be used as an alternative to the traditional assessment tools, with better and more reliable results, since they can be administered in contexts more similar to the familiar ones, where the child can feel at ease.

Examples of play-based assessments are the Play In Early Childhood Evaluation System-PIECES [391], the Penn Interactive Peer Play Scale-PIPPS [243], and the Transdisciplinary Play-Based Assessment-TPBA [435, 436]. They all are "observations of cognitive, social, emotional, communication and sensory-motor development in play situations, alone or with peers" [573]:22.

Looking at the issue of play assessment in a more general way, the cited authors state, with Bundy [138], the need to consider always five facets of play: (a) child's play preferences; (b) child's play skills; (c) playfulness; (d) physical and social environment; and (e) play activity.

Each of these facets can be investigated by using direct and indirect information sources. Direct sources are mainly based on observation that requires devoted techniques, tools and settings and counts on specific materials; the observer's role should be precisely established and maintained during the ludic event; very often the event is recorded, to give the opportunity to reduce biases and to have data double coding. Indirect information sources are manly represented by interviews and questionnaires that can be proposed to parents, caregivers, and professionals, but should also always involve children themselves, and, in that case, adaptations should be provided to let them express in the best way their feelings, emotions, and ideas.

2.10.2 Two Thorny Descriptors of Play

Two descriptors of play are frequently adopted in the related research because they are directly connected with the characteristics of play and therefore demonstrate to be consonant with the issue and particularly insightful for possible improvements. However, both have non-secondary critical aspects, which should be taken into consideration.

Play for the Sake of Play

The first descriptor proposed for careful consideration is *play for sake of play*. This descriptor is meant to clarify which kind of goal/objective the practitioner and/or the researcher intend to purse with the play activity they are planning.

When play is organized and planned by adults, or by professionals, it is generally used for its extraordinary capacity to recruit the player's motivation and attention; in these cases, it gains pedagogical usefulness, but undoubtedly it loses some ludic features, e.g., freedom, transgression, autonomous initiative, autotelic spirit, etc.

The Italian pedagogist Visalberghi [731] clearly systematized this difference; these activities, despite being fun—they can in fact be continuous, challenging, progressive just like real play activities—do not end in themselves, do not find their main purpose in themselves, but rather, they are "controlled" by the professional and by the educational goal; he defined them *play-like activities*. These differ from the pure (or real) *play activities* by the fact that they do not end in themselves, but have educational objectives and a final scope, in many cases learning or developing skills. Useful signs to recognize that a player is in a playful, but "controlled" or "goal-oriented" context can be identified by the presence of precise frames, such as well-structured relationships among players and the presence of expressly indicated rules. In these cases, the professional often provides stable guidance to the play activity, essentially dominating it, defining times and procedures.

In the field literature, the expression play for the sake of play is often used to indicate play as such, for the purposes of the play itself, devoid of preordained extrinsic purposes, but not fixed, immutable, or downright messy. It is certainly a free activity, but also a very specific one, which can be framed in a particular type of play or made up of a set of types. If one purpose can be identified with it, it is to make players feel "inside the playful frame".

On closer inspection, play for the sake of play is the play defined by Burghardt. It is the playful activity of Visalberghi. It is the play of the socio-constructivist model, which makes the child develop and create contexts and opportunities for this may happen. Simply calling it "free play" is not completely correct, and it impoverishes and misrepresents it: in fact, play for the sake of play is never without limits, rather it seeks them, to become more challenging and engaging, and, in some cases, it makes use of strict rules. Play for the sake of play contains the exact degree and type of fun and challenge that the player expects. Undoubtedly it 'produces' learning in many developmental areas, but it does not pursue this aim and it is impossible to predict or determine what players will learn. For sure, players will learn a lot about themselves—their own preferences, abilities, inclinations—and about others—how to recognize their intentions and feelings, build relationships with them, deal with the unpredictability of their emotions, negotiate rules with them.

Play for the sake of play happens in life simply because somebody decides to play, but when the play activity is expressly designed (particularly for research purposes), it should be really clear the role that will be assigned to play in relation to the objectives pursued, and therefore to the characteristics of the activity. This step is really crucial, on a methodological level, because the whole structure of the activity follows from it:

modalities to propose and to carry it out, constraints that will be introduced, contexts where it will be performed, roles taken by the various participants, etc.

A radical and explicit choice is required, so as to construct a precise and correct research design (or, for example, an educational-didactic planning): on the one hand, there is the organization of a play activity as a support to (or background of) a major and predominant activity, with its own objectives; on the other hand, there is the proposal of a playful activity in the form of play for the sake of play, to the purpose of observing it, studying it, or even contributing to its improvement and growth. It is not at all a choice of value, rather a choice of design orientation by the researcher/professional, but this choice is decisive, in order not to overlap or confuse the objectives to be pursued.

Playfulness

The second descriptor to be clarified is *playfulness*. The construct of playfulness has been first systematically pursued by Lieberman[61] (1977), who stated that "behaviourally, it could be seen in the play of young children and, at later developmental stages, as a personal trait of the individual" [282]:3.[62] Lieberman designed an assessment tool to measure five areas in which playfulness could be represented: physical, social, cognitive spontaneity, manifest joy, and sense of humour.

Since inter-rater reliability of the tool was not demonstrated acceptable, Barnett and her colleagues [40]—who defined playfulness as an individual "disposition to play"—revised and scaled it, and created the *Children's Playfulness Scale* (CPS), retaining the previous five areas; they also concluded in favour of the adequacy of the construct validity of CPS. Later, playfulness was introduced within the Occupational Therapy field as an eventually fruitful construct to evaluate these professionals' work in supporting playing of children with some kind of impairment.

To replace other play evaluation tools that were found unsuitable, and to substitute Barnett's scale that was not considered valid for children with disabilities, Bundy [137] (1997) developed the *Test of Playfulness* (ToP), which culls "three elements of play: intrinsic motivation, suspension of reality, internal locus of control. [Furthermore] it also incorporates a fourth aspect of play called framing", extrapolated from Bateson's play interpretation [48]. The validity and reliability of ToP

[61] Playfulness in play was already introduced at that time in studies concerning the adult (Deutsch in 1958, underlined the important role of combinatorial play in the creative process [216]), while with regard to children it was cited as a differentiated trait in comparing the most creative boys and girls [707] and as a "playful attitude toward theme" by Getzels and Jackson [282].

[62] She testified, in that occasion, the way she came to her conclusion, during long observations in the kindergarten: "A look to Susanna's behaviour tells of her using realistic props for a flight of fancy, including her playmates; moving spatially out of the prop situation [...]; switching to an act of physical exuberance; elaborating the fantasy; and returning to the original place and original activity. All this suggests physical, social, and cognitive mobility in a spontaneous manner. [...] What emerges, then, is Susanna's way of acting in a play situation: the quality of her play or her style of play. I labelled this behaviour 'playfulness"' [425]:4.

have been then demonstrated [139] and the tool "shows promise as an assessment from which members of professional disciplines could gather valuable information that could be used to contribute to a growing body of knowledge in play theory" (ivi:290). Then, why should playfulness be a thorny descriptor of play? The first elusive element of the construct is—as usual in this field—the imprecision of its definition.

Well-meaning authors in play use it in an original, decontextualized way, as an expression that could be synonymous with pleasurable, or fun, joy, "ludicity". Russ [597]:131, for example, within an article devoted to play in psychotherapy for children, reports, among others, the following guideline for a play intervention programme, proposed by [331][63]: "Be alert to the 'playfulness' of the intervention and the pleasure it should be evoking". Gray [300] also, in his studies on hunter-gatherer societies, seems to use the term as an attribute of the activity—"If the focus were on competition, the pressure to win could reduce the playfulness and fun of the activity" (p. 514)—or of the societies—"[Hunter-gatherer] maintained playful attitudes in their hunting, gathering, and other sustenance activities" (p. 476) and "the playfulness of the indigenous inhabitants" (p. 479).[64]

Playfulness can also take, with small variations, collateral meanings, with an utilitarian outcome for the purposes of a research; this is the case in the study by Arrasvuori et al. [24] (2010) who, involved in Nokia videogame research field, stand that it "can be regarded as the attitude of a person when he or she is engaged mentally and physically in the state of play": not a personal trait, then, but something that arises in everybody whenever the "play mode" has been activated.

The second critical point with the playfulness construct is a less formal-linguistic and more epistemological one. Is "playfulness" to be considered a personal trait—an innate pre-disposition[65]?—or should it be better positioned between the individual and his/her life context? This means: where the individual lives and was born, where the play activity takes place, with the related tools and companions, according to the adopted play types, etc. This seems to be a possible new interpretation of the construct, still hidden but perhaps promising. Briefly, Henricks states that "playfulness is contextual" [332]:164. And Lieberman herself seems to admit to have in some ways eradicated the construct from its natural groove: "I went beyond the play setting. I attempted—and to some extent succeeded—to cull from play what I perceived to be its quintessence and labelled this 'playfulness'" [425]:23.

The reflection that playfulness, conceived merely as an individual trait, is insufficient for professional purposes is perhaps also confirmed by the development, by

[63] This last text is not available in the most popular databases.

[64] He does not include the definition of "playful"—although announced—and uses the word as a mere adjective derived from the noun "play".

[65] On this trace of reflection, it should just be noticed that Burghardt and Pellis speak of some "most playful" species [143]:11. Similarly, the reference to the "neurobiology of playfulness" contained in an article of Siviy [644] actuates an interpretation of the term in the sense of "previous experience of playing" in the animals studied.

Bundy, of another Scale (the *Test of Environmental Supportiveness* (TOES), [137]),[66] to address more specifically the ways in which the environment influences play. This was due to the need to evaluate the user "within an environmental context [also to] encourage interventions focused on the person in his or her environment" [117]:242. Bulgarelli and Bianquin [135] also reached similar conclusive reflections after use of the ToP in a series of experimental tests with children with disabilities; the authors, in addition to finding the ToP not suitable for studying playfulness in the case of solitary play, state that the tool was not sensitive to evaluate many characteristics of the activities carried out, which were decisive to determine their quality and came from the context, e.g., the type of toy, the play partners, and the severity of disability. Therefore, interpreted as an individual trait, playfulness does not appear adequate in the experimental context. The strict and unavoidable interaction between the "individual playfulness" and the environment is also acknowledged by Lieberman again, in at least two aspects: (a) when she argues that playfulness is not innate, but it derives from concrete play experience[67]; (b) when, to deepen the quality of playfulness as a child's behavioural component, she proposes to study the childrearing modes and the teachers' personality and methods.[68]

So, playfulness can be learnt and/or be expressly taught: this is the thesis supported by Barnett [41], who explored whether the construct of playfulness is sensitive to cultural values and discussed about playfulness as socially constructed.

To conclude: on the basis of the experimental research findings, as well as on the examined controversial aspects, it may be time now to delve into the construct of playfulness described so far as a personal trait.

By adopting an eco-systemic model, as Bronfenbrenner [116] has suggested for a long time now, it would probably be much more productive to look at the play activity as a system (and thus also as a possible unit of analysis, with many sub-units to be defined from time to time), in which the player is the protagonist, but what happens around him/her, or is available around him/her, is an integral part of the system and contributes to determining outcomes, failures or successes of the activity itself.

Could a new interpretation of the construct of playfulness be the operational parameter to measure the quality of this outcome? Therefore, could it also guide the assessment of the quality of the interventions of each system component in determining this outcome? In this respect, the play research area appears to be a promising, up-to-date challenge.

---

[66] While also TOES has demonstrated validity and reliability, the correlational study conducted on the magnitude of its relationship with the ToP is not satisfactory and still requires further research development [117].

[67] "I hypothesized that playfulness as a quality of play would developmentally transform itself into a personality trait of the player in adolescence and adulthood" [425]:23.

[68] More precisely: "While in and of itself quality of play or playfulness was important as part of the behaviour repertory of the child, its significance was seen to involve questions of a much broader nature: [...] 3. What some of the childrearing antecedents are that influence playfulness; 4. What some of the variables in teacher personality and methodology are that influence playfulness" [425]:24.

Chapter 3
Play and Disabilities

Serenella Besio

Abstract The UN Convention on Children's Rights has stated the right to play for any children, including children with disabilities. For them, play possibilities may be affected by not only the lack of tools to play with, considering the specific impairments, but also by the need for the presence of peers and caregivers to play with. Above all, their right to play may be denied by the unavailability of adequate play contexts, lack of methodological knowledge as well as unawareness of the importance of play. Not only children with disabilities but also adults with developmental disorders often do not have access to play, while play may have a relevant role in their life, as for everybody. Playful activities may improve the motivation to participate in therapies since play is an intrinsic need for everybody. Moreover, play for the sake of play, independently from therapeutic protocols, may make interesting aspects emerging, as well as functional evolution. Appropriate design of playful activities may obtain important improvements but needs to consider the different impairments. In this chapter, we motivate the need of play for everybody, we review how the different types of play may find obstacles in the different types of impairments and we discuss how these obstacles could be removed.

3.1 Play and Children with Disabilities. A Right Claiming for Accomplishment

3.1.1 Children with Disabilities are Children and They Do Play

In the last decades, a novel interest in the theme of play for children with disabilities has awakened, together with a new awareness of its centrality in the life of this part of the population, and consequently in the involved research areas: psychology, pedagogy, medicine, law, and technology. Within this cultural stream, the already-mentioned Action entitled "LUDI Play for Children with Disabilities", developed within the COST European Program, was entirely dedicated to it, resulting in

A. Bonarini and S. Besio, *Robot Play for All*, Research for Development,
https://doi.org/10.1007/978-3-031-05042-8_3

volumes, collection of best practices, scientific statements, and political stances.[1] A simple, but not trivial, syllogism was established at the basis of the action itself, as follows.[2]

a. *The play is the child.* The exclusivity and unavoidability of play in childhood for the full and harmonious development of the individual no longer require any confirmation because it has been deeply ascertained by research. Moreover, the UN Convention on the rights of the child (UNCRC, 1989)[3] enshrined it, in its Article 31, forever and universally: the right to play concerns all the children indistinctly, regardless of gender, wealth, ethnicity, or physical functioning. It addresses above all those children that—due to economic, sanitary, psychological, and political conditions—are at risk of suffering from deprivation of this powerful and unique experience.[4] A generalized awareness exists about the importance of this right, but often it is merely theoretical or superficial and does not transform into coherent (educational, political, cultural) actions; the theme of play is still very lively in the research and application areas—for instance, in the educational and technological fields—thus demonstrating its inexhaustible vitality and its capacity to arouse curiosity. Play is still a fruitful field of study, as evidenced by the wide contemporary literature in the sector, as well as by the intense activity of dedicated international associations.[5]
b. *The child with a disability is—first and above all—a child.* The statement is easy to understand, but not as easily applicable, and certainly not applied. The life of these children, and their childhood itself, are pressed, invaded by: the medical directions and the rehabilitation activities; the emotional, psychological, and relational tensions often experienced by parents in search of certainty and future perspectives; the vital thrusts towards full participation into communities; the natural propensity to enter social contexts. Children with disabilities often emerge more for their difficulties, the type and severity of their impairment, the correlated health elements, the numerous problems they face, and the needs they present to their family and to society at large. Their childhood, despite being a

[1] In 2017, during the Triennial World Conference held in Calgary, the Action has been attributed the International Play Association Award "in recognition of their implementation of the Article 31 of the UN *Convention on the Rights of the Child*" http://www.ludi-network.eu/successful-stories.

[2] This part of the text is inspired by Besio [71].

[3] https://www.ohchr.org/en/professionalinterest/pages/crc.aspx.

[4] The psychiatrist Stuart Brown is the researcher who first highlighted the risks related to play deprivation; he studied the possible psychological and affective consequences after the collection of more than 6,000 individual interviews with play details. Despite they were not conducted on a rigorous methodological basis, he sustains that the volume of the information allows credible hypotheses. His conclusion is that "sustained, moderate to severe play deprivations particularly during the first ten years of life, appear linked to major but virtually omnipresent emotional disregulation". He then states the need for the development of basic science of play and play deprivation [120].

[5] The breadth of the literature in the field and of its various lines of study has been demonstrated in the previous chapter. As to the associations, it is worth mentioning here the International Play Association (IPA; https://ipaworld.org) and the International Council on Children's Play (ICCP; www.iccp-play.org).

prevailing characteristic, that should emerge as priority, remains instead in the background. What prevails is the urgency perceived by family members, rehabilitation professionals, educators, to obtain functional, physical, and psychological, improvements due to adequate interventions; as a consequence, infancy, with its needs and prerogatives, is suspended, neglected, in an attempt to build a better future, maybe a perfect one. The specificity of the condition of the child with disabilities has been recognized also by the UN *Convention on the Rights of Persons with Disabilities* (UNCRPD, 2006),[6] with special emphasis.

c. *The play is also the child with disabilities.* Play is still, in the concreteness of everyday life, an activity that is not easy to carry out in the case of children with disabilities. This is mainly due to the fact that unfortunately their life contexts are not yet well prepared (due to cultural, socio-economic, political, and structural obstacles) to address their needs, to respond to their particular modes of functioning. This dramatically restricts their opportunities to grow and equally take part in social life. Particularly, Article 30 of the UNCRPD—devoted to Participation in cultural life, recreation, leisure and sport—states that it is up to the States parties "to ensure that children with disabilities have equal access with other children to participation in play, recreation and leisure and sporting activities, including those activities in the school system". Perhaps even more interestingly, the point has been authoritatively confirmed by the General Comment No. 17 to the aforementioned Article 31 of the UNCRC, accepted by the UN in 2013.[7] Among the documents supporting it, there is the *Position Statement* of the International Play Association, that cites also the work of LUDI: "IPA believes that no child should be excluded from the joyfulness, friendship and benefits that come from a childhood filled with play. IPA members around the world have voiced their concern that many disabled children face multiple barriers to exercising their right to play. IPA has therefore developed this *Position Statement on the Play Rights of Disabled Children* to re-assert the play rights of disabled children, growing up in all circumstances and living environments".[8]

The publication of the General Comment provides a unique opportunity to further raise awareness on the importance of Article 31 with the State parties, government departments, civil society, and the general public across the world. The right to play of children with disabilities is therefore a fact for everyone and nobody can now question it. The link with their health, well-being, and development makes children's play fundamental, not optional. Family members, caregivers, professionals, policymakers, and governments have the responsibility to ensure its accomplishment [79].

---

[6] www.un.org/development/desa/disabilities/convention-on-the-rights-of-persons-withdisabilities.html.

[7] https://ipaworld.org/ipa-position-statement-on-the-play-rights-of-disabled-children/; the General Comment is reported here: https://www.refworld.org/docid/51ef9bcc4.html.

[8] The LUDI *Position Statement* cited by IPA can be found here: http://www.ludi-network.eu/wp-content/uploads/2017/11/LUDI-Position-Statement.pdf. The LUDI *Manifesto* can be downloaded here: http://www.ludi-network.eu/wp-content/uploads/2018/04/LUDI-Manifesto.pdf.

3.1.2 What Is Disability?

After more than 20 years of work on this issue,[9] the World Health Organization published the International Classification of Functioning, Disability and Health (ICF; WHO, 2001).[10] ICF is today the most widespread and authoritative available framework for interpreting disability, but certainly, it is not the sole existing one.

The conceptions of disability, in fact, have alternated over time, building a significant body of studies, that is still full of debates. The huge cultural work conducted by the Disability Studies[11] made the two prevailing models emerge, the one defined as medical-individual and the other known as social; they have reached a degree of theorization such as to be able to construct interpretations of reality and clearly polarized intervention perspectives [64].

The pivot of the medical-individual model is located in the biological causal agent, disease, or deficit intrinsically provoking disability, thus interpreted as a deviation from a norm, and as a carrier of social disadvantage and even of tragic destinies.

On the contrary, the central axis of the social model is the overthrow of a passive vision of disability, which is interpreted as a condition of oppression operated by an "ableist" society; the social model claims for greater visibility and participation of persons with disabilities, and for a new world finally free both from structural and social barriers.

If the medical-individual model makes the impairment an object of study, even fixing it in prototypes, the social model, at least in its initial versions, excludes it from any consideration—leaving it to very private personal experience—since disability, the product of an oppressive society, has no causal relationship with the impairment.

As Bernardini maintains, by prescribing that the impairment remains confined within private experience and not led to real thematization, the social model actually consigns the body to an "epistemological invisibility" [64]:36, ending up provoking just the opposite of what the model aims at, namely the concealment of disability, if not even its return to medical interpretation [352], lived in silent solitude.

The contradiction has been highlighted for some time within the Disability Studies and has generated a revival of studies, from a social perspective, on the concept of impairment and the interpretation it should assume within the model [580, 626]. The debate is still very animate; but the challenge now requires to design an innovative scenario, that may grasp together the need for specificity brought about by the individual impairment and the need to take fully part in a welcoming and inclusive world; an intermediate paradigm that takes into account the different concurrent factors in

[9] This work elaborated the first international framework for disability, and it produced the International Classification of Impairment, Disability and Handicap (ICIDH; WHO, 1980). https://apps.who.int/iris/handle/10665/65990.

[10] https://www.who.int/standards/classifications/international-classification-of-functioning-disability-and-health.

[11] Born in the sociological area, the Disability Studies originated in the eighties as a critical academic perspective, after the Disability Rights Movement of the sixties; they share the core theme of their studies, the working methodology, based on a participatory model, as well as the multidisciplinary approach. Research and political action have always been intertwined in their evolution.

determining a condition of disability, and at the same time knows how to recognize the different directions towards which a life can unfold [70].

The bio-psycho-social model refers to systemic thinking and proposes a relational idea of health as an intertwining of biological, psychological, and social factors. If on a theoretical level the model maintains an uncertain reputation, its main operational application in the disability sector does not: the ICF incorporates it and it represents "a synthesis of the medical and social approaches to disablement"; it also wants to be a response both to the hypermedicalization of the previous model and to the tendency of the social model to "detach disability from its biomedical basis" [81]:1183.

This result is obtained through the interaction between four different components, which organize and describe the functioning of each person, in relation to the contextual factors in which he/she lives and by which he/she is determined. These components are *Body Structures* and *Body Functions* on the one hand and *Activity* and *Participation* on the other hand; it is thanks to their strict intertwining with the other components—the *Environmental* and *Personal Factors*—that the individual's functioning becomes true: therefore, the ICF model envisages the individual as active and participating. Within this relational frame, the body and the contextual factors come into contact with each other and they give rise to a functioning, which can be more or less effective—with respect to the needs and the objectives of the individual—in activity and participation.

Disability is defined in ICF as the "outcome or the result of a complex relationship between an individual's health condition and personal factors, and of the external factors that represent the circumstances in which the individual lives". Because of this relationship, different environments may have a very different impact on the same individual with a given health condition. "An environment with barriers, or without facilitators, will restrict the individual's performance; other environments that are more facilitating may increase that performance. Society may hinder an individual's performance because either it creates barriers (e.g., inaccessible buildings) or it does not provide facilitators (e.g., unavailability of assistive devices)" (WHO, 2001:15).[12] Multidimensionality, interaction, universality, etiological and terminological neutrality are some of the characteristics recognized by the ICF [80], which shows a convincing applicability and operational effectiveness of the bio-psycho-social model, and makes this classification a powerful tool for intervention, from the perspective of the inclusion and construction of a life project that welcomes, enhances, and organizes every pertinent and titled protagonist, first of all, the voice of the protagonists.

But what about children? As individuals in an evolutionary phase, for which environmental and personal factors play a decisive role, their condition should be understood and safeguarded as part of a classification that intends to be all-inclusive. In 2007, the WHO published a version of ICF devoted to children and youth (ICF-CY),

[12] The definition of disability conceived by the UNCRPD is the following: "persons with disabilities include those who have long-term physical, mental, intellectual or sensory impairments which when interacting with various barriers, may hinder their full and effective participation in society on an equal basis with others". This definition, according to Kazou [388], is closer to the definition provided by the WHO than it is to the conception of disability supported by the social model.

that provides a comprehensive list of different aspects of child functioning together with environmental aspects, which co-exist and provide a holistic perspective of barriers and facilitators for child functioning.

As Simeonsson et al. [639] suggested, in this case, the model of interaction between person and environment should be reconsidered, taking into consideration the reciprocal influences and the evolutionary factors. The central element of this period of life is precisely given by the rapid and continuous changes not only of the child but also of the environments where he/she lives. Thus, the importance that ICF attributes to the life environments for studying the effectiveness of functioning, is also the key factor for planning successful action to support the child's development.

3.1.3 Disability Towards the Future: All Means All[13]

Children with disabilities are not invisible to the UNCRPD: their fundamental presence in societies and the necessity to consider them and their lives as a priority are already highlighted by the general principles which constitute the common and essential factor of the whole Convention.

Point 8 of Article 3 (*Principles*), in fact, reports the need to "respect for the evolving capacities of children with disabilities and respect for the right of children with disabilities to preserve their identities". Then, Article 7 is entirely dedicated to this population so that the States: (a) ensure their full enjoyment of all human rights and fundamental freedoms on an equal basis with other children; (b) in any action concerning them, treat their best interest as a primary consideration; (c) ensure the right to express their views freely on all matters concerning them, according to their age and maturity, on an equal basis with the other children.

The societies of the future, as outlined in the Convention, are therefore open to collect everyone's needs and wishes, allow and support the participation of all on an equitable basis, and favour the development of each one's autonomy and independence, supporting their choices.

Two principles contained in Article 3 represent the highway towards the achievement of this result: full effective participation and inclusion in society and accessibility. In what follows they will be shortly discussed according to the childhood perspective, as they are mainly discussed in the vast existing literature, that is in education.

Inclusion

The issue of inclusion, in particular of persons with disabilities, is at the top of the agenda of the majority of nations in the world. It constitutes one of the cornerstones on which the debate on the construction of coexistence and collaboration between peoples develops, and represents one of the greatest objectives of civilization.

[13] Some parts of this paragraph have been inspired by Besio and Bianquin [73].

Reference is made here to just a few examples of maximum representativeness: the UN *Disability inclusion strategy* launched in 2019[14] establishes a vision and commitment for the United Nations system on the inclusion of persons with disabilities at all levels. This action of course includes also education, one of the main areas where children can exploit their inclusive opportunities.

The 2020 UNESCO *Global Education Monitoring* (GEM),[15] has been devoted to *Education and Inclusion—All means All*, that does not only give a general overview about the implementation of inclusive education in the world but also identifies the practices in governance, curricula, textbooks and assessment, teacher education as well as relation with students that proved successful to unlock the process to inclusion. The initiative moves in support of the Agenda 2030, *Sustainable Development Goals (SDG)* of the United Nations, in particular of SDG4—*Ensuring an education of equal and inclusive quality and promoting opportunities throughout life for all*,[16] led by UNESCO again.

The term inclusion assumes today different meanings, according to the various research sectors, it applies [700]. In his *Think Piece* entitled *Defining the scope of inclusive education*, Sleep maintains that "inclusive education refers to securing and guaranteeing the right of all children to access, presence, participation and success in their local regular school. Inclusive education calls upon neighbourhood schools to build their capacity to eliminate barriers to access, presence, participation, and achievement in order to be able to provide excellent educational experiences and outcomes for all children and young people" [700]:8.

Inclusion has also different theoretical interpretation, and it is Slee again that tries to solve possible dilemmas in this respect, by sustaining that inclusive education (or inclusive pedagogy) has a double essence, being both a goal—that is, a political and social commitment of a global education community promoting inclusive principles—and a methodology—that is, a concrete activity which is built through the implementation of good practices, aimed at increasing pupil participation and reducing exclusion from common cultures and curricula [103].

However, inclusive practices do not constitute a homogeneous and recognizable group of modalities of intervention, and this gives the area a certain vagueness. *The Oxford Research Encyclopedia of Education* (2017) groups them together around three poles, (a) practices that derive from special pedagogy, such as Individual Educational Plans (IEPs), initially used in special classes, which are currently used in inclusive settings; in this way, a special educational practice found its way into the so-called mainstream schools; (b) inclusive pedagogical approaches that aim to eliminate or minimize the need for individualization of teaching; (c) critical discourse analysis, which questions institutional influences on thought and action and in particular the ways in which they reproduce power and inequalities in society [241].

Despite its fragmentation, inclusive pedagogy is understood as a proposal of substantial change in the teachers' pedagogical thinking, related to a didactic

---

14 https://www.un.org/en/content/disabilitystrategy/.

15 https://en.unesco.org/gem-report/report/2020/inclusion.

16 https://sdg4education2030.org/the-goal.

intentionality that supports the learning of all children [86, 257]. This new orientation translates into more flexible, global, and contextualized teaching practices [4], in which teachers and students work together to create a supportive and open environment that promotes social justice and allows each individual to participate fully in community life and to feel valued fairly with respect to peers [348].

A very interesting methodology favouring inclusion in schools comes from the proposal of *Universal Design for Learning* (UDL). Starting from the evaluation of the student's potential and the analysis of his/her learning needs within the context of the mainstream learning environment, it designs the learning environment including the tasks, the materials, and the technology that ensure that all students can learn to the maximum extent possible" [330]. UDL states that all curricula should be intentionally designed "in a way that: (a) give all learners an opportunity to acquire information and knowledge in a variety of ways; (b) engage (motivate) all learners by tapping into their interests, aptitudes and prior knowledge; (c) provide all learners with alternatives for demonstrating what they know" (ivi:3).

Accessibility

Accessibility can be considered both as a theoretical concept able to describe and assess the world we live in, and as an objective to achieve, or a standard to respect, to ensure everyone the real possibility to take an active part in the collective social life and to be included.

According to the International Standard Organization (ISO, 2011), accessibility is "the extent to which products, systems, services, environments and facilities can be used by people from a population with the widest range of characteristics and capabilities to achieve a specified goal in a specified context of use". Article 9 of the UNCRPD indicates two main fields of application: "(a) buildings, roads, transportation and other indoor and outdoor facilities, including schools, housing, medical facilities and workplaces; (b) information, communications and other services, including electronic services and emergency services".

Making an accessible world means adopting an accessible or universal design, "design focused on diverse users to maximize the number of potential users who can readily use a system in diverse contexts".

Universal Design is sustained by UNCRPD which is defined as "design of products, environments, programmes and services to be usable by all people, to the greatest extent possible, without the need for adaptation or specialized design".

Accessibility to education, in all its aspects, is the unavoidable basis for inclusion. First, this means that the national educational systems are clearly addressed to apply the idea that "with adequate support all children, irrespective of their different needs, should be able to learn together in mainstream classroom in their local communities" (UNESCO, 2015).[17]

To reach this goal, the educational physical environment should be interpreted in a broad and creative sense. An inclusive educational system should guarantee not

---

[17] http://en.unesco.org/gem-report/report/2015/education-all-2000-2015-achievements-and-challenges#sthash.qU3TD28b.dpbs.

only that mainstream schools are accessible but also that territories should not be underserved by schools or that effective and free transport services are organized. An accessible and inclusive education requires that all the spaces frequented by children for learning and leisure time are safe and inclusive so that children with disabilities can be engaged not only within their own communities: the various school facilities but also playgrounds, open spaces, natural environments, and routes. Among the basic aspects of accessibility of educational contexts, mobility should always be considered together with lightness and acoustics issues. The overall classroom's design, including desks, seating, and objects, should respond—e.g., as to dimensions, shape, positioning, flexibility, etc.—to the functional needs of children with disabilities and should consider the devices and the systems they might use (for mobility, communication, writing and reading, learning, etc.). Furniture and products on the mainstream or specialized market can respond to the most common needs, while in some cases, personalized tools should be realized, either for specific individual requirements or for particular educational activities. Also, the space organization of the premises is of utmost importance to facilitate the children's participation to the class activities, extend their learning opportunities, and favour their free expression. Specialized material and aids—e.g., textbooks in Braille, tables for communication or for daily activities schedules, simplified books, modified tools for writing, drawing, calculating, etc.—must always be available and easy to reach by children.

Technologies are one of the most prominent support for the learning of children with disabilities within the framework of an inclusive perspective, giving them alternative solutions to access learning materials and taking part in educational activities. Assistive Technologies (ATs)[18] proved to be more significantly effective, being particularly designed based on specific users' needs and with the precise purpose of improving or making it possible some activities otherwise unattainable. The right combination of ATs and ICTs is very often the basis for achieving the best learning results: "Using computers and related assistive technology in educational activities helps children gain self-confidence, social skills, communication skills, gross and fine motor skills, problem-solving skills, and a wide range of abilities and knowledge needed to function in society" (UNICEF, 2012).[19]

Ultimately, accessibility to education and to society at large is not feasible, without a coherent change in social attitudes, which should be accompanied and supported by the right policies, social measures, and communication procedures. Social negative attitudes and systems, societies that discriminate against persons and children with disabilities still exist: accessibility measures shall apply to both the physical and the

[18] According to the International Standard Organization (ISO Standard 9999:2016), AT concerns "Assistive products for persons with disability, as a group of technologies including devices, equipment, instruments and software, especially produced or generally available, used by or for persons with disabilities for different purposes". The Global Cooperation on Assistive Technology (GATE) initiative has been recently established by WHO to support spreading information and access to AT: https://www.who.int/news-room/feature-stories/detail/global-cooperation-on-assistive-technology-(gate).

[19] The right of children with disabilities to education: A rights-based approach to Inclusive Education. Position Paper www.unicef.org/ceecis/IEPositionPaper_ENGLISH.pdf.

psychosocial environment. Education is vital for children with disabilities not only in itself but also as a major experience in participation, but inclusive education is also vital for all students since the contact with disability favours familiarity with differences and reduces prejudice.

3.1.4 Play and Children with Disabilities: Relation is the Key

Encouraging or supporting a child with a disability to play is not easy, nor is it easy to guarantee the maximum possible fun. It is not easy with respect to the reflections that have been presented in the previous chapter.

It is not easy, especially if play is considered a characteristic of the child development that exists in itself, and not an opportunity to achieve other goals. For example: to guarantee the maximum possible fun for him, to ensure that she can play with her companions, to the full satisfaction of all; to allow him to play at the highest possible level of his possibilities so that the play challenge is really exciting; to ensure that she explores the various types of play, developing them according to her wishes, her plans, and her preferences. Making sure that he feels free, that she can get lost like her peers in her personal "play frame".

Children with mild-severe intellectual disabilities have difficulties in communication and social interaction and in the development of imaginative activities; therefore, it is difficult for them to interact through play with their peers, preferring to play with the youngest and in any case proposing repetitive activities. For many of them, the symbolic type of play phase remains unattainable due to its complexity and the same can be said for the rule-based games. Children with autism spectrum disorders find it difficult to participate in a playful activity: they are reluctant and distrustful of interpersonal relationships, if not even fearful and do not show a natural propensity towards unusual environments and unknown persons, while on the contrary, some objects sometimes attract their attention in an exasperated way. It might be difficult to approach them, interact, share an object of interest, and build together a playful event. Visual impairment causes a serious decrease in the quantity and the quality of the possible play options, which ends up converging on sedentary activities, based on pre-formed materials or on the use of devoted apps; however, later on, visually impaired or blind people can also practice sports, such as skiing, thanks to some technical measures. The visual component, moreover, is very important in almost all types of rule-based games and this requires, especially in the case of group activities, adequate support, and materials to allow their full participation. Children with motor impairments often, quite paradoxically, love playful activities that involve movement, even if passive. Their playing skills, however, are generally impaired by the severity of the motor functional limitation and the possible association with other types of impairment. If their possibilities of action on the world and on objects are very limited, they are often proposed a passive play activities: for the little ones, sound and visual games, toys in motion, perhaps operated by others. The difficulties are also accentuated with the older child: the most accessible toy implies only basic elementary challenges and, conversely, the most exciting and interesting ones are not usable or accessible. Furthermore, while the symbolic type of play is above all experienced in an internalized way, the construction play can be unattainable, even if in some cases it is replaced by digital versions of real competition with peers, for example, in the responsiveness sector, is obviously not realistic.

Faced with these obstacles posed by functional limitations, family members, and professionals often lose naturalness in their ludic interaction with the child. The dyadic relationship—the child with a counterpart: an adult, a child, a group—from which the play can arise and develop seems impoverished and weakened. The playful dialogue with the child with disabilities must be refounded, its code, related to his/her needs, and functional manifestations, must be deepened and known: but its primary function, pure fun, and self-driving, should never be forgotten. Its vicarious function, that of acting as a useful but ancillary background to educational and rehabilitative proposals, can reveal useful, but should not become preponderant, under penalty of changing the paradigm and transforming the "child" into "the disabled".

The naturalness of the playful intention, therefore, in the case of children with disabilities, must be re-conquered in order to make it available to them. How? Four pillars, described below, are involved; however, separating them in a list is not correct, since they overlap and intertwine to compose a unique framework, the framework of playfulness.[20]

The child

The first pillar concerns the change of perspective on the child's participation to play: she must be considered—since she is—the protagonist of the play activity. Every child, also a child with disabilities, shows preferences and needs in the area of play and they must be known; and, as said, he/she has the right to express them and to have them taken into consideration.

This means also a change of gaze on the child's proposals. A consistent approach based on the systematic observation of his/her behaviours, preferences, and possibilities that he/she brings into play in relation to different contexts and proposals, should be the common patrimony of the professional in the sector, education, rehabilitation, and a research setting. This refers to a precise knowledge of the functional limitations pertaining to the impairment, to be able to interpret the reactions, the proposals, and the communicative signs; the professional must acquire an expert competence to look, listen, perceive, and manage distances and approaches, not only to grasp or guess the moment in which the relationship is possible and the proposal can be fruitfully accepted but also to advance the right proposal, which constitutes the exact degree of perturbation or imbalance in the direction of fun and challenging play. The competence, one would say, to create and act within the Zone of Proximal Development.[21]

The variability implied by the presence of companions must always be considered, both because it can completely change the observational results outlined with a single

---

[20] See also Sect. 2.10.2.

[21] See definition on Sect. 2.2.5.

individual, and because it is always desirable that play takes place in social and inclusive situations, that promise greater learning and fun.

The tools and the toys

The second pillar requires being experts in the choice, adoption, and use of tools, toys, and play methodologies that facilitate playful behaviour. Studies in this area derive from the most recent awareness of the role played by environmental factors in determining the degree and quality of the activity and participation of the child. Most solutions have been proposed in the fields of Assistive Technology—specially designed toys and adapted toys that respond to specific needs—and also of Universal Design. These last concerns are the initiatives addressed to evaluate the accessibility and usability of commercial toys and materials but also the development of "toys for all", an approach intending to develop toys and material usable by a wider population. Assistive Technologies can be used also to mediate the interaction with objects, toys and robots since they are can be used to accomodate to the abilities of the child (e.g., joystick, keyboards, switches, eye control, etc.). They should be carefully chosen according to the needs of the single child [188].[22]

Knowledge and awareness should be exerted by the professionals and the adults in general to analyse and evaluate these tools according to their affordance qualities—with respect to the particular child they are playing with—and possible elements that make them non-usable or non-accessible. Skills for applying adaptation strategies are also required and/or knowledge of alternative possibilities to adopt for giving the child the opportunity to play as she wants. Furthermore, tools and toys should be consonant to the type of play and also to the type of activity that is going on or is planned, especially for the difference between solitary play, or play in dyads, or in group, with peers.

The play activities and their contexts

In their turn, play activities and related toys should be considered with respect to the environment where they are or will be carried out, that must be accessible not only according to the standard rules but also for the peculiar needs of the play situation. Playing a symbolic activity or a game with rules requires a different organization of the space, and, as Périno suggests [541], in the same wide space more organized areas can co-exist, so as to favour the child's choice and expression of wishes and attitudes. Also, the environment must give the opportunity to change one's own activity from the solitary to the group play and vice versa, and also from the play to the non-play situation, to give the child the opportunity to have a rest, to break temporarily the "play frame", to express his/her feelings of tiredness, anger, disappointment or disagreement, and letting them settle.

Play activities may involve few or many children, may occur indoor or outdoor, they may have a long time or a short time available. The quality of the relationships and the related feelings is of utmost importance for the success of play and for general fun; the presence of a child with a disability should be carefully considered and

[22] See Sect. 2.9.2, particularly the TUET tool.

appropriate measures should be applied (to accessibility, availability of the right tools or needed support) so that she can happily participate, bring her contribution, establish friendship with peers. Environments should also take into account the possible presence of adults in the same space and identify their position and their roles. The play activity can be done "for the sake of play", as it should be also within educational contexts, or it can be the background to activities that have different purposes; these are the "play-like activities", which are aimed at pursuing, in a fun way, objective in education or, in the case of children with disabilities, often in rehabilitation.[23]

Obviously, an educational or rehabilitation exercise conducted in a pleasant way is highly preferable to a purely technical one, which risks exaggeratingly tiring the child and making her lose concentration and motivation. Therefore, the play-like activities are certainly interesting and welcome, in the panorama of activities faced by the child with disabilities in their daily life. However, much of the discourse that takes place in this volume is aimed at livening up greater attention to the play for the sake of play, because this activity helps him to live outside and beyond his impairment, or to live better with his impairment, and also because this activity allows peers, parents, relatives, and educators, to make the child emerge behind the veil created by disability.

The role of adults

As it is written in Sect. 2.9, the adults have many important opportunities to exploit within the play activities, thus making it more fun, more challenging, more satisfying to the group relationships, clearer to the rules, etc. These roles have been identified in builder of rights, promoter of inclusion, and scaffolder (observer, activator, partner). All these roles, carried out by the adult in any play situation, require the activation of expert skills when in the group there is also a child with disabilities; peculiar methodological skills are required to the professionals for choosing, selecting, adapting the tools, for organizing the environments and well as the activity itself.

Methodological, technological, scientific, and clinical knowledge and competence might be called into action. A characteristic of the play activity of many children with disabilities is worth mentioning here because it should be carefully considered both in planning concrete play events and in making research in the field. Often, these children need long time to get accustomed with new situations and to learn, they go through phases of consolidation, they risk somehow to "get stuck" in rituals, or repetitive behaviours. A new play proposal, even if appreciated, will require to them understanding and adjustment times and specific exercises to become acquainted with. This situation may provoke obstacles to progress towards subsequent developments in play and can also contribute to creating relational frictions with peers. The adult may be responsible to balance the needed time for exercise—necessary to fully manage the executive process—and the child's autonomous initiative, which guarantees his/her free playful expression, even in the case it is apparently sole repetition. Acquiring new skills, consolidating them, and fostering further development

[23] See also Sect. 2.10.

are different, overlapping phases whose management requires experience, intuition, and empathy by the part of the adult.

The following sections present the characteristics of the play of the five most common types of impairment during childhood.

The ICF approach has been adopted as an inspiring background for the structure of this work, thus considering disability—in this case, the difficulty to play, develop play, and have fun from play—as the product of a relationship between the body functions and structures on one hand and the environmental factors on the other hand.

Thus, each type of impairment has been described according to (a) body functions, that is their main characteristics and pointedly the impact that the specific impairment might have on the play activity; (b) environmental factors, including the barriers and the facilitators that can hamper or favour the play activities; these ones are always described according to the four LUDI types of play,[24] as well as to the play mediators (tools, environments, play companions).

The contents are based on the most recent literature in the field, with the intention of favouring new research based on the state of the art. Although the investigation carried out has tried to be exhaustive, some research may have inadvertently escaped. While the whole work is aimed at inspiring new studies in the field of play for the sake of play of children with disabilities, each paragraph includes also a section called "current trends in intervention" that intends to give information—albeit concise—about the state of the art of education/rehabilitation in the specific field, on gaps and ongoing debates to the reader who is interested in inventing and developing new play-like activities with (and in favour of) children with that particular type of impairment.

3.2 Children with Physical Impairments

3.2.1 Physical Impairment, its Characteristics, and Current Issues[25]

Physical impairments may prevent the child from acting in an autonomous way in his/her daily activities, and in their turn, these limitations cause insufficient development of his/her sensory and perception capabilities, as well as low self-esteem and self-efficacy. A physical impairment—both congenital and acquired—creates substantial limitations to physical ability or motor skills.[26]

When it is related to a problem of the central nervous system—as in the case of Cerebral Palsy (CP), ataxia, or traumatic brain injury—it may be accompanied, at

[24] See Sect. 2.6.3.

[25] This paragraph is also inspired by Besio and Amelina [72].

[26] Between motricity and mind, there is a complex interrelation, which could be described as cyclic: a movement can exert some consequence on the surrounding environment, and due to the perception

different degrees, by intellectual and neuro-psychological impairments,[27] language and speech disorders,[28] sensory disabilities, as well as emotional and social difficulties [704]. Thus, the motor component is no more the only variable to consider, but it should be analysed together with the others: perceptive, attentional, motivational, cognitive, and emotional affective.

When the physical impairment is related to a damage to the peripheral nervous system and/or to the effector organs (muscles, joints, and bones), it often provokes a severe functional movement limitation—as in the case of some types of muscular dystrophy, and of spinal muscular atrophy—with rapid worsening. When it is less dramatic—as in the case of juvenile rheumatoid arthritis—it limits the children's movement, thus restricting their ability and also their willingness to be active and participate.

Other developmental disabilities, e.g., due to genetic syndromes, cause movement disturbances, difficult coordination, problems in fine- and gross-motor control; in some cases, children prematurely born may experience problems in physical development and complex motor skills. Very often, these children need the adoption of various assistive devices and supports for movement and for communication. Of course, this implies a special organization of their daily life, because they need to be trained in the use of these tools for long periods, and in turn, this may create restrictions in social participation as well as difficulties at the psychological level, mainly with respect to self-construction and self-representation.

Current trends in intervention

Damiano et al. [204] recently published a systematic literature review concerning existing national Guidelines on the care of persons with cerebral palsy; the study has been developed within an initiative, inspired by ICF, of the WHO "to develop a global package of interventions for rehabilitation", as the title of the article says. The authors selected 339 recommendations from 5 final guidelines, whose prominent interest was devoted to body functions (mainly mobility); surprisingly, "no guideline focused specifically on physical or occupational therapies to improve activity and participation, despite their prevalence in rehabilitation" has been found.

---

of these consequences, new, modified movements can be produced; this relationship appears very clearly in a newborn [39]. According to this approach, it is not the movement that satisfies the mind's needs, but it is the mind that performs the actions [512]. Some authors recently sustain that motor control resides in the nervous system, body, and environments "viewed as dynamical systems in continuous interaction"[718]:3.

[27] Some Italian researches have highlighted the high presence (the two-third) of an intellectual disability in children with CP with a mean lower performance of one standard deviation [180]. According to the clinical literature, slowness of thought processes and inertness of thinking are typical of children with CP. Insufficiency of the highest cortical functions can also be shown in a delayed development of the representations of space and time, of the processes of phonemic analysis, and synthesis and problems of astereognosis [465].

[28] Speech development of children with CP is characterized by disorders on many components: lexical, grammatical, and phonetic or phonemic. Most frequently, they suffer from dysarthria or even anarthria.

So far, cerebral palsy and severe physical impairments still seem to be dominated by the medical approach, and so are the persons involved.

A historical examination of the studies in this field [205] shows that the initial research was aimed at refining the diagnosis and understanding the disease. Then, classifications and functional evaluations were developed so that the same language could be used worldwide. Now, it is the time for studying in-depth multidisciplinary, new treatment approaches, most of them ultimately are addressed also towards quality of life. This last aspect is confirmed by another systematic literature review (covering the last 10 years), that found growing emphasis also on activity, exercise, and treatment options, rather than on diagnosis and pathology. Moreover, studies are now oriented towards providing guidance for the persons' needs over the course of a lifetime [395].

A further more detailed review, covering the Australian territory only, appears more skeptical regarding the effectiveness of rehabilitation techniques, while instead arguing that "health care professionals can change the natural history of cerebral palsy and improve participation and quality of life for [these] children" and highlighting also the importance of early identification "which has become of paramount importance in the management of cerebral palsy". Furthermore, they refer to the "six Fs Framework, which provides a guide for developing shared goals with families; they are: function, family, fitness, fun, friends and future" [298]. An intriguing list for those interested in play and children with disabilities.

In their institutional paper about cerebral palsy, Gulati and Sondhi, after a systematic examination of the most important aspects of this neurological condition, conclude their review by adding, as a future development, that "robot-assisted activity can improve upper-arm function in adults with impaired mobility after stroke. Preliminary data suggests that this type of therapy also improves motor function in the upper and lower extremities that are caused by CP or other acquired brain injuries. These data suggest that use of such interventions in children with CP can improve movement and function as they do in adults with stroke" [306]:1014. In the same vein, Yazici et al. [772] within a controlled study involving 24 children with hemiparetic CP, found that a Robot Gait Training can give many benefits to the muscular system and it improves functional walking performance. More directly located in the field of play, an integrative review concerned "ludic strategies focusing on the fine motor skills, gross motor skills, balance and gait of children with cerebral palsy", reporting satisfactory results in this area [540]. Toys and play tools used in the analysed literature were very different in nature: virtual reality game, robotic prototypes (2), a wooden sword, a horse (alive), Nintendo Wii and other various videogames (10), a rotating platform, and an adapted toy car.

3.2.2 *Impact of Physical Impairment on Participation to Play*

The impairment can make movement management and control very difficult for these children and can deeply challenge the effectiveness of the professionals' support and to empower their play abilities.

There is also a dramatic conflict between rehabilitation objectives, such as obtaining a stable and comfortable physical positioning, which allows the adoption of correct postures and supports the child's gaze, and the spontaneous ways to finalize one's own actions, which often are based on the exploitation of "pathological" patterns and have to deal with the interference of uncontrolled movements, such as dystonia, athetosis, etc.

"Children with physical impairments may be relatively more impaired at some aspects of coordinated play actions than others, but limitations in one aspect of a play-action tend to have cascading effects on other aspects of play that can be adjusted to compensate for those limitations" [195]:600. The physical impairment manifests its major impact when these children attempt to actively relate to the environment; in fact, even simple play actions may be affected by their limitations in proprioception, i.e., poor awareness about the position and motion of their body parts during play.

"Precise control of play actions such as stacking blocks requires not only range of motion and the ability to grasp and release objects but also dynamic judgment of the position of one's own hand in relationship to the target and ability to adjust that motion in response to sensorimotor feedback throughout the play event. Poor trunk control or independent mobility may restrict potential play positions or locations more than expected for a child's chronological or developmental age" [195]:601. This poor kinesthetic and proprioceptive feedback may compromise the awareness of the cause-effect relationship,[29] that is between one's own body movements and the play action. "For instance, a child with cerebral palsy who has involuntary movement of multiple body parts and production of sounds may find it hard to distinguish which of those body movements has caused a play result or which behaviour is the cause of a desired result in a play partner" [195]:602.

These observations highlight the need for rehabilitation to implement objectives related to the increase of their awareness and enhancement in control of finalized (e.g., in playing) body movements and skills [375]. Coordinating gaze with play actions and partners may be influenced by possible associated sensory limitations, since the neurological preservation of primitive reflexes may interfere with intentional movement, resulting in frequent failures.

The evolutionary triangulation (person-object-person) that is at the basis of symbolic communication onset [749], is in this case limited by poor gaze control and coordination, as well as difficulties in head/trunk control [20]. Complex functioning situations may also end in communication difficulties as well as in expressing one own's preferences, that sometimes should be disambiguated through the eye gaze [419].

Speech disorders may disadvantage their communication with peers, as it might be difficult to understand them, or an Augmentative Alternative Communication (AAC)[30] system should be adopted. Olswang and Pinder [513] found that these

[29] Even if the onset of the cause-effect mechanism in the individual cannot be attributed only to the development of movement coordination [617].

[30] Augmentative and Alternative Communication (AAC) includes all the communication methods used to supplement or replace speech or writing for persons who experience difficulties in the area,

children are able to show a wider variety of play strategies if coordination between movement and gaze improves.

Contrary to the difficulties and obstacles presented up to now, there are interventions that proved effective: for instance, Ryalls et al. [600] demonstrated significative changes in play skills through physical therapy addressed to improve independent sitting, in 3–6-year-old children with CP. Okimoto et al. [509] worked effectively on both coaching parent-child interactions and carrying out direct neurodevelopmental treatment of 3–18-month-old children with CP and verified what they call "improved playfulness ratings". Interestingly, receiving communication intervention addressed to produce messages improves appropriate motor movements more than intervention addressed to understand others' messages and behaviours [751].

All these aspects, together with the possible difficulties in the emotional sphere reported in the clinic literature, can result in social participation restriction [415, 769] if appropriate inclusive contexts are not established. This seems to happen even more in other disability groups [358]:363. Variations are very high in this cohort of children; whenever interpersonal engagement and task persistence are higher components of the children's behaviour, they will be more motivated to try to compensate their physical limitations. As expected, "they can have very different preferences for types of play including structured or unstructured interaction, physical or social activities, and solitary or partner-based play" (ibidem).

Assessment of play

Assessment of these children's play requires adaptations, because they might show difficulties in using and moving objects, to coordinate movement, to orient and fix their gaze, to understand, and/or answer to questions.

Some tools exist in the field even if they do not address specifically the issue of play in-depth, rather treating it as one of the areas of a child's development: it is the case of the *Pediatric Evaluation of Disability Inventory* (PEDI [313]), which tests particularly cognitive and social abilities in this population.

Other tools might prove useful to get an insight into the impact of the impairments on the child's functioning. For example, the *Communication and Symbolic Behavior Scales—Developmental Profile* (CSBS-DP [749]), can offer information on the progressions in communication skills, by using play samples as normative indicators of them; in this case, the "play temptations[31]" for the CSBS have been adapted for assessment use with infants and toddlers with physical impairments [196]. Finally, the *Transdisciplinary Play-Based Assessment* [434] can be adopted too for assessment purposes; as the other cited ones, it is a play-based assessment tool.

---

due to impairments in the production or comprehension of spoken or written language. AAC makes use of different codes for communication—pictures, symbols, graphic, auditory cues—and is based on the adoption of a variety of support devices, from low- to high-tech.

[31] "Communicative Temptations" is a technique used within the framework of Applied Behaviour Analysis for "tempting" the child to communicate with the interlocutor; the idea is to make the effects of child's communication desirable for him/her through reinforcement of his/her positive answer [564].

As regards the implementation of the assessment phase, in order to gain the best possible knowledge of the play skills of children with physical disabilities, a specific mediated assessment method should be implemented. "This should focus on providing optimal play environments (special adapted positioning, visual and sensory environment), adapted play materials and clear awareness of the child's aided and unaided communication [methods and tools]. Therefore, the motor, sensory, cognitive, social and emotional strengths and limitations of each child must be acknowledged to best adapt the mediated assessment process. In addition, it is important to have a clear understanding of the parents' perspective on their child's play, as they have a crucial role in facilitating play experiences" [573]:44.

3.2.3 Factors Affecting and Favouring the Play Activity[32]

Types of play and their tools

The areas of Assistive Technology and Assistive Robotics have deeply explored the issue of play and children with physical impairment. Some solutions and many studies have been produced, following the idea that supporting these children in manipulating and exploring toys and objects and their relationships though play can have important consequences on their cognitive development. Despite this promising scientific interest, many obstacles and difficulties have been faced; for examplle, the cognitive complexity required to manipulate an object by means of a robot might be cognitively challenging, while it is still not available a "theoretical approach to the assessment and quantification of the complexity of children using the robot as a tool, rather than directly manipulating an object with their arm and hand" [233]: 228. These tools-mainly products of experimental research—are available for all the considered types of play (an exhaustive review is contained in [ibidem]).

The identification of the type of play activity is related to the specific preferences of the child as well as to his/her abilities and competences and the subsequent choice of toys depends on their physical features.

Due to their physical needs, issues such as slowness, fatigue, motor inaccuracy in effectiveness, and coordination impairment, are to be addressed; and, altogether, all the other possible existing impairments and their impact on the play activity.

As to the toys, it should be considered, in particular: "(a) how the toy can be used: with which parts of the body, if it is possible to use it by means of other parts of the body; (b) which kinds of action are needed (grasping, pulling, pushing, inserting, plugging, sliding, picking up, combining, and so on); (c) which precision and coordination of movements are required and also to what extent strength should be adopted" [542]:191.

If a sensory impairment is associated, it should be reminded that these children prefer hard toys and vibratory toys [201] to soft furry ones [573]:39.

[32] This paragraph is also inspired by Périno and Besio [542].

Modification to traditional and mainstream toys, different for each child, should be adopted by substituting the activation systems, introducing handles, buttons, grasping solutions, and other possible devices.[33] "More elaborate dedicated or computer-based devices can provide integrated control of multiple play actions and messages, sometimes organized around particular play schemes" [195]:600. Picture symbols and boards can be introduced too to facilitate and mediate communication exchange.

Practice play

In these, children play can be delayed, regardless an associated intellectual disability, because they find it difficult to act on the world around them and to socially participate. Children who cannot experience the expected types and amount of physical interactions can show delays in play skills[34] and are particularly disadvantaged in practice play activities.

Moreover, even if some authors [130] sustained that the concrete motor act is not decisive to determine the child's development, rather it is important the intention to make it, it seems proved that "the inferential processes [...] proceed from the motor abilities, and particularly, from their use within the play activities" [195]:599; so, a reduced motor experience in turn may cause a reduction in the ability to control play objects. "For instance, infants require repeated experiences at reaching and touching objects to build perceptual-motor mapping and cognitive conceptions of object relationships in their world, particularly during middle infancy" (ibidem).

Due to their functional limitations, some physically impaired children cannot reach, manipulate, and use play objects and are only onlookers of their peers' play activities. To elicit play abilities, to favour curiosity, and to increase relationships of the young motor-impaired children, some solutions have been experimented [144], mainly technology-based, that try to give them as much mobility as possible, as early as possible.

Toys for these children should be solid, easy to hold and to be used, and steady for sensorimotor and gross motor skills play. They should be of good quality for lighting, musical, tactile, and other effects.

The ludic idea they inspire should be well defined and easy to produce even if physical possibilities are reduced in terms of strength and gestural precision. The use of these toys should also be carefully considered in relation to the children's motor devices to facilitate play and make it as safe as possible. Outdoor play activities should also be included because kinesthetic discovering is important to create awareness of one's own body as a whole.

Symbolic play

Severe physical impairment is often accompanied by a deep impairment in communication and/or speech acquisition and use. The development of the symbolic

[33] Information about these modifications is available in the related literature and on websites devoted to Assistive Technologies. See for example, www.eastin.eu;https://www.who.int/news-room/feature-stories/detail/global-cooperation-on-assistive-technology-(gate).

[34] For example, Soares et al. [12] reported less active exploration as mouthing of objects in preterm infants than full-term infants between 5 and 7 months.

functions is a complex issue in the case of physical impairment since its delay can be caused both by the motor impairment and the intellectual/cognitive difficulties; the possibilities and the limitations for developing an "internal" linguistic code without the related speech skills is a matter of discussion since many decades [160, 533].

Some findings in literature [464] describe cases of symbolic play in the absence of a completely developed speech capability, where the appropriate strategies of alternative communication were implemented.

If some studies indicate significant differences in play abilities between children without and with developmental language difficulties, being lower in this last case [163], other ones demonstrate that pretend play does not show a stable correlation with the use of verbal language [452] even if language seems to have a pulling role for the development of the symbolic function as a whole.

Moreover, play is improved when multiple communication modalities and play schemes are adopted [695]. Pfeifer et al., studying the pretend play of 20 preschool children with CP, found significative negative correlations between their motor severity level and their elaborateness of play with conventional imaginative and symbolic play materials and a number of object substitutions in symbolic play.[35] They comment that "this indicated that children with greater motor limitations (65% of the sample) had diminished [symbolic] play ability" [544]:10. These results seem partially disconfirmed by another study [19], according to which, even if play performance of children with typical development was superior to those with cerebral palsy (a sample of 30 + 30 was adopted), "the degree of impairment of functional mobility and manual function was negatively associated with play exploration but did not relate to pretend play or social interaction in play".

Anyway, caution should be adopted in doing a comparison with the previous one, since in this second case another tool to assess a child's play has been used, with a different concept and articulation of pretence/symbolic play.[36]

Some members of the same research group, in the same year, published another article, in which a sample of 4–7-year-old children with CP were studied in their symbolic play abilities by using the ChIPPA test; the obtained results demonstrated that qualitative aspects of the children's pretend play were satisfactory since they showed typical play indicators in all the categories, but one: in fact, the "Story" area requires that the child invent a brand new narrative; most of them were able to create a scenario, but the majority was not able to construct a story; an in-depth hypothesis on possible causes of this result is not presented in the work.

Cress sustains that in case of older children with physical impairments "multi-step symbolic play is not independently demonstrable [. . .] who cannot control multiple actions or objects. On the contrary, symbolic play actions are often co-constructed with partners. For instance, instead of independently stirring, scooping, and feeding pretend food to a doll, a child with physical impairments might need a partner to hold up play items to choose the spoon, then ask about possible play locations where the

[35] The *Child-Initiated Pretend Play Assessment* (ChIPPA) test was used in this experiment [545].

[36] The *Knox Preschool Pretend Play Scale revised* (KPPPSr) test was used in this second experiment [398].

spoon might go and actions to take with the spoon, as a multi-step partner-assisted alternative to independent doll feeding. These play choices can be presented through a variety of object choices gestures, symbol selections, voice output, words, and signs" [195]:606.

Symbolic play can be greatly compromised by the physical impairment itself, e.g., when the fine use of tools and toys is involved. Assistive Technology products can be of great help if they are designed accordingly to these children's possible needs: play activities can be organized along with sequential steps—like within a narration—and, in case speech is poor, augmentative communication symbols can be implemented on their toys and play objects.

Research demonstrates that the adoption of suitable ATs to support symbolic play can enable learning and associated development.

Toys for this type of play "should be realistic and easy to use; they allow children to take on roles and enter situations to experiment in play what they cannot do and live in their real life. Symbolic play is the way for children to express their emotional life, fears, dreams, and satisfactions. Dolls and other traditional toys for symbolic play (puppets, theatre characters, miniature objects, etc.) can be chosen or modified for being easy to use. Costumes and disguises should also include wheelchairs and other movement supports to give these children the possibility to fully take part in play sessions together with their peers" [542]:192.

Constructive play

Smilansky's [650] idea to introduce this specific type of play into her classification is particularly productive and rich in new ideas for the play of children with physical impairments because it facilitated the raising of research projects in the field of engineering and robotics.

As to the toys, to facilitate the use of the available tools for constructive play, "it is essential to choose them according to the size of pieces and their weight, nor too small nor too heavy. [Even most important,] it is to consider carefully the mechanism to assemble the elements; magnetic or Velcro links are preferable, so that construction play becomes possible even in case of imprecise gestures or jerky movements. In some cases, mainstream toys can be modified, so that they can be manipulated and used: handles and various kinds of systems to take the pieces and assemble or disassemble them can be adopted" [542].

Commercially available Assistive Robotic tools, such as CRS A465™, Microbot TeachMover and Lego Mindstorms RCX, from the pedagogical point of view might be included, according to the different ways of use by the child, as tools for practice play and/or for symbolic play [233]:230–235.

Rule-based play and games

In many cases, children with physical impairments can approach this type of play by recurring to the support of Assistive or Information Technology products, or a mixed solution between the two. If the accessibility issue is correctly solved and the suitable game is chosen in relation to their cognitive abilities, it is possible to offer them a virtual environment that is adaptable and usable.

This kind of game has been already experimented successfully [577, 747]: for example, adolescents with CP showed appreciation and enjoyment in using these tools, in strict correlation with the cognitive workload requested by the game.

Reid and Campbell [578] reported a successful use by children with CP (with non-disabled peers) of a Virtual Reality environment—managed by a video camera as a device for capturing and tracking—for playing games of volleyball and snowboarding. The perceived virtual reality as an "equalizer" of abilities with their peers, and this fostered feelings of competence and acceptance by the others. One of the main problems of mainstream videogames for these children is their requirement of playing fast and being action-oriented. Hernandez et al. [339] created a specially designed "exergame" to avoid the need for time-sensitive actions and to keep the game pace slow, which have been tested with children with CP, both to achieve the right physical activity and fun. Speed in this type of play is an issue for these children; to give them the opportunity to participate, this variable should be modified, or their role within the game should change. Sport games' rules can be adapted so that participation of many persons with different needs is facilitated.

Commercial board games may be not usable, due to the shape and dimension of their components, but some modifications may be undertaken to improve their usability: for instance, a magnetic base can be added to the pawns, while big dice can substitute the traditional ones. The duration of the play should be shortened when possible, for decreasing the fatigue due to a prolonged motor engagement that may create difficulties in controlling movements thus adversely affecting the motivation and the quality of the child's involvement in the game.

Physical and social environments

Due to these children's movement difficulties, the best possible interaction—specific for each individual—with the environment should be accurately prepared, so that they can feel in control of it, thus increasing their motivation [90].

Accordingly, first of all to the child's preferences, the type of play to be activated, as well as the suggestions also contained in this text, the right tools and toys should be found, tested, and used. Of course, all the possible AT tools they use, as supports for movement and communication, should be available and included effectively within the environment, so that they can be used easily without disturbing or hindering the play activity. In this regard, it is important to notice that, in case of complex communication needs, the introduction of a simple voice output device within the interaction with the child provokes greater attention to the child's needs during the play activity [474] and this encourages the adoption of AAC strategies as facilitators rather than barriers for communication development [416].

The space where the activity takes place must be totally accessible to their AT devices, and it must assure the best and complete relationships with play tools and companions. For instance, a wheelchair imposes some distance from the floor, or it requires the suitable height of the tables or work surfaces where the activity takes place; if the play activity or tool needs the use of the floor, the right positioning of the child on the floor too should be adopted: the most important thing is that he/she can have a complete visual and motor control on the toy or game and can easily reach and use them as he/she wants [542].

The onset of locomotion in children is accompanied by many developmental achievements [156]: new forms of practice play can be tested, and social issues are involved [383]. The fact that children with physical impairment may have delays or are unable in walking acquisition can cause further losses in play engagement, for example, in outdoor spaces: the need to avoid this risk reinforces the field research supporting early adoption of tools for independent mobility [28, 105, 703], despite the child's limited walking skills (e.g., with the aid of canes or walkers).

As to the duration, usually, a shortening of the activity might be considered, to guarantee the child's interest and commitment; nevertheless, attention and motivation are strictly related to fun and engagement, and duration can vary a lot according to the single event and the effectiveness of its components. It should never be forgotten that the playfulness of the single play event springs from the more or less effective relationship between the three elements—child, context (space, tools, toys), play companions[37]—and that making this relationship interesting, fascinating, fun, is often the responsibility of the adult, who introduces his/her awareness, competence, sensitivity, and also his/her drive (playful, educational, or rehabilitative).

Inclusion also is mainly a matter of adequate educational planning, in the various contexts of life. Anyway, literature reports a worrying situation, in this regard: "activities are more passive, mainly organised at home and lack variety [634]; [...] the intensity of participation is influenced by some determinants of the child and his or her family: higher participation is related to higher gross motor function, higher enjoyment, younger age, and higher family orientation; moreover social supports and environmental services also play an important role in increasing the degree of participation" [196]:598.

Moreover, the cost/benefit imbalance (between high motion cost of controlling a play action and benefits of play) may limit active engagement in play and provoke the adoption of those passive interaction strategies [194]. The degree of social engagement experienced by these children is also related to the creation of an experiential baggage that they can reproduce in play with peers, for example, within symbolic play: in fact, lack of exposure to peer play and limited participation in daily life routines and community activities might produce a poor repertoire of schemes that they can imitate [195].

Adults' participation as play mediators in the case of children with physical impairments is important; current literature has interpreted this fact in a contradictory way. Brodin [115] warns that parents may adopt a "diagnostic" attitude, mainly focused on recovery and rehabilitation of the impairment, thus disqualifying play for the sake of play as a waste of time. In addition, according to her, they should be supported in acquiring the needed competence to liven their child's concentration on the scope of the play activity.

On this point, Yoder and Warren [773] do agree, since parental responsiveness to the child's play needs should be improved. Lower parent responsiveness or higher

[37] See also Sect. 2.9.

parental directiveness in play for children with developmental and/or physical impairments has been found (e.g., [316]). Furthermore, "if children require physical or procedural support from partners to manage play interactions, they may actually experience fewer play events than in typical development, without the advantage of independent trial-and-error play practice separate from partner-scaffolded play" [195]:602 as well as fewer successful play actions in physical or social play compared with typically developing peers [654].

Nevertheless, professional intervention in parent-child interaction during play has demonstrated to improve the responsivity quality in the case of infants who were preterm with physical and/or developmental delays [238]. Parents trained at improving their interactive modalities in daily activities become also less directive and more participative in child activities [692].

Another productive line of research and intervention concerning adults' involvement in children's play is conducted in a less-strict technological area, and it is aimed to increase the awareness of teachers and professionals and to improve their knowledge and competence in assessing and choosing products, toys, and technologies for the play of children with physical impairment.

The child and his/her play companions

In older research, children with severe disabilities were described usually as passive or frustrated by their motor impairment: they tended to adopt subaltern roles in the group, and also with their siblings [203]; they acted better in a play dyad if they were the youngest, thus benefiting by control behaviours adopted by the other child [471]; they poorly trusted in themselves as players and play companions [556]. They have been also described as snivelling and emotionally unstable, not very friendly [665]. More recently, social interactions with peers have been still demonstrated as poor for children with physical impairments [525]. This may strongly depend on the related norms concerning the socio-educational services and institutions of the various countries, with particular reference to the implementation of the inclusive processes[38]; nevertheless, the problem seems strongly rooted, since Whittingham et al. [752] demonstrated that even as early as 18 months, over 70% of children with cerebral palsy were more than one standard deviation poorer than the mean on measures of social development [195].

However, these research results are contradicted by others, such as in the case of Clarke and Wilkinson [184] who found that school-aged children with physical impairment were contributed to activate non-serious interaction elements, such as laughter and shared activity.

Specific characteristics related to the impairment can greatly influence the acquisition of play competences: children with good verbal competences are more likely to be involved in the peers' play activities [320, 674]. Higher ability to be independent in communication creates the possibility of more participation in social play and recreation [183]. The cognitive competences also influence the associative and collaborative types of play, because sometimes these activities prove to be

[38] See Sect. 3.1.3.

too complex for an impaired child. Furthermore, children who are not autonomous in their movements and need some support for moving tend to rely on adults for entering the peers' group [72]. "Some of the limitations in peer play for children with physical impairments involve the speed and flexibility of play and communicative behaviours produced. If peers are quicker at producing and adapting play behaviours, then children with physical impairments may take a relatively passive role during interaction" [195]:605: for instance, they spend more time as onlookers of play [654], they use to initiate less the interaction and respond more, through their AAC electronic device, than their peers [182].

Technology seems to confirm its pro-active function for their social participation: Spencer-Cavaliere and Watkinson [663] sustain that they feel "included" in a physical activity when they gain entry to play, feel like a legitimate participant, and have friends. According to Skär [645], they improve their own perception if they use ATs that can give them more autonomy in play activities, without recurring to the aid of an adult. Interestingly, children expert in the use of augmented communication systems were able to manage play situations in an effective way, supporting their peers in building an original structure of the play activity [50].

Yet, in general, children whose physical impairment leaves the possibility to recur to gestures, speech, or other communication strategies were more successful in establishing relationships with their peers [195]. On the other hand, cooperative behaviours in siblings (one of them with CP) increase in time as well as pro-social and care behaviours; a different chronological age probably increases the awareness about the reciprocal needs and supports in building a good relationship: the non-disabled sibling becomes more and more competent in interpreting the sister or brother's wishes and in complying with them, maintaining attitudes of support and physical proximity. This also results in increasing the impaired child's participation and attention to the play activities [72].

3.3 Children with Intellectual Disability

3.3.1 Intellectual Disability, its Characteristics and Current Issues

Intellectual Disability (ID) is "a disability characterised by significant limitations in intellectual functioning and in adaptive behaviour, which covers many everyday social and practical skills. This disability originates before the age of 18 years" [14]. "These significant limitations: (a) reflect an inability or constraint in both personal functioning and the performance of socially expected roles and tasks; (b) represent a substantial disadvantage to the individual; (c) are influenced by contextual variables; (d) can be mitigated (i.e., reduced or alleviated) through interventions and supports, or by reducing barriers that preclude opportunities, equity, and inclusion" [611]. Deficits in intellectual and adaptive functioning are the main characteristics of intellectual disability with a reported prevalence between 1 and 3% of the population with some regional variations [530]. Significant impairment measured through IQ rating is usually located on two standard deviations below average (IQ below 70); standardized measures for adaptive behaviour include conceptual, social, and practical skills [211].

The abilities of persons with ID may vary a lot, and the related difficulties will significantly influence the way they interact with the community; according to the WHO the various degrees of intellectual disability can be categorized as follows: (a) Mild (IQ of 50–70)—the ability to communicate effectively and live relatively independently with minimal support within the community; (b) Moderate (IQ of 35–49)—individuals who, with lifelong support, will have significant relationships, can communicate, handle money, travel on public transport, make choices for themselves, and understand daily schedules; (c) Severe or Profound (respectively IQ < 34 or < 20)—individuals who are almost totally dependent on those around them and will require lifelong help with personal care tasks, communication, and accessing and participating in community facilities, services, and activities [766].

A wide range of aetiologies can provoke intellectual disability: chromosomal anomalies,[39] environmental factors can also be involved such as intra-uterine infections, peri-natal trauma, nutritional deficits, maternal alcohol abuse, and childhood neglect and deprivation. In approximately half of cases, no cause has yet been identified [211]. "According to the *Diagnostic and Statistical Manual of Mental Disorders* (DSM-5) [14], the deficits in intellectual function include reasoning, problem solving, planning, abstract thinking, judgment, academic learning, and learning from experience. The critical components of intellectual functioning included in the DSM-5 criteria are verbal comprehension, working memory, perceptual reasoning, quantitative reasoning, abstract thought, and cognitive efficacy" [530]:S25. Comorbidity is reported with reference to possible problems with vision [239], and with hearing [472], that may provoke worsening of skills in mobility, learning, and behaviour; some persons with ID can also experience risks of obesity, cardiovascular and respiratory diseases, and epilepsy [211].

Different types of impairments—that are considered within this volume—can be associated with ID, first of all, autism spectrum disorders and cerebral palsy; in this last case, ID adds complexity and may increase health and mortality disparities [579]. All the developmental areas—movement, language, cognitive, academic, and socio-emotional skills—are usually delayed, but they are impaired in a wide heterogeneous ways [420]. In particular, all persons with ID have communication difficulties; when this ability is severely compromised, they can make use of AAC techniques and tools.[40]

Learners with Down syndrome frequently have speech and language impairments, although their difficulties may vary; usually, they show relative strengths in understanding the others' language, but they experience problems in phonology,

---

[39] The list of monogenic forms of ID has increased rapidly in recent years thanks to the implementation of genomic sequencing techniques [15]. Among the ID caused by chromosomal anomalies, the best-known and most widespread in the population are the Down, the Williams, and the Willi-Prader syndromes.

[40] See note on Sect. 3.2.2.

vocabulary, and grammar. In some cases, they make use of gestures to support their communication.

Some of them may also incur behavioural problems, such as being antisocial, anxious, dependent, depressed or withdrawn, and social difficulties [690].

Current trends in intervention

Recent literature in the field of ID is prevailingly concentrated on deepening the theme of the adults with ID and accomplishing results for them; therefore, issues related to work, employment outcomes, and vocational rehabilitation are mainly considered.

Another well-represented area of studies concerns the predominant social representations of intellectual disabilities and the eventually existing attitudinal and prejudicial barriers to social inclusion [400, 501, 640].

However, the novelty in the field might come, in the future, from the critical analyses on Evidence-Based Practice (EBP)[41] within the existing literature, which will help to give comparative value to the research results accumulated over time and to highlight, consequently, the studies that should be considered more significant and reliable.

Sturmey has accurately worked on this topic: "there are at over 100 meta-analyses of psychosocial treatments for people with developmental disabilities and a similar number of systematic reviews" [677]:29. The author's final statements, after a detailed presentation of the results obtained, despite being interesting, were not homogeneous; in the case of effects of Early Interventions, he comments that "it is possible to intervene to achieve large improvement in broad Adapted Behaviours for at least some individuals with developmental disabilities. All share the common feature of a massive environmental design to remove barriers to learning and foster learning" (ivi:41). In the case of specifically adapted behaviours in the field of social skills, he concludes: "these six meta-analysis studies reached different conclusions and appear perplexing and contradictory [...] A closer examination of these papers, however, suggests that these differences reflect different research questions and the databases searched" but, "despite these limitations, there is sufficient agreement [...] that social skills training is an EBP" (ivi:44). Unfortunately, a comprehensive study of this magnitude on play of children with ID has not yet been conducted. On the contrary, in the case of persons with ID, the topic of play therapy—i.e., the use of play as a means as well as an intervention technique for reaching results other than play itself—is quite represented since decades.

According to Astramovich et al. [26], play therapy has been suggested to support children with ID to develop adaptive behaviours and fix social relationships. The authors identify four historical approaches: (a) structured and unstructured play therapy; (b) imaginative play therapy; (c) "Theraplay"; (d) child-centred play therapy.

[41] Many definitions of EBP exist and are reported by Sturmey [677]:4; the author adopts the one by Sackett et al. [603]: "the integration of best research evidence with clinical expertise and patient values", used also by the American Psychological Association's (APA) Presidential Task Force on EBP (2006). Evidence-based approaches are characterized by systematic reviews and meta-analyses.

An additional type is the "cognitive behaviour play therapy", based on the cognitive behaviour therapy, that has been "used with some success in the treatment of various types of behavioural problems in individuals with ID" [637]:146, but at the present time, there is insufficient evidence to support the use of this therapy in clinical practice. Two studies conducted by Iranian researchers—a meta-analysis on 18 studies and a quasi-intervention study on forty 8–12-year-old children—support the effectiveness of an intervention based on this method, but the two works contain many cultural and scientific biases.[42]

For what concerns more general aspects, the comprehensive frameworks in ID study and interpretation have been recently analysed by Schalock et al. [612], who propose to overcome the four previous co-existing perspectives—the biomedical, the psychoeducational, the socio-cultural, and the justice—since "they do not explain the complexity of ID, nor do they individually provide a holistic theoretical framework to understand ID and guide efforts to mitigate its impact" [612]:79. Then, the authors propose and discuss what they call a holistic theoretical approach to ID.[43]

3.3.2 Impact of Intellectual Impairment on Participation to Play

The severity of ID influences the nature and characteristics of children's play. Some of them are reported in what follows. John Langdon Down in the nineteenth century first documented the ability to learn by imitation of the children whose syndrome he discovered [770]; this attribute is still considered a powerful strength of these persons and a powerful asset within inclusive contexts, as a basis for shared activities.

Apart from individual characteristics, that can make further differences, visual supports for learning are usually an effective strategy for students with ID with respect to auditory ones [193]. Gross motor development is delayed when compared with typically developing, mainly for normative in the case of more complex physical movements [159]. Clumsiness of movement is a pervasive feature of Down syndrome and it produces slow, less efficient gross motor movements in addition to high velocity, inaccurate fine motor movements [730]. While physical education and sports are highly recommended, the degree of fine motor impairment may suggest the adoption of Assistive Technologies for complex academic activities such as instrumental writing of letters, texts, numbers, and arithmetic operations.

Some behavioural characteristics may strongly impact these children's involvement in activities: for instance, they prefer to adopt avoidance strategies to refuse

[42] In the first—written in Persian—it is not clear which kind of play activities the authors did include in their research, being the works cited in the references very eclectic; in the second, some methodological aspects have not been discussed exhaustively.

[43] Whose components are: a holistic view of the explanation of ID, the locus of the disability, the significant risk factors leading to ID, interventions and supports for prevention or mitigation of ID, and the elements of a multidimensional approach to subgroup classification [36, 485]. They can be applied to various areas of intervention by adopting practices consistent with them.

engagement in other tasks (e.g., scholastic and learning) that they consider challenging [757]. Linn et al. [437] also found that children with Down syndrome were more likely to show passive behaviour in unstructured play than developmental age-matched peers. A difference in the limbic system [780] provokes longer lasting emotional responses that lead to strong long-term memory associations.

Another aspect that may provoke distressing behaviours is the age-related poor language proficiency that reduces the individuals' ability to negotiate so that they may appear stubborn or defiant [244]. However, the main causes of delay and difficulties lie in the cognitive functioning of these persons, which has been the subject of in-depth and passionate studies since the sixties.

The important role of memory in all intellectual pursuits has been singled out as well as the consequences of its deficit in the case of ID.[44] Particularly, it was found that, in addition to having difficulties in memory skills, these students experience difficulties in adopting the correct strategies to efficiently store the material and to recruit the information necessary to solve a task [670]. Glidden and Warner [289] found no differences following training between adolescents with mild intellectual disabilities who were taught a cumulative rehearsal strategy[45] and others who were not. This has been interpreted as a failure in adopting the right metacognitive capacities, that gives the opportunity to use the appropriate strategies: for instance, students may develop competence in the use of the learnt strategy at the time of presentation, but they may fail to acquire the vital retrieval strategies necessary for the completion of the task [25].

The rigidity in applying strategies only to the training task has been called "welding" [633], and it is still recognized as an important barrier to overcome in strategy training interventions and also, in a wider sense, to adopt planning, generalization, and self-regulation strategies. Some studies concerning training activities report that students with mild ID did not achieve generalization. Parmenter [526] explained this lack in terms of their inability to use the new taught strategies instead than the ones previously adopted; he concluded that generalization is a specific problem for persons with ID. Self-regulation capacity refers to flexible problem-solving which includes the development, selection, connection, and monitoring of effective strategies to maximize learning [25]; it is also one of the key factors of behaviour in a social context [51, 349]. Self-regulation of thoughts and behaviour stands out as a long-term and high-level goal of educators and researchers [524]. The ability to

[44] With special reference to children with Down syndrome, this impairment can be described as follows: visual-spatial working memory (images, objects, their location) is quite preserved; verbal working memory (that holds speech-based and acoustic information) is significantly weak; long-term memory seems to be preserved too, but its quality strictly depends on the quality of the material that has been stored [244]. Recently Zimpel [780] suggested that heightened memory records of persons with Down syndrome may be due to strong emotional responses caused by increased activity of the brain's limbic system (ibidem).

[45] "Rehearsal" is the literal repetition of the exact words that a person wants to remember. It can be oral, visual, or written. It influences the attention and storing of information in memory. Various rehearsal strategies are known, i.e., simple repetition, cumulative repetition, copying/note-taking, and text markup.

engage self-regulation capacities is due to metacognitive capacities [670] that enable the selection of behaviour regulation strategies.

Social competence difficulties and self-regulation might be a function of working memory deficit; Dučič et al. [224] through an experimental study including 41 participants with mild ID confirmed a direct correlation between self-regulation scores obtained with a devoted scale and social skills, that were also dependent on the results obtained at working memory initial tests, in the leisure time part. "These and other studies have demonstrated that once trained in specific areas, students with learning and intellectual disabilities are able to control their own learning [and behaviour]. This is an important finding that indicates that self-instruction and self-control procedures have an important part" in ID students' learning process [25]:110. All the references presented until this point belong to a cognitive neuropsychological approach, that is addressed at a more static analysis of detailed aspects of learning; this is considered unsatisfying by the neo-constructivist approach, according to which "basic-level deficits have subtle cascading effects on numerous domains over development", and suggests rather to "embrace complexity by establishing large research consortia to integrate findings at multiple levels (e.g., genetic, neural, cognitive, environmental) across developmental time" [223]. A developmental approach "posits that number processing is an emergent property of a self-organizing system that interacts with the environment" and this will provoke an earlier and more convinced focus on the intervention efforts, by targeting "those basic-level processes with the aim of improving developmental processes and outcomes" and identifying "possible protective factors (factors that improve outcome) and risk factors (factors that worsen outcome)" (ibidem). Of course, this positioning is very highly promising for persons with ID and also for all practitioners working in the field.

Assessment of play

Allen (1980) reports that play in children with ID may not emerge so naturally and informally as it does with typically developing children and may need to be encouraged. Some studies pointed out that—even if usually delayed—the patterns of play in children with ID, within the same context, were similar to those of children with typically developing ones: in fact, both groups of children spent nearly equal time in functional, constructive, and pretend play during home-based independent play situation [459, 460].

Moreover, Linn et al. [437] stated that despite the frequencies of passivity and repletion, children with ID spent the majority of their time engaging in spontaneous, nonrepetitive play. Similar findings emerged in a study [458] in which mothers were requested to describe play in their children with ID [136]:88.

The evaluation of play, as already stated elsewhere in Sect. 2.10.1, is mainly carried out through the adoption of tools devoted to play itself—or to specific types—or it is part of a wider assessment process, thus making use of developmental scales that include only some items devoted to play skills. In both cases, the tools are standardized and therefore measure the individual's ability with regards to its distance from the mean age-related competences or with regards to the imbalance among the various developmental areas that contribute to achieving that specific ability.

Macy and Bagnato note that such norm-referenced tests used in the case of children with ID are problematic "because (a) they have low treatment validity, (b) they are not universally designed or adaptable, (c) it is difficult to capture the real life behaviours/skills of young children, (d) they do little to facilitate collaboration with parents, (e) they lack sensitivity to changes in the child's development and learning, and (f) children with disabilities are often excluded from group data" [454]:1.

Then, they introduce the "authentic assessment, which promotes a natural context to best understand what a child can do" and that favours events, materials, and individuals who are familiar to the child. (ivi:2). More precisely, they propose the REAL tips to apply the authentic assessment, that include (a) Role of data collectors: the assessment team should consist of informed caregivers who know the child's skills; (b) Equipment and materials, such as common toys or household items, and also normal moments in daily life; (c) Assessment tools should bring together interdisciplinary and interagency teams—e.g., curriculum-based tools to connect assessment and educational planning[46]; (d) Location; assessment should reflect the real-life experiences children may encounter in the contexts they live in, and during the real-life times and conditions [32]. This methodological proposal gives clear insights into the more recent interpretations of ID, in which life contexts have a prominent role, and the person's adaptive functioning is considered the driving force for his/her actual performance and the more reliable basis for planning appropriate activities.

Nevertheless, authentic assessment can be associated with a further assessment method that highlights the role of the adult as a promoter of development and that for this reason reveals specifically adequate to the needs of children with ID. In fact, through expert interactions with the child, the assessor can identify and appreciate the evolutionary areas that are undergoing change and therefore promise immediate growth.

Dynamic Assessment is "an umbrella term that refers to various approaches to interactive assessment, including learning potential assessments" [133], aimed at intervening in the individual's cognitive development through the experience mediated by the relationship [176]. It relies on the Vygotskijan construct of Zone of Proximal Development[47] and it is based on "forms of support designed to influence student performance and thus to reveal their potential for change" [155]:151. "From an epistemological point of view, the DA contrasts any fixed and stable interpretation of intelligence as well as any theoretical framework built on rigid stadial concepts. Human thinking should not be measured on the basis of defined data, predictive of an unavoidable future" [73], but rather on developing skills, in continuous transformation, that should be considered "malleable and flexible rather than fixed" [669]:1. From these considerations, the importance of the quality of the experiential contexts assumes clear evidence; two main modalities to build up such productive relationships are envisaged within this model: scaffolding [48] and intersubjectivity [719].

---

[46] This "tip" is associated to a specific methodology suggested by the author to identify the more appropriate assessment tools in the framework of this proposal [32].

[47] See also Sect. 2.2.4.

[48] See also the note on Sect. 2.9.3.

3.3.3 *Factors Affecting and Favouring the Play Activity*[49]

Types of play and their tools

As already noticed, the development of play in children with ID proceeds similarly as for typically developing children, but the complexity it reaches is related, at every age, to the child's cognitive functioning. Delays are usually present and the symbolic play, which demonstrates the child's entrance in the world of abstraction and imagination, appears later [53, 179, 250, 345, 355, 424, 490, 717].

Moreover, these children love to indulge—more than others—in repetitive behaviours and they easily incur distractibility [417, 488]. Notwithstanding, their ludic attitude—revealed by attitudes of curiosity, initiative, pleasure, spontaneity, and participation—did not demonstrate a correlation with the IQ level and the cognitive functioning not to their social competence and participation [437, 449, 476].

For what concerns toys, any category can support their play activity, depending on their interests and kind/degree of impairment. To choose the appropriate toys, the first step is to bear in mind the types of play the child would be able to be involved in, and consequently to propose the toys that can suggest such an activity. Secondly, within the specific activity and type of play, the choice is related to the player's interests and preferences for some aesthetic aspects (colours, dimensions, etc.), sensorial effects (texture, smell, etc.), and also for the type of use and the affordance of the tool (types and complexity of the actions to make, etc.).

It should not be overlooked that the choice depends also on the toy's power to facilitate the play activity and to make it particularly attractive to the child.

Practice play

Infants with developmental disabilities showed lower levels of play complexity than the same developmental age peers at 6, 11, and 15 months, and the duration and frequency of object play were greater for children without disabilities than those with disabilities, even in conditions such as Down syndrome in which physical skills may not be severely restricted [297].

Toys for practice play should be as realistic as possible and should not be displayed as part of a group of toys but rather in an isolated way, and shown one at a time, to activate exploratory behaviours [108] and the pleasure of deep understanding. Toys must provide strong stimuli and require simple or few successive actions by the child; each sequence of the play activity should be short enough to allow him/her to keep enjoying play, without losing interest, which is frequent in this case.

Unpredictable effects of the use of toys or non-visible mechanisms of activation should be avoided because they can be frightened and, above all, they will not have the opportunity to verify and understand the cause-effect connection. In addition, this may prolong the time of "magical thinking", that will not invite them to explore and solve problems.

[49] This paragraph is also inspired both by the works of Bulgarelli and Stancheva-Popkostadinova [136] and by Périno and Besio [542].

In addition, in order to avoid stereotyped sequences of play and to help them evolve and adopt new different kinds of gestures and more complex movements, it is useful to provide different objects to make the same ludic activity, e.g., pop-up toys that are operated in different ways.

Symbolic play

In literature, numerous studies on practice and symbolic play in children with ID can be found, mainly because they are considered indicators of cognitive development. Hughes [353] stresses that children with ID are more interested in the physical characteristics of play materials rather than in their representational possibilities; they are more likely to simply manipulate and handle play materials [417] and prefer structured materials—such as puzzles and jacks—when their peer prefer open-ended materials (e.g., art supplies) that allow them to be creative and imaginative.

As said, the emergence of symbolic play is delayed and it will not reach the same levels of complexity of the peers [136, 353]. Messier et al. [476] reported that in a group of children with ID between 6 and 8 years of age, play age was about 2.5 years. While their practice play, involving gross and fine motor skills, as well as their interest in exploration and perception of sensory elements of play, were well-established, aspects related to imitation, imagination, and dramatization were delayed. Singh et al. [643] found that 12 2–5-year-old children with Down Syndrome mainly performed functional play[50] and less complex symbolic play. Children with ID between 8 and 12 years of age displayed level of symbolic play homogeneous with their mental age (3–6 years) [53, 345, 490, 499]. When involved in structured situations, in which, for instance, play objectives are defined by adults, children with ID showed higher pretend to play level [499].

For what concerns the choice of toys, the shape and the size of the toys for symbolic play should be as realistic as possible to favour the process of mental representation; it is also preferable that they concern tools and situations related to the real and daily life environment. To suggest comprehensive scenarios of symbolic play, they should be proposed inside a restrained area with complementary objects (for example, a doll and a cradle to play "mummy", or fruits, dishes, and pots to play "cooking").

Make-believe play can be difficult for children with ID who find it hard to understand the abstract concept of using an object as it was another one, or that a person can play a different role from his/her usual and real own. The use of realistic objects within a thematic area simplifies their participation in the play group and makes it possible for them to establish reciprocal exchanges, to recognize the various individuals' roles. The use of costumes needs appropriate and timely preparation and should be accompanied by adult support as well as by explanations, since the unusual situation created by masks and other analogous objects may be frightening to some of them.

[50] Intended in this study as practice play. See an interesting discussion on the terminology concerning the expression "functional play" in Sidhu et al. [636].

Constructive play

Studies about constructive and rule play in this population are uncommon because these types of play pose many challenges to children with ID: definition of goals, imagination, planning, adoption of strategies, problem-solving.

Due to the specific cognitive and meta-cognitive difficulties and their motor clumsiness, these children find it difficult to assemble objects appropriately in play. [353]. This task in fact asks the child to pay attention to the various play sequences, maintain in mind the final goal with the various steps to reach it, thus to recruit concentration (to avoid lack of interest), and, finally, adopt a monitoring feedback to check the evolution of the planned action.

In the case that these toys are made of parts to be assembled, the connection between them should be simple and easily achievable, these children can meet some difficulties, since they may have impairments in psychomotor coordination.

Rule-based play and games

In this case, games should be appropriate for the child, with respect to the cognitive capacity of the player, particularly regarding reasoning, making hypotheses, deduction, and time of concentration required.

Physical and social environments

Parents usually have the most important responsibility to prepare the play social environment for their children. Mothers of children with ID tend to be more directive and supportive than mothers of typically developing ones [327, 586]; this is probably due to the fact that direct and clear feedback proves effective to initially support children's play—e.g., used by the adult with great emphasis in association to vocalization and attention recruitment on a tool or a toy—and as a consequence it tends to become a frequently adopted behaviour in the relationship with the child [586]. Landry and Chapieski [411] in one of their studies found that mothers used fewer strategies for eliciting higher level play from their children with Down syndrome than expected for parents of premature infants that were mental-age and motor-age matched, and they related this less expert behaviour to differences in infant attentional capacity.

The adults' role is a very important issue to support children with ID in finding a way to express their creativity and wish to explore the world within an emotionally secure environment; it has been shown that play unfolds on a lower level, without their intervention.

Teaching basic play skills to individuals with ID can be a challenging task: for them in fact play does not always appear a natural activity, rather it seems to require express teaching [360, 376]. They may do obtain this result while acting as play partners, in a gentle, patient, non-judgmental, enthusiastic mode, and determined at the same time. They support them in maintaining attention, entering a ludic sequence, respecting and sharing the roles and the rules, accept the influence of chance. When play is taught in a structured way, children might be able to develop even more advanced types of play such as pretend play [376, 631]; therefore, the role of adults is crucial in supporting these children reach their full potential [631]. One of the best ways to obtain this result is to teach to some extent the mechanics of play (e.g., how to push a car into the garage, dress and undress a doll), but fostering an environment able to support the child's intrinsic pleasure to play for the sake of play is challenging and difficult, even more in case of association of Autism Spectrum Disorders [629].

Adults should be prepared to continuously act as models, not only in using objects in a functional way both for simply exploration and for role-play and make-believe activities but also in showing how game rules should be used, accepted, and applied, how play roles should be personified. They must be aware of the importance to give a quality and timely feedback, respondent to the child's preferences, his/her right behaviours, so that they can be fixed in his/her repertoire. Adults must be also competent in giving the child the right and needed prompts (including the physical guide), to support their approach to the objects and to the scenarios, and to favour the exploitation of all his/her play potential.

Repetition in learning these practical aspects of play can be useful; and, on the other hand, children with ID do like to repeat. Imray and Hinchcliffe [360] claim that play should be taught everyday both in and out of the classroom, going far beyond the designated limited play time at school and involving the teaching of literacy and numeracy [359] "The role of schools is crucial, as it is the schools' responsibility to provide breadth of choice and depth of experience in terms of play and to forge strong partnerships with parents and carers" [359]:570, to ensure consistency of approaches and generalization of skills.

Another point of attention in preparing effective environments concerns the need to avoid undue infantilization. As Giangreco observes, individuals with ID are too often in contact with "environments, social expectations, verbal interactions, clothing and accessories, educational materials, books, movies, toys, games, and activities associated with much younger individuals" [283]:56. Age-inappropriateness lowers the expectations of the interlocutors, and encourages to perceive them as "forever children".

The child and his/her play companions

With respect to the social dimension of play, children with ID show a higher proportion of solitary play [307, 309, 310] than the typically developing ones and, in general, social interactions are more restricted than those of comparable groups of children [307]. Furthermore, they interact less with peers, exhibit lower levels of complexity in engagement [308, 449], show some problems in co-operating, and have specific problems in ludic interactions with them: particularly, in initiating play activities with them [449, 476].

As Bulgarelli and Stancheva-Popkostadinova stress, "playing with peers is a high-demanding activity from a linguistic, cognitive, and social point of view: it implies self-regulatory strategies, achieving interpersonal goals, sustaining and coordinating play sequences, resolving conflicts, processing complex social information, and so on" [136]:90. As a consequence, social inclusion of children with ID is more effective within structured activities in kindergartens [449], where the role of the adults as mediators can be decisive again.

During play interaction, if they are not adequately supported, they tend to adopt passive behaviours and disengage from the group activity [404, 417, 437]; another important variable that may cause their abandonment is the play duration since they need to rest and restart the activity [437]. Moreover, they find it difficult to quickly shift from an activity to another one as well as to alternate the play companions; rapid changing in contexts, roles, and tools risk to confuse them. If on the one hand they tend to isolate themselves and move away from challenges, on the other hand, the environment sometimes risks subjecting them to undue infantilization. Usually, children with ID can count on smaller social networks than their peers; this increases the amount of play and leisure time they spend with adults (parents, teachers, educators) or siblings [491], who are more likely to adapt to their cognitive-level and interaction mode [212, 449, 655].

Since the mid-eighties cooperative learning has been introduced as a new form of teaching and learning; now it is widely recognized as a valid methodology not only to mediate problem-solving but also for the significant social gains it has demonstrated [132]. Two common approaches, within this framework, have taken the floor: peer tutoring has demonstrated its effectiveness in supporting children to teach to their peers with mild ID [410], but not always; reciprocal teaching, in spite of some criticism, has collected enthusiastic comments for some time [118], for being mainly based on two meta-cognitive techniques (scaffolding and self-questioning). Both approaches, in any case, seem very promising for they apply and disseminate inclusive methodologies within the educational contexts: their adaptation also to the play activity could be the result of a challenging program of applied research, and would in turn be hailed as a real innovation in the field.

As to the supports provided to children with ID to let them fully participate to the play activities with peers, they should be as natural as possible, i.e., they should be based on materials and technologies that are usually adopted in that specific context. An often-overlooked natural support is the student with ID him/her-self: the student can in fact give "an insightful perspective about his or her own needs while learning self-determination skills" [283].

3.4 Children with Autism Spectrum Disorders

3.4.1 Autism Spectrum Disorders, its Characteristics and Current Issues

The peculiar communication and social difficulties of this specific group of children were discovered and analysed first in 1943 by Kanner who used the word "autism" for labelling them. Since then, the history of the identification of this particular functioning mode of some individuals has never stopped, developing various proposals for diagnosis and intervention.

At present the *Diagnostic and Statistical Manual of Mental Disorders* (DSM–5) [14] defines it as a continuum of symptoms, combined in many different ways and with different severity levels: this is why the expression adopted is Autism

Spectrum Disorders (ASD) [732], stressing a wide heterogeneity of manifestations and of causal factors. DSM–5 concentrates the diagnostic criteria on: (a) the areas of social communication and interaction across multiple contexts (social-emotional reciprocity; nonverbal communicative behaviours used for social interaction; developing, maintaining, and understand relationships); (b) the presence of restricted, repetitive patterns of behaviour, interests, or activities.[51] Then, additional criteria about symptoms are: they must be present in early developmental period; they cause clinically significant impairment in social, occupational, or other important areas of current functioning; they are not better explained by Intellectual Disability (ID).

The incidence of the disorder in the population is currently a very controversial topic that collects extremely varied data from country to country and that nevertheless reveals a generalized tendency to a constant increase, due to some interpretations to methodological changes in the diagnostic methods [260], even if the topic is not fixed [473]; WHO declared in 2021 that one in 160 children has an ASD,[52] but it also clarified that other well-controlled studies report substantially higher figures and also that the prevalence of ASD in many low- and middle-income countries is unknown. Comorbidity with ID, albeit being another controversial topic of discussion, is highly represented. First studies in the mid-sixties reported a 75%, while later studies provide variable percentages ranging from 26 to 40% and a review reported by Papoudi and Kossyvaki [522]:564 further widens this gap from 15 to 84% [232]. According to the Autism and Developmental Disabilities Monitoring (ADDM) Network—that integrates data from 11 American states—31% of children with ASD have an intellectual disability (IQ $<$ 70), 25% are in a borderline range (IQ 71–85), while 44% obtain average or higher data (>86). On the contrary, Fombonne [259], in another review, found that 29% of the sample had mild to moderate intellectual disabilities and 42% had severe to profound intellectual disabilities. The real cause of these uneven data may be found in the difficulty of applying usual standardized tests with these children, since their particular behaviour and relational modalities make it difficult to detect their cognitive profile (delays and oddities in communication, lack of attention skills, difficulties in behaviour control, poor tolerance for the duration of the sessions).

Regardless of the degree of intellectual impairment, a characteristic of the cognitive profile of these subjects on which scientific observers agree, is that the performance component is always, and often significantly, superior to the verbal component, since it implies how skills based on visual-spatial processing are better than those based on verbal processing. However, having a reliable cognitive assessment available is essential to be able to plan adequate, timely and effective interventions. In fact [778]:229: (a) the IQ is prognostically predictive of the adult's competences; (b) higher IQ scores predict better daily life skills in adulthood; (c) the presence

[51] These "may manifest as preoccupation with one or more stereotyped and restricted patterns of interest, as inflexible adherence to specific, non-functional routines or rituals, or as stereotyped and repetitive motor mannerisms (e.g., hand or finger flapping or twisting or complex whole-body movements) as well as the persistent preoccupation with parts of objects" [522]:566.

[52] https://www.who.int/news-room/fact-sheets/detail/autism-spectrum-disorders(June 2021).

of intellectual disability is expressly indicated among the diagnostic criteria in the DSM-5. ID is perhaps, at the same time, the most common co-occurring disorder with ASD, and a strong predictor of poor prognosis [467]; Maguire et al. [455], after a wide scoping review, concluded that "older adults with ID/ASD may have reduced functional independence, increased psychiatric comorbidity and psychotropic prescribing and more behavioural presentations than the older population generally or those with ID only".

By using the *Quality of Life* (QOL) Scale of Schalock and Verdugo [613], Arias et al. [22] compared two groups of children with ASD and ID and children with ID only and found that scores were lower for ASD+ID individuals in several QOL domains, and particularly for interpersonal relationships, social inclusion and physical well-being. Miot et al. [484], in another work, studied the association of ASD-ID condition with premature ageing, finding a large range of medical comorbidities, including mental and neurological diseases, that was positively correlated with age, decreased autonomy, and polypharmacy.

A particularity within this population that should not be overlooked to understand its characteristics concerns the so-called "islets of capacity[53]", extraordinary abilities shown by about 10% of these individuals [778] that involve such areas as art, painting, sculpture, calculation, calendar knowledge, mechanical and spatial skills. These special memory skills are maintained over time and sometimes manage to transform themselves into real, always specialized activities [708].

The domain of relational and social skills is the most compromised in the case of children with ASD. In severe situations, they are unable to show interest or affectivity even towards family members, nor to recognize the effects of the others' emotions and affectivity on themselves. They find it difficult to recognize their own emotions and feelings, and even more so in attributing emotions and feelings to others as individuals different and separated from themselves. They are unable to effectively relate to others, often do not share the gaze or turn it away, use only a limited amount of facial expressions suitable for the expression of their emotions (e.g., social smile) and have difficulty decoding the others' facial expressions. Usually they prefer aloneness, do not make friends, nor ask for comfort. In social situations they feel often uncomfortable, since they don't know or are able to control body posture, and gestures to regulate social interaction, nor to infer the rules that are in place within them.

Deficiencies in communicative and linguistic development are another central area of their functioning profile. A first indication of these problem is that from the earliest stages of life, they do not recur to gestures—in particular to indication—for communicative purposes. Prominent studies have identified the inability or severe deficiency of these children in joint attention behaviours.[54] The pivotal role of joint attention in the development of children with ASD has been demonstrated by many

[53] The expression was already coined by Kanner.

[54] Joint attention behaviours emerge in typically developing children between 6 and 12 months and concern the triadic sharing of attention between the infant, another person, and an object or event; such behaviours include gaze sharing, showing and pointing objects. Imperative triadic exchanges serve an instrumental or requesting function, whereas declarative triadic exchanges serve to share

lines of evidence: (a) early symptoms reported by parents and relatives; (b) retrospective analysis of home videos including children before diagnosis; (c) studies have demonstrated [33] that early lack of gaze and of pointing for interest, together with absence of simple pretend play were highly predictive of autism; d) other studies [492] found that joint attention behaviours were associated with subsequent language ability [171]. Nevertheless, joint attention impairments do not necessarily imply autism, rather it is an early 'alarm bell' about possible brain psychopathology. Joint attention, together with the use of symbols (gestures, mimicry, words, and play) are the two major developmental milestones in children with ASD's development [748].

In the most severe cases, verbal language is absent; when it exists, it manifests some very specific characteristics, such as echolalia, the stereotyped use of some linguistic forms, the inversion of personal pronouns, the use of neologisms and idiosyncratic forms. Tager-Flusberg [689] supported a positive interpretation of their communication modalities, noting how they represent a way, albeit unusual, of keeping in touch with the interlocutors. The use of language in conversational situations (pragmatic aspect) is particularly affected; these children (even in the case of high functioning) tend to find narration very difficult, replacing the story with the description; their stories are short, lack cause-and-effect sequences, do not relate events to the characters' roles.

The etiology of ASD remains still uncertain. Research in the last years studied in-depth both neurophysiological and genetic factors, after total abandonment of the previous psycho-dynamic hypotheses. Some evidence exists (e.g., studies including twins, the high prevalence in males, etc.) on predominance of genetic factors. The discovery of mirror neurons[55] has led to the hypothesis that: (a) they are the basis for understanding the actions of others, and for the recognition of the underlying intentionality: in fact, they are activated even when the action of the others is not completed, but its purpose is known; (b) in the case of autism, they can be compromised [382]. Mirror neurons are therefore crucial for developing the ability of imitation, which in turn is the basis of the overall development, including the acknowledgement of the others' desires and intentions. Some now available studies confirm that mirror neurons are compromised in subjects with ASD, highlighting particularly an absence of activity in the inferior frontal gyrus; this would explain the deficits in imitation, Theory of Mind (ToM), social communication [778]. Thus, the social behaviour deficits of individuals with ASD might be caused by a dysfunction in the mirror neuron system [207].

However, some authors are skeptical on these conclusions as: (a) laboratory research contains methodological criticalities; (b) the imitation ability depends on the involvement of other brain areas too and not just of mirror neurons; (c) the

awareness, or the experience, of an object or event [171]. Individuals with autism are impaired in the development of both imperative and declarative acts, although impairments in the latter are more severe [43].

55 "Located in the opercular part of the inferior frontal gyrus and in the rostral part of the inferior parietal lobule of the brain" [778]:242, they are activated when an action is performed, or when one observes another that completes it [585].

impairment of mirror neurons would not explain other manifestations of ASD such as repetitive behaviours [508].

Current trends in intervention

ASD is still considered an "enigma", as Frith stated in 2003 [273]. To the purpose of trying to explain this phenomenon so as to intervene in the best way, some interpretations are now contemporarily active in the related literature [778]. Altogether, they represent the edges on which the discussion unfolds today around the ASD.

In 1985, Baron-Cohen et al. [43] sustained that children with ASD have a lacking in the ability of Theory of Mind—usually showing at 3–4 years—, which means they experience many difficulties in attributing to oneself and the others mental states related to thoughts, desires, intentions, thoughts and beliefs. Leslie [418] added that this difficulty may be explained by a more general meta-representational impairment. This interpretation is able to explain the disorders of socialization, communication and imagination, but it does not appear adequate, for example, to account for all social difficulties, nor the onset and manifestation of obsessive and repetitive behaviours, rigidity, etc.

The weak central coherence theory, mainly sustained by Happé [317] and by Frith [273], holds that these individuals have a problem that prevents them from processing information as a whole by hindering access to higher-level meanings; central coherence in fact consists in the ability to process information in its context, putting together different elements to the purpose of giving a whole meaning, even to the detriment of the details. This hypothesis then sustains that individuals with ASD have a natural propensity to focus on details, that has consequences in perceptual, linguistic, cognitive, problem-solving tasks. The theory would explain many language deficiencies, stereotypies and narrow interests, but it also accounts for some positive characteristics, such as some excellent performances where attention to detail is decisive.

The executive function deficit theory calls into question "the skills involved in planning and organizing actions, in inhibiting automatic responses and in anticipating the progression of an event" [778]. As with prefrontal lesion deficit, people with ASD often adopt inflexible behaviours, are obsessed with daily routines, pay attention to details, can be impulsive, and sometimes fail to inhibit responses [599]. However, these deficits are also present in other types of disorders and therefore give a too general response, not sufficiently convincing in the case of autism.

The theory of primary socio-affective deficit develops entirely within the psychological discipline, and tries to identify causes of the autistic condition in events or aspects that occurred during the development of these persons. Hobson [347] sustains that these individuals find it difficult to consider the others as bearers of their own subjectivity; then, the author proposes that the inability or difficulty in intersubjective engagement with others is the primary nucleus that explains this attitude and the other disorders. Thus, these children have an innate inability to forge emotional contacts (much less relationships) with others: as a consequence, the others move away. This vicious circle would finally compromise social reciprocity processes.

Another lively theme in the contemporary debate on ASD concerns the play of these children; for this reason, it will be treated in-depth in the following paragraphs.

3.4.2 *Impact of Autism Spectrum Disorders on Participation to Play*[56]

Many aspects of the physical functioning of children with ASD may have a negative impact on the development of playful and satisfying activities. Their behaviour is often characterized by a certain fixation: they exhibit "preoccupations ranging from a fascination with objects to an intense focus on arcane topics" [759]:57.

Some authors [590, 742] suggest that this might be a result of sensory integration dysfunctions, that are frequently associated with ASD: in fact, difficulty in processing sensory stimuli involves 45–96% of these children [58, 412], thus affecting participation in play activities [609]. In some other cases a low threshold in response to stimuli is present—e.g., in the case of over-sensitivity to noise, light, smell, or touch—may provoke avoidance of movement, restricted preferences to only some play tools or activities [610] as well as reduced social interaction. On the contrary, sensory insensitivity or high threshold may induce behaviours aiming at provoking self-stimulation, such as excessive movement, manipulative play, sounds production, etc. This inaccurate functioning of sensitivity might also be at the basis of inattention, that makes it difficult for the child to concentrate, while he/she prefers to switch from various activities, and this may interfere with play [412].

Furthermore, it should be reminded that according to the enactive mind theory [396], the perceptive apparatus of typically developing children is naturally oriented to focus on the information salient for survival. In the case of children with ASD, it has been demonstrated that, on the contrary, they show shortcomings in identifying quickly the relevant aspects of social information. This might be responsible, for instance, for their difficulties in perceiving the human faces and other social aspects of the environment; this could also be responsible of some difficulties they meet in social play.

Cairney [150] underlined that children with ASD have also motor coordination difficulties "such as poor balance, eye-hand coordination, and decreased ability to plan and execute motor tasks, create social isolation and restrict participation in play" [574]. Some studies stressed [393] that motor coordination skills are an important source for participation in physical play and children with such type of impairment show a lower developmental play age and engage less frequently in play than their typical peers (ibidem).

As known, some basic skills to start and develop play behaviours are lacking in children with ASD: impaired joint attention, decreased imitation, and social imagination that give rise to both sensorimotor and symbolic play, especially in their social and shared application, are then seriously compromised [498, 696].

Moreover, the difficulties in the development of communication, social interaction, and symbolic thinking [519, 521, 709] are associated with difficulties in these children's play. Also, severe verbal linguistic impairment heavily affects both pretend play and symbolic play, for at least two reasons: because they represent high-level

[56] This section is also inspired by Ray-Kaeser et al. [574].

conceptualizations (pretending that one object is another one is a cognitive act; representing and participating to play scenarios require control of executive functions) and because internalized verbal language is one of the main ways of imagination; in addition, the impossibility to communicate adequately seriously limits relationships [759].

An impairment of the Theory of Mind might be co-responsible for the hard implementation of the symbolic play competences; this is true also in the case of other types of play, such as the 'hide and seek' game, that involves decentration skills and mental representations of oneself and of the other ones in the shared space [701]. Disorders in activating and monitoring one's own executive functions may impact on all the types of play that require a planned series of actions or sequences, taking and changing turns, as well as when the play is based on rules that should be applied but also negotiated, or changed [701].

Assessment of play

"Despite the importance of play in both the diagnosis and treatment of toddlers and preschool-aged children with ASD, there is little research on the effective measurement of play in this population" [551]. In addition to really assess their play competence, an observation and collection of their behaviours both at home or in other contexts (rehabilitation or school settings) should be needed [387, 630].

Pierucci et al. [551] studied the relations between four commonly used standardized diagnostic instruments which nevertheless, include but are not limited to, the measure of play skills. Play is frequently measured within the ASD assessment batteries,[57] but the definitions and classifications of play they adopt are unclear and are not the same through different tools. The authors analysed and compared the play composites included within four existing scales,[58] to the purpose of identifying possible correlations between them. They concluded that "play composites from these diagnostic evaluation measures were not all significantly correlated. This [. . .] suggests that (a) these global measures assess different aspects/types of play and (b) the context of play observations matters" [551]:41. Thanks to their work, and after further analysis on their data, additional reflections on the concepts of play adopted in these scales can bring to light a truly uneven situation: (a) the value and importance attributed to play through the scales is not equivalent (as well as its "weight" within the whole scale); (b) the scales measure different types of play (functional, with objects, symbolic, activity level, etc.); (c) they leave the examiner wide margins for interpretation about them, since they are not associated with specific definitions of the considered types; (d) in some cases a generic type of "playful behaviour" seems to be required for examination: e.g., activity level, imitation, object use; (e) different degrees of complexity between the various types are not considered: "object use"

---

[57] In a wider perspective, few studies exist that compare different assessment tools used in autism evaluation [517].

[58] They are: *Adaptive Behavior Assessment System* (ABAS-II [322]); *Autism Diagnostic Observation Scale* (ADOS [440]); *Child Autism Rating Scale* (CARS2-ST [618]; *Communication and Symbolic Behavior Scales-Developmental Profile Infant-Toddler Checklist* (CSBS DP ITC; [749].

might involve very different behaviours that imply perceptual, psychomotor, cognitive and social abilities (for instance, knocking an object on the table, throwing it into the room, pulling the rope of a toy car, fitting two or more Lego bricks and also feeding a doll); moreover, a possible evolutionary progression between the various types does not seem to be envisaged.

As Pierucci et al. underlined, assessment scales in the field of ASD usually include play among the areas to be evaluated; since this activity evolves through social exchanges, is hugely responsible for the child's overall development and is widely recognized as one of the main points of difficulty of individuals with ASD.

Other scales do exist that are more directly addressed to support an overall assessment of the child's play activity and behaviours, or that devote a part of the more comprehensive tool expressly to play. Some of them are applied in the assessment of children with ASD or have been incorporated within programs aimed at teaching play behaviours.[59]

Among these, some are shortly presented below, without the intention of being exhaustive.[60]

Child-Initiated Pretend Play Assessment (ChIPPA) [666] is a standardized assessment that measures 3–7-year-old children's ability to initiate and engage in spontaneous pretend play for a limited time. It assesses both "symbolic and conventional-imaginative pretend play using a standard set of toys" (ibidem). It is administered one-on-one in a location free from distraction by excessive noise or other children. The ChIPPA measures three aspects of pretend play in children: complexity, elaborateness and organization. The standardized scores compare the child's cognitive pretend play ability to that of their peers [723]:36.

The *Penn Interactive Peer Play Scale* (PIPPS) [242, 243] rates a child's social competence based on their interactive peer play and is completed by the child's classroom teacher. It differentiates children with accomplished peer interaction skills from those who encounter some difficulty while interacting with their peers. Its items include positive and negative play indicators, providing insight into the child's strengths and weaknesses regarding interactive peer play (ibidem).

The *Developmental Play Assessment Scale* (DPA) [427, 429] consists of eight play levels, and 15 play categories within them; categories and levels relate respectively to types of play and the various phases inherent each of them, including the toys and the ways to use them.

While this instrument did not have any further editions, a promising new version, the *Developmental Play Assessment for Practitioners* (DPA-P) that has been just published [428], aiming at "assessment of naturally occurring play activities

[59] Additional assessment tools with respect to those already cited in this paragraph, are available for evaluation of ASD development, and some of them have a substantial part devoted to play behaviours. Among them, it is worth citing the *Screening Tool for Autism in Two-Year-Olds* (STAT) [672, 673].

[60] Other tools to be considered because used in the field of ASD are: *Questionnaire for Play Observation* [77]; *Revised Preschool Play Scale* [397]; *Protocols for Play Behaviour* [642]; *Scale of Organisation of Play Behaviour* [357]. See also Ziviani [781].

for evaluating young children's developmental progress accurately, so that useful interventions can take place as early as possible".

An adapted version of the DPA has been successfully used by Thiemann-Bourque and coll. to explore possible differences in some types of play between children with ASD and typically developing children, finding that the first group may have comparable functional play skills and struggle with the transition to some, but not all types of symbolic play (2012) and between children with ASD and children with other types of difficulties, finding that the first group showed engaged in more conventional play, and that there high correlations between play, language, and cognitive measures (2019).

Two innovative studies, both from Taiwan, take into consideration an important aspect in the playful behaviour of children with ASD. In fact, the authors study the correlation between the Theory of Mind (assessed with the ToM test [247]) of a group of children with ASD and: (a) on one hand, their play skills, in particular in pretend playing, assessed through the *Child Initiated Pretend Play Assessment* test (ChIPPA [666]) ; (b) on the other hand, the playfulness attitude, assessed with the *Test of Playfulness* (ToP [137]). From the first experiment, involving 20 children (from 3 to 7-year-old), they report that ToM significantly predicted pretend play variables, but not playfulness, and conclude that: (a) "children with ASD who have better ToM might be able to develop better pretend play, but not better playfulness, which might be more strongly related to their autistic severity" and (b) severity of autistic behaviours seem to prevail on ToM in maintaining play themes, sequences, and narrative during play, thus impeding children to feel joyful and free during play [169]:44.

The second experiment concentrates on the pretend play characteristics with respect to the Theory of Mind and findings demonstrate that it "has a predominant role in the quality, not the quantity, of pretend play of children with ASD, when the children's autistic behaviours and verbal comprehension are considered" [433]:1187. Particularly, better verbal comprehension was positively correlated both with quality and quantity of pretend play, children were able to initiate pretend play by themselves and did not need any cues; worse comprehension occurred in children with more autistic behaviours, and this caused difficulties in initiating play, as well as in imitation.

3.4.3 When Play Becomes a Means of Intervention Programs to Teach and Learn to Play[61]

The huge difficulties children with ASD meet in naturally developing pleasant and complex play activities are first and foremost linked to their difficulties in social interaction: from face-to-face contacts and spontaneous play with their mothers [493,

[61] This paragraph is also inspired by Ray-Kaeser et al. [574].

494], to the acquisition of joint attention and object sharing, to the enjoyment of fruitful exchanges with their peers and the engagement in ludic relationships [762].

In general, these children seem less playful than their peers, showing repetitive behaviours with objects, and restricted play interests [59]. As it has been described in the previous paragraphs, additional and specific impairments contribute to defining an overall condition that may explain the serious difficulties these children encounter in playing. These considerations brought researchers and professionals in the field to give play a special place in the education and rehabilitation programs for these children. On the one hand, in fact, on the basis of psycho-educational theories consistent with this approach, in particular those related to Vygotskij work, play has been interpreted as an unavoidable area for their development, due to its power to drive the child's cognitive and social evolution. On the other hand, play has been considered a proper and irreplaceable context of these children's life, within which the reparative activities could be located, proposed, carried out, in a pleasant and useful way.

As a consequence, devoted psychoeducational programs of intervention that address play—or highly based on it—have been developed, aimed at teaching and promoting play in children with ASD.

In what follows some of them will be presented; anyway, for the purposes of this volume, it is appropriate to specify[62] that these applications of play must be considered play-like activities. In fact, they have the express purpose of using the play context to achieve purposes other than the play itself, for example, social or cognitive improvements, and they do not respond to an important characteristic of play, which is self-organization, the intrinsic drive of playful activity. The play programs presented to the children with ASD are usually on individual base; group play will be proposed later, where the generalization of learning may occur. Studies based on the principles of applied behaviour analysis have shown that children with autism can be taught to achieve basic acts of play through games and their functional use [385].

Within such framework, environments for learning skills to play should be specially prepared for these activities; this may happen by adopting a very structured space, were the activities as well as the external cues are really strict [693] as in the *Applied Behavioural Analysis* (ABA) method [443]; however, this kind of too high relations with the specific setting can lead to difficulties in the generalization of learning [764].

Argyropoulou and Papoudi [21] applied the principles of *Intensive Interaction*[63] and interactive play as an educational approach in a case study of a boy with autism to evaluate its effectiveness in the improvement of his interactions with a pupil in the same nursery. The program showed useful for reciprocal social interactions and provided evidence of inclusive practice. Before they can correctly express emotions in daily life, children with ASD need to learn to understand emotions and recognize

[62] See also Sect. 2.10.2.

[63] Intensive Interaction [341, 342] is an approach to teaching to persons with learning difficulties which is aimed specifically at facilitating the development of the most fundamental social and communication abilities. It is based on the model of caregiver-infant interaction and makes use of caregivers' playful style in the interactive process. According to Nind [505] there are some reasons for applying this approach also to persons with ASD.

them and their meaning. For this reason, *emotional recognition* and *Theory of Mind* are frequently taught to these children before work can begin to improve play for the sake of play [702]. Many studies investigate the impact of such interventions; according to behavioural strategies, new skills should be taught in an environment where the antecedent stimuli are clear and systematic reinforcement should follow a correct response [189].

For example, Ingersoll and Gergans [361] explored the impact of *Reciprocal Imitation Training* on spontaneous imitation skills, employing three mothers and their young children with autism and intellectual disabilities. Kasari and her associates [386] explored the effectiveness of a parent-mediated intervention on play skills of children with autism, focusing on joint engagement, joint attention, and found an increase in children's play diversity and higher play levels. Although such practices have been generally shown to have positive results, i.e., improvement in interpersonal communication, play, and language development, they must be applied to a larger number of children with autism and to corresponding control groups in order to confirm their effectiveness and examine these outcomes in relation to learning [522].

Playing with others requires multiple skills, especially at social level; through social play, children with autism learn about social interaction, but they need support and facilitation to accomplish this result. Through social interaction, interactive play, and peer play, they may learn how to play and how to create positive relationships and, as a result, become less isolated, by playing as equal members of a group. "It is interaction and connectedness with others that generate developmental benefits in communication, in reciprocity during social transactions, in imagination and thought flexibility, and in the strengthening of the relationship between parents, educators, and children, as well as among the children themselves" [522]. Many psycho-educational models and programs address this specific topic—the role and importance of social interaction in the development of children with ASD and their play—by encouraging interactive play between parents and children. According to Luckett et al. [444], these interventions are the most effective for developing play skills because they use the child's strengths and seek inner motivation through activity more than external rewards.

In the *floor time approach* [753], the adult follows and supports the child's initiatives while using language, gestures and emotional expressions to elicit more complex communication.

"Rogers [589] and her associates introduced the *Denver model* as a developmental intervention model that focuses on (1) the development of interpersonal, constructive, and symbolic play; (2) the establishment of relationships characterized by positive affect, reciprocity, and imitation; and (3) the development of speech" [522]. Also, in this case the adult should follow the child's lead, interpret his/her proposals giving them communicative value; appropriate organization of the surrounding environment and assuring strong affect-laden relationships is important to obtain the needed involvement [361].

The *Integrated Play Groups model* is instead based on the child's participation to social peer groups. More originally, it promotes the design of specific play areas that offer opportunities for construction and socio-dramatic role-play; opening and closing ritual are also organized to facilitate the understanding of the 'play frame' context by children with ASD [761].

The role of technology in supporting teaching the play skills to children with autism should not be underestimated, since they usually like technology for the digital environments offer structure, visual supports, control, and opportunities for repetition. The technique of *video-modelling*[64] has been largely adopted, for instance to teach pretend play skills in children with autism, to teach toy-related conversational skills [694], social initiation and toy play [504], appropriate verbal and motor play [531], play dialogues [496], and verbal compliments given to peers during group play [453, 522]. However, it is worth noting that studies focusing on technology-mediated interventions to teach play skills are considerably fewer than studies focusing on skills pertaining to the core difficulties seen in autism (e.g., social skills, communication) and academic skills.

3.4.4 Factors Affecting and Favouring the Play Activity

After the review of studies and considerations, however brief, presented in the previous paragraphs, an important question arises against this background: "to what extent this indeed constitutes play, given that flexibility, creativity, and fun are not often observed [in these programs]? [385, 762].

Any intervention aiming to unfold play should stem from the child's developmental level, the play of the children themselves, and their individual needs, instead of being based on a predesigned program" [522]:569. The two previously cited studies from Taiwan have something to add in this regard, and they appear enlightening. On the contrary, one could object: if these children do not autonomously and freely manifest the urge to spontaneous and self-regulated play, and if play is confirmed as one of the liveliest expressions of childhood and in human life, how can the professionals in education or in rehabilitator, how can the parents face such a problem?

It will be necessary to pursue, in the years to come, the goal of teaching these children to play, avoiding to make play one of the numerous daily routines they must repeat and perform following exercise, rather by triggering the spark that allows play to become a personal property, a private and necessary desire, that claims to be self-guided. It is a matter of pursuing a balance, not at all simple, between skill teaching and supporting the child's free appropriation and expression of a need.

As is it clear, the field literature is strongly influenced by the fact that "play", in the case of children with ASD, means prevailingly "skills to be taught" and it has been mainly studied within the framework of the cognitive approach. The development of play in infants and young children with autism and, most importantly, the social, interpersonal, and emotional dimensions of play have hardly been studied [521]; it

[64] Video-modelling is a technique to teach new skills or behaviour to autistic children. The video shows someone doing an activity or a behaviour. The child watching the video copies them.

is very difficult to find studies and materials that are more directly and consciously dedicated to play for the sake of play, above all in the case of these children.

In this section, it was then decided to include reference to some studies which seem to offer information that might give rise to new ideas and new perspectives in the field, once reworked and rethought in a freer design perspective.

Types of play and their tools

As it is well-known nowadays, children with autism approach play in a different way to that of their non-autistic peers. "Using the specific skills of children with ASD to increase their motivation in play seems essential. Specific skills related to the characteristics of ASD, for example, the ability to perceive details or even the restricted interests of a child, could then become assets in some play situations" [574]. Furthermore, they show excessive preoccupation with certain toys and an interest in a very limited number of toys [522]; in some cases, they are fascinated by their appearance, or by their immediate sensory characteristics, or the opportunities they might offer for simple manipulation, while they remain indifferent to the cultural or symbolic meaning the objects may carry [574].

The thematic content of the play of children with autism is characterized by a lack of coherence and creativity and by repetitiveness to the point of ritual [519].

As to the concrete choice of toys and games, they should not be replaced every day. To protect the players' emotional well-being, a balance should be found between already known toys and games, and new ones. In order to guarantee continuity to the play activity and to increase gradually its complexity, toys and games should vary slightly over time, according to their functionalities.

Practice play

Some research reports that toddlers with autism at 20 months exhibit functional play and pretend play at the same level as infants with developmental delay and their performance in pretend play is at a lower level only compared with that of typical toddlers of the same age [172]. But other studies contradict this statement, and it is important to underline also that the expression "functional play" [636], widely used especially in this specific field of play studies, is highly inaccurate and gives raise to scientific misunderstanding.

Sensorimotor (or practice) play in the case of ASD is not so much treated in the sector literature; it is known that these children tend to play by themselves, engaging in the same play routines, and indulge in self-stimulatory behaviours that include flicking or spinning objects (visual), tapping and clicking (auditory), licking (taste), feeling different textures (tactile), spinning themselves, climbing, and balancing (vestibular), and getting into odd body postures (proprioceptive) [522]. Some research makes a comparison between the ability of these children to explore and use objects functionally and the serious difficulties in acquiring spontaneous symbolic and pretend play during their preschool and school years.

For what concerns toys for practice play, children with ASD are not attracted by the overall shape of the objects, as they are more interested by some specific aspects, or small details. When proposing toys to attract their attention, weight is an interesting element to consider, due to proprioceptive sensations and the body consciousness it provokes; texture of the object is also important, as well as sensorial feedback it can produce (visual—light is usually appropriate—or auditory). Sometimes, this feedback is only provoked by the particular way adopted by the child in using the toy. The cause-and-effect relationship is also a positive element of toys for children with ASD, if it is immediate and easy to be perceived. Some toys for practice play are particularly interesting as they can initiate social connection, for example, by throwing, catching, giving, and giving back.

Symbolic play

It has been found that in children with autism who have developed understanding and production of speech, as well as in children with secure attachment, functional and symbolic play occur more often and at a higher level. There is also evidence that the use of joint attention is connected to the ability for symbolic play in children with autism [385].

Nevertheless, a lack of varied, spontaneous make-believe play or social imitative play appropriate to the child's developmental level is also often reported in the field literature; according to Kasari et al. [385], these children are not very likely to develop symbolic play, or they may do so only to a limited extent and after instruction.

There is also evidence that in relation to symbolic and pretend play, limitations in creative, playful pretend play among children with autism is related to their restricted interpersonal communication and engagement [346].

In choosing the best toys to support this type of play, it should be reminded that the difficulties in symbolic play encountered by children with autism are linked not to the ability for play, but rather to performance of play [89]. When it comes, for instance, to role-playing, that is particularly tricky for these children, they often feel challenged by representing and changing roles, and find it difficult to adopt the point of view of another person, or to act for them. This play activity is then initiated by adults who help in simplifying roles and activities and break it down into subsequent steps, each of them corresponding to one specific isolated action with objects (for example, interpreting 'being a musician' only by playing drums). As to the symbolic play with figurines and miniatures, tools should be preferred that match social interactions to real life [31].

In addition, isolated toys are more appropriate than ensembles: for example, playing with a car and moving it forward instead of managing a whole garage. Once effective play sessions with one object are obtained, it becomes possible to use toys that can be related to the same topic to expand the children's play. The adults can act as models of symbolic play, can initiate role-playing and encourage it by reminding the children stories and tales they already know and proposing to interpret them.

Constructive play

In this case the duration of the play activity can be decisive; these children are not able to remain concentrated for a long time on an activity that pursues a complex and distant goal. These children need to finish their purposeful action quickly so as to feel successful.

Assembling toys can be chosen on the basis of the mechanism that holds the pieces together; these children may be fascinated by this aspect of the play activity and reveal experts in this type of toys. In this case, they may spend a lot of time in assembling small elements, even if it is not always clear and recognizable the final project they have in mind. Putting together pieces, completing a puzzle as quickly as possible, repeating for the sake of repetition may seem, in these cases, the only scope of their play. More complex toys in these cases can be proposed to interrupt a sterile repetition of gestures and activities, if this reiteration is perceived as devoid of joy. The adults may show examples of how to continue the construction and avoid the children with ASD to repeat always the same sequence or propose the children to explain their project.

Rule-based play and games

Rule-based play can be challenging for these children, especially if an intellectual impairment is associated. It would be useful in this case to simplify the rules, as well as to shorten the mean game duration. Specific attention should be posed, in addition, to the give the instruction in the clearest way. They usually appreciate very much games that require comparison and differentiation abilities.

Children with ASD need simple rules because the play social situation is challenging for them and they are mostly concentrated on monitoring this aspect of the activity. Furthermore, rules can be contemporarily a problem and an advantage for children with ASD: in fact, they facilitate understanding of the play activity, because they put clear limits to control the situation; on the other hand, they increase the tendency of these children to act in a well-regulated and repetitive manner.

Adopting shortcuts or flexible solutions is not possible for them and this might reveal a difficulty in the social context, in case other children propose to change the rules, to adopt alternative ways for using the game, etc. In case they start to appreciate this type of toys and games, this could be a powerful and joyful way, for them, to face human relationships. One of the roles of the adults is to simplify the play situation to avoid or minimize frustrations; for example, within games such as snakes and ladders, by taking the dice off so that each player's turn is respected [350].

Physical and social environments

The social environments where these children live and spend their time should be aware of their special and specific functioning characteristics. The whole environment/s—physical, social, cultural—should be informed at this scope, and change appropriately. For emotional comfort and well-being, the number of toys presented at the same time should be reduced to two or three, and the overall environment should be quiet, without sudden noise or changes in lighting.

Some children prefer to play alone and may find play with other children uncomfortable or even distressing, and this, according to Calder et al. [151], should be respected, above all during assessment phase or specific activities. As social relations with non-familiar people are not easy for these children, adults may promote parallel play between players by putting in place more thematic play areas and supporting children with ASD, so that they can feel secure, imitate and play on their own, but alongside other children.

On the contrary to this statement, other studies stress that it is particularly important for them "to participate in playful environments, to be encouraged to play, to practice playful activities, and, through interaction with adults and peers, to 'unfold' play itself" [522]. In gaining this level of involvement, they can be supported by adults or peers, as demonstrated by Kasari et al. [385].

Adults—educators and parents—must be able to design appropriate environments that will address their play needs [740], by mediating within interactive play events and by providing guidance that leads to higher levels of play; adults should be aware of the best relational style that favours collaboration and adjust themselves accordingly. And children will develop empathy, social understanding, greater tolerance toward different forms of communication and play [760].

Environments surrounding the child with ASD should be informed at a sort of 'play culture', that gives access to and support for peer play and discourages isolation [762]. The existence of a framework—in the family, the school, the community—which enables a 'play culture' and a 'peer culture', can contribute significantly to the improvement of social interaction and communication as well as to the development of creativity, imagination, and symbolic thought, thus opening to fun and happiness [522]. Happiness and well-being have not yet studied adequately in the field of autism [726], while the quality of life among adults with autism has been found to correlate with regular and meaningful recreational activities [85].[65]

The child and his/her play companions

Children with ASD's behaviour is very often described as avoiding playing with others, preferring aloneness, and showing serious difficulties in engaging in spontaneous, socially acceptable play, as well as participating in dyadic play and, later, peer play. Furthermore, they often take refuge in lonely stereotypical behaviours [376]. Some studies found them rejected by their peers, if they are not considered as equally able playmates [21, 520]. Interactive play [625] and peer play [762] should be explicitly supported by adults, by setting up appropriate environments able to contain their restlessness and fear and by favouring a delicate, secure, pleasant contact with the peers.

Within the needed and desirable inclusive contexts, this setting must include also the right information for the other children, so that they can become aware of their own communication styles as well as on the reciprocal and eventually different needs—to play, to have fun, to collaborate. For example, Kasari et al. demonstrated [385] that an integration intervention focused on the group of classmates was more fruitful than an intervention addressed to the children with ASD, since in the first case children with ASD were considered as members of the social network of the class and more involved during the rest of the activities.

[65] This reflection introduces also the—neither trivial or predictable—discussion on the fact that according to some authors the 'normative benchmarks' [698] are likely to be challenged in the case of play and autism, for instance by considering that having fun should not be sacrificed in the name of age appropriateness [359].

A harvest of educational literature in the educational field do exist nowadays on how to make contexts more inclusive for children. The fact that play is not yet so much represented in these studies must not be considered as a problem but rather as a stimulus to proceed intensively in this direction.

3.5 Children with Visual Impairments

3.5.1 Visual Impairment, its Characteristics and Current Issues[66]

A Visual Impairment (VI) may be due to a reduction in visual acuity (central vision), or in the visual field (peripheral vision). The degree of impairment can vary from total blindness to low vision, in a continuum whose demarcation lines are often defined by national regulations (and determine, correspondingly, the dedicated supports). The WHO defines five categories of VI, based on the two parameters indicated above [766].

Despite these precise classifications, there are great individual differences in the manifestation of this problem, which results in a wide variability in the personal and social autonomy. Two factors may be responsible for this variability [158]: the first is the anatomical location of the impairment, the second concerns the time of onset. In particular, the differences between individuals who have a VI from birth, or have acquired it later, are substantial and involve many developmental areas: to manage spatial skills and competence, to socially participate (acknowledgement of the other's intentionality, application of the right 'social scripts' to the most common social events, etc.), the effectiveness of the language use (duration and alternation of turns in conversation, right interpretation of the suprasegmental traits of the verbal language, etc.) [277].

The causes of severe VI and blindness may be prenatal, perinatal, and postnatal. WHO reports[67] that there is a high variation in the causes between countries according to the socio-political and economic conditions, that reflect in availability and affordability of eye care services. For instance, the proportion of vision impairment attributable to cataract is higher in low- and middle-income countries than high-income countries. In high-income countries, diseases such as glaucoma and age-related macular degeneration are more common. Also in the case of children, although there are very few population-based studies on them, the congenital cataract is a leading cause in low-income countries, whereas in middle-income countries it is more likely to be retinopathy due to prematurity and uncorrected refractive error

[66] The first part of this paragraph is partially inspired by Zanobini and Usai [778].

[67] The report has been developed, together other documentation, within the "Vision 2020' program, which sets the aim to eliminate avoidable blindness by 2020. While there have been some positive changes in the reduction in the prevalence of blindness and MSVI, the main avoidable causes of vision loss, cataracts and refractive error are still the main causes of vision loss [389]:15.

remains a leading cause of vision impairment in the other countries.[68] According to Gilbert and Fosters [288], the prevalence of blindness in children varies according to socio-economic development and under-5 mortality rates.[69] In low-income countries with high under-5 mortality rates, the prevalence may be as high as 1.5 per 1000 children, while in high-income countries with low under-5 mortality rates, the prevalence is around 0.3 per 1000 children. More recent statistics at world level are not available only for children, but a WHO report [767] states that "globally, at least 2.2 billion people have a near or distance vision impairment. In at least 1 billion—or almost half—of these cases, vision impairment could have been prevented or has yet to be addressed".[70]

The classification of the degree of severity of VI ranges from mild to severe (partial blindness, total blindness), but their normative quantification in the various countries depends on the measurement methods adopted.

A major issue in children with neurodisabilities concerns the Cerebral Visual Impairment (CVI), whose most comprehensive definition—albeit controversial—is "a verifiable visual dysfunction which cannot be attributed to disorders of the anterior visual pathways or any potentially co-occurring ocular impairment" [514]. CVI can present in many combinations and degrees, and this depends on the timing, location, and extent of the causative lesion itself; it is common in children with cerebral palsy. A comprehensive neurodevelopmental assessment evaluation is needed, by a multidisciplinary team—including ophthalmology and neuro-disability/neurology—that works together with parents and teachers to reach an integrated and individualized perspective for the individual child.[71] Blind and severely VI people perceive the world by making use of different sensory modalities: this is often interpreted as their possibility to count on the brain's "compensatory plasticity", according to which they would develop "supranormal skills when using one of the remaining senses" [406] to interpret the world.

A huge and very specialized research on these elements collected some contradictory results, due to the various experimental frameworks adopted. Then, conclusive studies suggest that visual deprivation onset early in life does not lead to superior performance in all auditory tasks [164, 741], and that not at all touch is improved [671]. "The most crucial aspect [identified] is that "seeing" the world might be different for those with VI compared to the sighted, but that their perception is just as rich and varied due to the compensatory effects of practicing to experience the world through the other senses" [251]:29. "Research has found structurally different visual areas as well as different connections between these and tactile areas in blind individuals. [These findings] generalize across both sighted and visually impaired people and

[68] https://www.who.int/news-room/fact-sheets/detail/blindness-and-visual-impairment.

[69] "The under-five mortality rate refers to the probability of a child dying between birth and exactly 5 years of age, expressed per 1.000 live births" (https://data.unicef.org/topic/child-survival/under-five-mortality/).

[70] https://www.who.int/news-room/fact-sheets/detail/blindness-and-visual-impairment.

[71] The development of children with CVI may be deeply complicated by the severity and the type of the impairment. Although it is a quite recent topic in scientific literature, many studies have been devoted to its study, for example, the ones by Dutton and colleagues [226, 227, 779].

suggests that the cortex is highly plastic and able to re-route information displayed to the other senses or via sight restoration in just a matter of hours via existing multisensory neural connections" [251]:28.

Studies concentrated also on how the "blind brain" may differ from the sighted brain, as well as on the reasons for congenitally blind and late blind individuals significantly differ on cognitive tasks: this suggests in fact that visual input during the first few years of life plays a role in cognitive development.

Establishing fixed points on these themes is important for developing interventions, such as Assistive Technology (AT) and sensory substitution devices [567, 614] and could benefit employment and educational practice [477].

Current trends in intervention

The fields of most rapid knowledge development are in the medical area—pharmaceuticals, cell-based therapies, gene therapies—and in technology, that is still one of the liveliest and most promising branches of contemporary studies in the VI sector [740]. Assistive Technology (AT) have always been part of the habilitation process for persons with visual needs: sticks, long canes, acoustic canes, guide dogs, tools to support the use of the Braille code at different ages.

The recent explosion of new digital platforms and tools, the development of wireless devices and apps might be an interesting opportunity for blind persons to improve their quality of life, but the feedback from reality is not encouraging, and many critical issues emerge. Gori et al. [294], studying why such advances in AT for visually impaired are not taken up,[72] discovered many methodological critical issues: "they remain bulky and intrusive; they require extensive training [...], they mark a user out as different to their peers [...], they were trialled with a very small number of individuals, seldom scaled to larger numbers and [may prove] less applicable to those outside of the initial test group" also due to the wide heterogeneity of the interested population [740]:351. Furthermore, they need to block a sensory route that is used only for the device, while during their daily life blind persons need to count on a multiple flow of sensorial information. These tools require a significant cognitive load and thus are hardly usable by children, who have to deal with stimuli coming from the environment, and cannot yet count on an effective multi-channel processing. For these reasons, Gori et al. [294] argue that developers need to consider the needs of children and young people as distinct from those of adults and should consider their neuro-developmental characteristics.

The spread of some apps that are on ubiquitous smartphones, enthusiastically welcomed mainly by children, is also causing unwanted side effects, for example due to the fact that no effective relationship is established between the manufacturer, other specialists, and the users; the product can be created without any knowledge of the real needs of a person with VI, while the necessary information on the characteristics of the applications are not available as to evaluate their quality before

[72] They were of two types: first, those that compensate for the absence of sight by substituting visual inputs with sound and touch; and, second, where an additional strategy is proposed to circumvent a visual need [740]:351.

acquiring them [602]. Furthermore, the use of these apps may be related to a dramatic decline in the use of the Braille code; this requires practice and hard work to be learnt, even with new technologies, but it gives the opportunity to access the overall existing knowledge, in addition to supporting the process of normal literacy, which is cognitively irreplaceable in the individual's development. On the other hand, the use of smartphones, as well as web surfing, viewed as a requirement for modern living and, in some respects, a "right", would, on the contrary, claim for the acquisition of discerning and critical skills to face adequately the risk of fake news, exposure to traumatising behaviours such as bullying and abusive grooming [5].

The world around persons with VI is still widely designed "by the sighted for the sighted" [251]:29. Environmental accessibility is then one of the areas where research and development is hugely involved nowadays, together with AT design, that should take into consideration the particular way of sensing and perceiving the reality of these persons, by transforming the AT experience "into a format that other senses can process, and this is called sensory substitution" [30]. The key element of sensory substitution is the acknowledgment that perception ultimately takes place in the brain: thus, "turning images into sounds or into something that can be touched has demonstrated a fascinating potential of the brain for taking such sensory input and processing it in a meta-modal framework".[73]

Sensory substitution devices are—together with the bionic eye or vision prosthesis[74]—at the forefront or applied research in the field, and at the same time they are already objects of our daily life; they can be organized in: vision-to-auditory sensory[75] and vision-to-tactile sensory[76] substitution devices.

3.5.2 *Impact of Visual Impairment on Participation to Play*[77]

A congenital VI may influence all the areas of the child's development; the degree to which this influence can manifest in subsequent functional impairments and real

[73] Numerous researches have been done in this field. Fielder and Proulx [251] refer in particular the following ones: Brown and Proulx [120, 121], Haigh et al. [311], Proulx et al. [566], Proulx et al. [567], Bach-y-Rita et al. [29], Chebat et al. [173], Chebat et al. [174]).

[74] They are "implantable devices that use electrical currents to stimulate the residual healthy components of a damaged visual pathway. The technology is analogous to cochlear implants [...]. However, as the eye is anatomically more complex than the ear, the technological challenges are significant in the quest to develop a high-resolution vision prosthesis. [...] Most electronic vision prostheses are based on a video camera that captures the visual scene, which is then converted to electrical signals via an external processing unit. The electrical signals are then transmitted to the implanted electrodes, which stimulate the residual visual pathway to provide artificial vision" [27]:390–391).

[75] They include "seeing with sounds", a prosthetic system in which "images from a glasses-mounted camera are converted into a "soundscape", with a consistent mapping between visual location and auditory information" [740]:404.

[76] They include glasses which provide visual augmentation to persons with some remaining sight, by converting the visual scene into a high-contrast representation [740].

[77] This paragraph is also inspired by Ray-Kaeser et al. [574].

developmental delays depends on many variables, mainly environmental, as this short review of studies intends to demonstrate. Motor skills are certainly delayed by the absence or severe impairment of vision: they develop late, and sometimes result in severe disability. Not only the gross-motor skills are involved—moving, walking, running—but also fine motor skills [266], which concern the contact with objects, their exploration, their finalized use. According to Tröster e Brambing [711], congenital blindness acts on motor development both directly—i.e., in establishing an optimal and functionally effective relationship with the environment, its spaces and contained objects—and indirectly: blind children are less naturally inclined[78] and less secure to move their own body around and more uncertain in exploration and they develop a delay in the mental representation of reality and space. This last aspect transforms, later, into the academic learning difficulties manifested in various disciplines based on spatial notions (geography, geometry, technical drawing, etc.). To underline its importance, Sleeuwenhoek et al. [649] proposed a conceptual model of representation of these children's disability that also includes motor capacity as a contributor to the generalized developmental delay of children with VI.

Hearing and vision are two primary senses whose development intertwines during the first year of life and become integrated around 9 months of age [515]. The evolutionary triangulation that relates the child to an object through the adult's mediation that is responsible for initiating the symbolic process, is highly regulated by senses: seeing—and touching—an object while simultaneously hearing a speaker pronounce the word representing the object (the semiotic "triangle of reference") is the basis for originating both verbal language [128, 744] and pretend play [470]. When a novel toy is shown to a visually impaired child, visual cues may not be sufficient to captivate the child's attention or to see and recognize useful details; furthermore, maintaining attention is guaranteed by socially driven interaction, and facilitated by eye-gaze monitoring, eye contact and facial expression recognition: all these activities might not be efficient enough during the interaction between the adult and these children. Tadic et al. [688] studied the attention skills of children who have visual profound and severe impairment from birth. The two groups scored significantly lower in attention tests (regulate their attention between people and objects, in terms of establishing, maintaining, and shifting attention) with respect to the sighted children, while the profoundly impaired showed significantly low performance than the other two groups in attention shifting (that were similar on this component). Furthermore, overall cognitive ability influenced too the shift attention performance of profoundly impaired, but it was not the sole cause of this deficit. These results are important for the concerns about joint attention in this population [84, 202, 576] and support the idea of devoted intervention, since the demonstrated developmental potential should be capitalized on using alternative non-visual techniques [202], albeit children with severe VI remain a vulnerable population.

[78] In the absence of the incentive represented by sight, and since there are no vicariant modalities for recognizing reality, "the child with visual impairment cannot venture towards an empty, mysterious, unknown reality, full of obstacles and dangers" [245]:124.

To guarantee these children become able to use the objects according to their own function, they must recognize and categorize them. Rickard et al. [584] proposed a wonderful experimental trial demonstrating how categorization may (and should) arise from the interaction with the adult (particularly, in this case, within the dyad mother-child). While sighted children may count on a "gestaltic" visual resource for categorising object, in the case of blind children this ability starts from a manual search of the representative and typical parts of an object (the beak for a bird, or the snout for a pig). The study demonstrates how through "a sequential complex interaction, the mother guides her daughter to an accurate perception of a criterial property (udders) to recognize a cow" (p. 9), by naming them, recognizing the cow by tact in a pile of toys, finding it by searching the distinctive udders, etc., through a careful scaffolding support precisely correlated to the child's behaviour; then, in a second phase the mother assures that the daughter establishes the categorical label "cow" to all the toys with udders, and this is made thanks to the use of a phonological "generalizing cue" (the sound "moo"). The authors conclude on the need that research in the field of blind children, instead of focusing on what they lack compared to their sighted peers, should concentrate on "how they make use of the resources to which they do have access in order to achieve interactional and communicative goals" and that, as a consequence, "a more comprehensive model of the development and acquisition of embodied cognition must necessarily include haptic and other sensorimotor pathways as partially contributory or singular alternatives to the visual modality" (p. 12; see also Struiksma et al. [676]).

Another critical developmental area for children with congenital VI has been reported in the delayed Theory of Mind; this would be very critical for their quality of life, because it might result in social skills difficulties, that in turn would impede the plain and full development of social and play activities with their peers. Nevertheless, this is disconfirmed by an experiment conducted by Pijnacker et al. [552], addressed "to explore whether children with a broader range of congenital VI have a delay in more advanced ToM understanding, in particular second-order ToM (i.e., awareness that other people have beliefs about beliefs) and non-literal language (e.g., irony or figure of speech)" (p. 2440). They found that performance of children—with and without VI—of similar age and verbal competence, on the second-order ToM and non-literal stories was alike. What changed in this experiment with respect to the previous ones, is that tasks submitted to children to the purpose of exploring the studied ability were presented in verbal mode and not based on visual materials: this fact radically changed the performance they were able to demonstrate.

Cognitive development in these children may incur in delays and deficits, especially in the case of CVI, when the central nervous system is involved. In the case of low vision, the experienced difficulties are related to the severity degree and the extent to which the substitute role of tactile, auditory and proprioceptive senses prove effective to overcome difficulties to the maximum level possible. On the contrary, the experience of the blind person has totally different characteristics and his/her representational construction of the world has peculiarities that distinguish it.

The grasp of the sound object occurs much later than in the sighted child [106], the blind child does not show defense reactions with respect to a moving object perceived through the air displacement, the notion of permanence of the object, which according to Piaget [547] starts representative intelligence, seems to be reached around 20–22 months [83] compared to 9 months of typically developing children.[79] Hatwell [326] found a delay in infralogical notions, such as the conservation of weight, quantity and substance; in inherent tasks, blind children show greater rigidity and resistance to adapt to changes, probably failing to visually "imagine" such changes as quickly as a sighted child [221]. Their prevailing difficulties however reside in the spatial representations, since the blind person tends to anchor the spatial and orientation localizations on his/her own body. As said, this may result in consequences at academic level.

Assessment of play

Although a research has been done on the most common databases in the fields of education and rehabilitation, no specific tool to support the assessment of the play of children with VI has been found. The use of the play assessment tools already mentioned in this text can be done, within certain limits; however, adaptations of both materials and questions as well as work settings need to be developed. No data were found on existing standardization of these forms of adaptation.

3.5.3 Factors Affecting and Favouring the Play Activity

Literature on the child with VI is not very rich for what concerns play, particularly early play. On the contrary, research suggests that the problems experimented by the blind children manifest above all as delays in skill and competence acquisitions, while their development is highly receptive to the stimuli coming from the environment, that must be informed at the right appropriateness and accessibility, by focusing systematically on vicariant senses; on this background, the play of visually impaired children can be supported, improved, made more alive than it is today. "There is an urgent need for new assessment paradigms to evaluate their symbolic development. Larger cohort studies are required to provide a broader picture of their intervention needs" [123]: 583. Never, perhaps, as in the case of this type of impairment, the joy related to play depend on the features of the toys, together with the play activity created and the support of the social environment.

Types of play and their tools[80]

Practice play

Practice play is hugely influenced by the sight absence or impairment. Parents' and caregivers' support is essential for its development, since they are not attracted enough by the surrounding environment: thus, also practice play does not initiate

[79] Fraiberg identified it at an early age; nevertheless, she indicated that only starting from this developmental phase does the child also manifest walking behaviour. "As long as the child has not developed an objective, stable and permanent external space, he/she cannot move from only voluntarily because he/she has nowhere to go" (cited in [469]).

[80] Among the other sources, this paragraph is also inspired by Tzvetkova-Arsova and Zappaterra [720] and by Périno and Besio [542].

and evolve according to an autonomous drive, rather should be sustained within the relationship, first and mainly by imitation. This is one of the possible causes for significant play development delay; for instance, Fraiberg found [266] that imitative play is not performed by these children before 30–36 month; Tröster and Brambring [712] reported that sighted children engaged in more complex levels of play at an earlier age than the blind children; furthermore, these last preferred tactile-auditory games and toys and rarely engaged in symbolic games.

A study conducted by Brambring [110] that compared children with and without VI on skill development reported—among a huge amount of other data—the following delays between the two groups in some basic play activities: beating a drum with two drumsticks (37 months versus 11); building a tower with three toy blocks (29 months versus 15); finding two identical objects in a set of five (26 months versus 42).

Other studies underline that the blind child remains engaged for long in play activities that include exploration of own body, undifferentiated manipulation of an object, in a nonfunctional modality, without specific purposes [423, 527, 705]. Some of these activities may assume the form of repetitive and stereotyped solitary play. Similarly, Hughes et al. [355], found that when 40-month-old children with VI played alone at home, more than half their play was exploratory or sensorimotor—typical of sighted children of 12–14 months of age—and symbolic play accounted for a mere 4%. And since other studies found that blind children of 20–30 months of age can be engaged in symbolic play by parents [175], it can be concluded that without the adult's support, play regresses to earlier immature forms.

Tröster and Brambring's [712] study, which compared questionnaire responses of a cohort of parents of 48-month-olds with and without VI, discovered that VI children were more likely to engage in solitary play using noisemakers and less interested in complex construction toys than were their sighted counterparts. All this taken into consideration, the sensorial—tactile, hearing, olfactory, kinaesthetic—effects offered by the toys are of utmost importance.

Toys must be steady, easy to manipulate, with a consistent design, easily understandable by touch; they must be safely put inside the mouth to let the child discover dimensions, shape, and appreciate sensorial features and textures, without the sight control. They should also offer unusual sensorial effects—vibration, magnetic—so as to arouse curiosity and surprise. They must be activated through precise gestures and offer precise feedback: this will implement children's pleasure and give them eagerness to succeed. Musical toys are particularly attractive when they give immediate and direct feedback to their activation. Toys should also support the child in exercising mobility, such as "walk and roll" objects that may offer an aid for walking—a sort of precursor of the white cane—a way to explore the floor and also a source for fun, due to the sound they produce while rolling.

Symbolic play

Visually impaired children demonstrate a delay in their symbolic play—at the age of 25,9 months [591], prolonged to 30–36 months of age [266]. According to Fraiberg and Adelson [267] the delayed acquisition of the concept of self in visually impaired children might be associated to the delay in their symbolic play; this opinion is supported by Brambring [109] who described the difficulty of the VI child's process of separation-individuation as the cause of his/her late speech development. Thus, both pretend and symbolic play are reported in literature for their delayed onset in the case of VI children.

Lewis et al. [423], nevertheless, examined 18 VI children (21–86 months of age) by distinguishing functional use of objects from symbolic (substituting one for another, pretending properties that the object did not have, etc.) use of them. As a whole, the group showed lower functional play test scores than expected for the age, while "symbolic play test scores which were at the appropriate level for their chronological age [...]. In addition, the scores among the group of VI children did not differ that much" (p. 449). This fact brought to the conclusion that visual access to play materials may limit their ability despite the severity degree of the impairment.

An interesting phenomenon in symbolic play of children with VI is the 'play' with words and sentences: they enjoy nonsense words and rhymes and often they use speech at a more sophisticated level than their peers [592, 754]. This might be also related to the qualitative differences found in fantasy play between sighted children and children with VI [527]; for instance, Andersen et al. [16] showed that they use to repeat and reconstruct past conversations between themselves and others.

For what concerns the play tools and toys, Tröster and Brambring [711] raise important questions about the use of substitute objects; for children with VI, in fact, it might be challenging to acknowledge that a toy car represents a real car, since they adhere more to their real experiences, coded through sound, touch, and language, rather than vision (in other word, the cannot count on a "gestaltic" overall shape of a car). Further, "they noted that imitation of adult routines was seldom present in children with VI, which form an important basis for later development of symbolic play scripts" [123]; this may support the conclusion that the symbolic development in these children is different rather than delayed, with respect to the sighted children, requiring adaptation of traditional assessment and intervention approaches.

For these children could participate to more complex symbolic play scenarios, that require adopting specific roles, toys must have realistic shapes and must be easy to understand by touch, and they cannot be too big for their hands. Symbolic play should always be introduced by an adult who describes the main play scenario (for example, kitchen, seller, jungle animals, garage) to facilitate that the child adopts the right role. More animated symbolic scenarios require that the objects and the furniture do not change position, once arranged, so that children with VI have no problems moving around and do not take risks. Haptic pens exist able to give the child a clear tactile feedback of what he/she is drawing on the paper or on the touch screen [236]. Other kinds of drawings can also be made with special coloured strips that can be positioned on a black base [6].

Constructive play

The constructive play, which requires a child place small pieces in relation to each other (e.g., to build a tower with toy blocks or to complete a puzzle), might prove challenging, and thus discarded by the child, for some related difficulties: in bimanual coordination, in spatial concept management, in mental representation of a final product to be constructed as a whole.

It is useful to propose toys whose elements are not too light in terms of weight, because these children need reinforcement by the tactile perception and to verify that the final constructions stands up and in a steady way. The connections between the elements (bricks, chopsticks, tracks of the train toy, pearls of the necklace, etc.) should be easy to accomplish, for example, through magnetic or Velcro systems; auditory feedback when elements are correctly connected could be useful. The pieces of puzzles should be well-designed and easily recognizable by touch—better if they are textured or in relief—so that children are motivated to complete it[81]; puzzles that are included within borders are preferable as children can better orient their actions and understand by themselves if they have terminated.

Rule-based play and games

According to Brambring [109], symbolic play appears in the blind children mainly within role-play games: perhaps the rules make it easier for them to manage the symbolization aspects of a play scenario, since the participants' roles are stable, and the events are more predictable. Many rule-based games are based on the use of language, and this area is one of the major strengths of these children.

Children with visual impairments, as all the other children, usually like to play games with rules. Of course, in order to find great pleasure in playing and possibly win the game, boards, pawns, dice and others pieces of the game must be explored by touch, or adapted to this purpose. The best known and most popular board games are often also available in a tactile version, while adapted homemade rules games are produced by families.

In case of low vision, all the aspects related to the management of colour and the contrast should be carefully considered. Once these children have understood well and experienced the rules of the game, they can also appreciate the value of turn-taking, of decentralizing their thoughts from themselves, by sharing and subjecting to an indisputable rule and also to the chance.

Physical and social environments

All the studies on the play of the child with VI support that it can start proceed in its early stages only with the support of the adult. In their turn, adults described their infant as unresponsive because of the difficulty in establishing eye contact, as well as the lack of vocal and facial responsiveness [561]. Furthermore, blind children are at risk of becoming stuck at lower levels of play and failing to move to more age-appropriate levels. All these children may need intervention to facilitate play and enhance their overall development [646], while, more generally speaking, parents need help to adequately observe and facilitate their children's play behaviour [340].

---

[81] For educational purposes, the Lego Foundation has launched the Lego Braille Bricks project worldwide in 2020 to teach Braille to blind children in a playful way, accompanied by examples of didactic activities that can be carried out with them (in addition to playing as usual): an interesting play-like idea. https://www.legobraillebricks.com/.

Early intervention with a focus on parent-child interaction can help to promote a secure attachment relationship,[82] to support the understanding of specific aspects of the child's behaviour and to strengthen sensitive responses of parents, may benefit the development of children with disabilities [619].[83]

Parents and other caregivers should encourage children to explore objects, facilitate exploration when necessary and teach children about persons and objects in the outside world [340]. Play in kindergarten and schools must be expressly supported and organized to be accessible for all. As children with visual impairments cannot mentally represent the space around them beyond their own body, toys and board games must be proposed inside demarcated areas to be easy to catch, find, take up again after having been thrown or located in a specific position.

The perception of the premise and of the situation where the play takes place should be very clear to the blind child, as well as to his/her peers. Facilitation of both outdoor and indoor spaces is usually done, e.g., through small mobility routes, that will encourage independence. Indoor play areas can be symbolized with shelving and mats to show, guide, and shield the play areas. Shelves and play boxes should have tactile labels so that a blind child can find necessary toys or play equipment without assistance. There must be a limited number of toys and permanent places for them; they must not 'disappear' far from the players, irrespective to the type of play they belong or to the child's age; auditory feedbacks whenever possible should be used and added. Auditory signals in the room must be carefully controlled, since they create noise, confusion and disorientation. On the contrary, technological solutions based on auditory signals might prove useful.

For pretending play and role-play, toys must be arranged inside thematic areas and consistent ensembles. It is very useful to propose complementary objects on the same theme to support exchange between partners, develop the theme, and explore several roles, expressions, and behaviours.

"Outdoors there must be an edge or a special texture underfoot near swings and climbing frames; paving or small trails with known features could lead up to different apparatus and the sand pit. Things must also be orderly here with permanent places for play equipment and tactile labels so all children can find what they need and put it back in the correct place" [191]:151.

The child and his/her play companions

Children with VI tend to be lonely, lazy, love to chat and tell stories, they are not attracted to sharing games, in which they often feel in danger and scarcely at ease. They are often described as not very sociable, they are not much loved by their companions especially in the first phase of childhood.

---

[82] "Secure attachment" is the positive parent-child relationship, in which the child displays confidence when the parent is present, shows mild distress when the parent leaves, and quickly re-establishes contact when the parent returns. The construct has been developed by Bowlby and Ainsworth in the seventies.

[83] According to the study of van der Boek et al. [340], Video-feedback Intervention to promote Positive Parenting (VIPP) [377] exploration proved successful in this respect versus attachment behaviour.

Some studies report the risk of children with visual impairment having difficulties with social relationships [647, 725]. Caballo's work [147] supports this finding, and claims for the need to provide educational programs to improve those skills—particularly play, cooperation, emotion recognition—to contribute to the quality of social interaction among children. A study by Crocker and Orr [197] found that, although engaging in mostly solitary play and less involved than their sighted peers in the activities, they willingly became engaged when encouraged by an adult to join in; during play, they tend to remain close to the adult; sometimes [166], they are able to initiate, but then stop to respond to peers.

Khadka's results [394] seem to suggest that educational styles may influence these children's willingness to be involved into social groups, showing themselves as "restricted in some specific activities; [but in some cases these restrictions] were imposed by those supporting them rather than their own abilities" (p. 182). On the contrary, the very promising study of Ozadyn [516] proved the positive effects that teaching play skills to preschool children can have on their abilities to initiate and respond to social interactions with their typically developing peers, in mainstream classrooms. Play skills were taught to the target students using direct teaching methods through small group arrangements outside the classroom; the analysis conducted proved effectiveness of these new skills in increasing the involved children's abilities to initiate interactions with their peers as well as their response behaviours. Moreover, the new abilities were retained 2 and 3 weeks after the completion of the trial. Even more interesting, after the skill training phase, the children's interactions with their peers in classroom were more stable and richer and the overall social atmosphere was improved. "They were also seen using the entire play area of the classroom and being more courageous in moving around independently" (p. 1035).

Corneliussen works in the same inclusive perspective. Starting from the consideration that any child wants and likes to play and this cannot be different for children with VI, she reminds that social play, with peers, is the most complete and challenging form of play, able to guarantee learning and growth to the child.

During play in an inclusive context, "they exchange roles and the organization of play, provide input, arguments and reject the input of others [...] Being included in play with peers means that blind children must be able to tolerate that their suggestions being rejected, and to adjust or change them, so they can adapt and continue playing" [191]:145.

To obtain this conclusive result, many aspects of the environments should be carefully and appropriately managed,[84] while the role played by the adult becomes prominent. He/she must act as a support during play, as an expert to compensate for the child's impairment, as a mediator for the creation of an inclusive climate in the classroom, and as a co-player him/herself and a scaffolder of the play activity.[85]

[84] The author, generous with practical examples, cites, for instance, the appropriate creation of permanent play groups, so that children can get acquainted in playing together. These group may grow over time, while the one of the blind children might grow more slowly [191].

[85] This organization of the author's discourse, coming from different literature references and developed in different professional experiences, echoes the LUDI list of the adult's roles in play. See

3.6 Children with Hearing Impairments

3.6.1 Hearing Impairment, its Characteristics and Current Issues

"Deaf children are those with severe or profound hearing loss, which implies very little or no hearing. Hearing devices, such as cochlear implants, may help them to hear and learn speech. In learning to communicate, such children may benefit from visual reinforcement, such as signs, cued speech and lipreading. [...] "Hard of hearing" is used to describe people with hearing loss ranging from mild to severe. At times, sounds (such as speech) are heard but not clearly understood. Such people usually communicate through spoken language and may benefit from hearing amplification with hearing aids and cochlear implants" [768].[86] Hearing loss affects individuals across all cultures; it is the fourth cause of living with a disability worldwide, since its presence concerns 6–8% of the population, while the burden of disease is growing [119]. It is more prevailing—both in child and adult—in low-income and middle-income countries than in high-income nations.

The WHO establishes a hearing loss as more than 40 dB in the better hearing ear in adults and 30 dB in the better hearing ear in children[87]; nevertheless, there are discrepancies in the various countries on this classification. The different degrees of hearing loss are also defined by grade—mild, moderate, severe, and profound—that range from 26 to 80 dB; "an individual with mild hearing loss might have difficulty understanding soft speech whereas an individual with severe loss will not hear most conversational speech" [123]:576. Between 20 and 30% of affected children have profound hearing loss, and about 30% of deaf children have an additional disability—most commonly, cognitive impairment [405]:1438.

Causes of Hearing Impairment (HI) include in utero infections (e.g., rubella, cytomegalovirus, etc.); in utero damage by drugs, jaundice, or lack of oxygen; genetic conditions and syndromes. Meningitis can leave hearing impairments; middle ear infections can cause fluctuating hearing impairments that damage development [769].[88]

While at birth the inner components of the ears are complete, the brain is immature and develops over many years. The child learns to differentiate the various stimuli coming from the environment, including the auditory, particularly the sounds, that are progressively recognized as phonemes, the mother's voice, a musical instrument, or

---

also Sect. 2.9.3.This consonance at a distance appears reassuring on a scientific level and seems to indicate that this new interpretative line of research on play is consolidating, finding feedback and new confirmations.

[86] http://www.who.int/mediacentre/factsheets/fs300/en.

[87] http://www.who.int/pbd/deafness/hearing_impairment_grades/en/.

[88] A detailed analysis of HI causes is presented in Brown et al. [119].

noise. From these first experiences, made in strict interaction with the environment, the child acquires perceptual, sensorimotor, and cognitive abilities.

Auditory input and communication are essential for the normal development of language, cognition, and behaviour; due to their loss, deaf children can incur in delays in many important aspects of development, such as visual attention and behavioural control [571]. Spoken language development requires auditory input and interaction with the environment. Thus, profound hearing loss provokes the lack of development of spoken language, with its impact on daily communication; this, in turn, risks to restrict learning and literacy, as well as to substantially compromise educational achievement and later overall quality of life [405]. This of course is said by considering exclusively the impairment's impact, without taking into consideration the many changes implemented—at least in advanced countries—by education, rehabilitation, technology, and society in general, to improve the inclusive opportunities of these persons.

The goal of giving deaf persons the opportunity to communicate, and therefore to lead a complete and satisfying life, is an ancient dream of humanity, that has its patently educational origins in the fifteenth century. Over time, two rehabilitative approaches have alternated, intertwined, and disputed: one based on the verbal spoken language and one based on the sign language. Nowadays the debate is still alive, sometimes radical,[89] and the two lines of intervention coexist, without being able to merge into a scientifically valid composition, that might correspond to "bilingualism", or to the adoption of one of the existing "simultaneous methods"[90]: think for example of the "bimodal method" born in Italy [733–735]) and of the "total communication" in the UK.[91]

Sign languages, finally considered as complete languages, became all over the world subject of educational and research interest in the seventies. "After decades of dogmatic oralism, communication was at last taking place"; then, simultaneous methods multiplicated, but none of them "seemed to be delivering the promised benefits in terms of academic attainment" [34].

A radical alternative proposal is "to abandon the attempt to reconcile two divergent languages in a hybrid form and work towards a bilingual approach, where sign language and English each has a role but they are separated" (ivi:79), and the balance of languages varies according to the individual need. "When these children have been given opportunities to become bilingual with a signed and a written or spoken

[89] Pressure groups and associations of deaf persons are determined to defend their language, which is strongly connected to their whole history of claiming a specific, unique culture, world, identity, for which they demand respect and social and political recognition.

[90] These methods proposed sophisticated and clever modalities for putting together sign and spoken languages to reach exhaustiveness and precision in discourse and conversation, attempts to optimize the combination of sign and speech [569]. The bimodal method, in particular, was also created as a more effective method to learn spoken language and includes special solutions for supporting academic learning.

[91] The term, mediated from the sociologist Margaret Mead, was first intended as "the full spectrum of language modes, child-devised gestures, the language of signs, speech, speech reading, finger spelling, reading and writing" (Denton, 1976, cit. in [34]:77).

language, it has enabled them to attend higher education, to have a qualified job and thereby a good life in the future" [560]:S39. "The philosophy underpinning sign bilingualism is based on a linguistic and cultural minority model of deafness and a social model of disability" [550]:89; nowadays more research is needed about ongoing developments.

After the recent technological advances that led to the development of Cochlear Implants (CI), and their increasing application especially in children, the oralist approach seems to prevail, while the debate between approaches has attenuated, despite critical aspects persist in supporting the language development of these children.[92]

Current trends in intervention

Congenital deafness changes the functional properties of the auditory system and affects both cortical development and mutual interaction of the cortical areas. Stimulation of the auditory system must happen during the sensitive periods in life to assure its normal development.

In addition, simultaneous auditory, visual, somatosensory responses are generated in real-world events; "deafness affects the functional coupling among the sensory systems: multimodal interactions do not develop, and other sensory systems completely or partially overtake some auditory cortical regions. [...] Information becomes to be represented in reference to other modalities, a process that has adverse cognitive effects.

Thus, deaf children have difficulty scanning and retrieving phonologic and lexical information in their working memory; they also differ from their peers with normal hearing in their ability to sustain visual attention and in visual sequence learning" [405]:1442.

Growing evidence suggests that sensory deprivation is associated with dramatic crossmodal neuroplastic changes in the brain; the areas normally associated with the sense that is lost (sight, hearing) are recruited by the brain to support the areas connected to the sensory modalities that are spared. The normal functioning, the consequences of sensory loss, or the possibility of resorting sensory functions through rehabilitation, might be understood only by incorporating the concept of brain plasticity. Nevertheless, neuroplasticity clearly affects an individual's rehabilitative outcome and novel strategies are needed to leverage cross-modal interactions in a manner that promotes functional adaptation in parallel to rehabilitative and restorative approaches: it is crucial to consider each individual's specific needs and goals within the context of his or her plastic brain interacting within a multisensory world [475].

[92] According to Bergeron et al., "contemporary speech and language interventions are not limited to disabilities but embrace the pragmatics of communication behaviours from the perspective of functional social participation. Accordingly, current speech and language therapies for deaf and hard-of-hearing children include a broad spectrum of approaches and techniques [and include notions and competence about] using hearing devices, evidence of their efficacy and how they are implemented in diverse clinical practices" [62]:378. An interesting systematic review about the use of sign and spoken language today by children with HI users of auditory aids is contained in Fitzpatrick et al. [254].

Cochlear implants have shown very promising in restoring auditory information to deaf children and concomitant improvements in speech recognition and production. Specific sensitive periods have been identified for implantation, which is now recommended in the first 1–2 years of life [405]. Sound localization is improved by 18, 5%, and an "average 20% improvement in the ability to hear speech against background noise" is reported.

The outcomes concerning the acquisition of spoken language are varied and still under evaluation; they depend on many elements: the type of communication input used before implantation, the effect of auditory deprivation, age of implantation, the child's cognitive level, the exposition to high-quality spoken language and a good quality support by parents and caregivers. "Measures of speech production after cochlear implantation confirm continuing improvements in the years after the procedure. Ten years after implantation, about 77% of children had speech that was intelligible to a listener. [...] However, many children continue to have difficulties with the more complex language constructs, such as syntax, semantics, and pragmatics" [405]:1446–1447.

Additional disabilities can worsen expectations for improvement. Quittner et al. [571], thanks to a wide multilevel trial, present their assumption that access to auditory information is likely to have profound positive effects on children's cognitive, behavioural, and social development. More recently, Strophal et al., after discussion about the wide variety of outcomes obtained by CI in post-lingually deaf, sustain that an important role is played by intra-modal and cross-modal reorganization; in fact, although cross-modal activation in auditory cortex is considered as maladaptive for speech recovery in CI, "a similar activation relates positively to lip reading skills and cross-modal activation of the visual cortex seems to be adaptive for speech recognition. [Thus,] an involvement of further brain areas" within rehabilitation methods might prove effective. Furthermore, "prospective longitudinal designs are needed to track the dynamics of cortical plasticity that takes place before and after implantation" [675]:128.

Through their extensive analysis of the current situation on contemporary speech and oral language care for deaf and hard-of-hearing children using hearing devices, Bergeron et al. [62] first of all recognize the tremendous change introduced by the CI in the care service area: there is a before and an after-CI era. Also, greater scientific certainty and more adequate technologies have significantly improved early diagnosis.

Parents look at CI not only as a mean to access normal language but also as a technical aid to guarantee a normal life. In addition, contemporary technology gives a great contribution to these persons' daily life (captioning of videos in sign or written language, virtual signers, communication software, apps and digital solutions for supporting independence), including AAC electronic devices[93] used in some cases. Nonetheless, "whatever future technological developments may bring, it is important to keep in mind that a CI does not restore normal hearing" [287]:18.

---

[93] See also note at Sect. 3.2.2.

Speech and language therapy has substantially changed in the last decade, to be up to date with the latest developments as well as with the most appropriate psycholinguistic and neurolinguistic theories. However, they "should never lose sight of the fact that the social participation of deaf and hard-of-hearing children is the targeted outcome and that communication is a key factor of this outcome, and communication is grounded on language development. Thus, regardless of the therapeutic approach, oral and/or signed based, language deprivation needs to be limited if not avoided" [62]:390.

3.6.2 *Impact of Hearing Impairment on Participation to Play*

Auditory, language and communication delays and difficulties are a not secondary obstacle in these children's life; as it is natural to expect, the related impairments during development cause and accompany the onset of further difficulties, both in the cognitive and social area. Generally speaking, deaf children have an incomplete and unsatisfactory access to a rich linguistic environment; the process of learning new words is slower, more unstable and more difficult than in the case of hearing children. The whole field literature reports delay in their vocabulary development, and in the use of the vocabulary they have [570].

The lexical and grammatical richness, the phonetic intelligibility as well as the conceptual complexity of their language is always lower, at every age, than those of their peers (and is in any case always lower than their own non-verbal cognitive abilities); this disparity can create significant difficulties with peers and other interlocutors, in sharing and regulating activities, in the implementation and explanation of one's own plans, in conversation and narration. Without adequate support and appropriate mediation, this can create a barrier to a fruitful contact with peers, especially in group contexts.

In case these children can use sign language—which, it must be remembered, is much more consonant with their cognitive skills, at every age—it must be ensured that the interlocutors are able to understand this mode of communication, and possibly respond in the same way.

The impaired auditory system may impact on these children's performances in many other areas. For instance, joint attention starts normally, but at the time in which language assumes its intermediating function between the mother and the object, they find it difficult to engage in "symbol-infused joint attention" [571]:549. Prezbindowski et al. [563] found that deaf toddlers of 20–24 months of age spent more time in coordinated joint attention than their hearing peers but virtually no time in symbol-infused joint attention compared with them.

Quittner et al. [570] verified attentional control problems at older ages, that they interpreted as related to the integration of multimodal sensory information, since sound is involved in regulating visual attention; in fact, 6–13-year-old deaf children performed worse than hearing children in attention tasks, but those with CI. Visual selective attention has been found impaired [571] and this may have an impact on academic learning. Moreover, a possible consequence of auditory impairment is that "short-term memory shows important processing delays in scanning and retrieving verbal information, and the working memory is characterized by a reduced rate of encoding phonologic and written information. Even on nonauditory tasks, such as sustained attention and visual-sequence learning, deaf children underperform as compared with their peers with normal hearing" [405]:1446.

Theory of Mind may also be compromised. A study involving 70 children 3–12-year-old with hearing impairments of different degrees of severity [7] refers that the severity of the hearing loss was negatively correlated with receptive language and ToM. These findings were confirmed by Peterson and Siegel [543], according to whose study deaf children, with hearing parents not fluent in sign language, often display a delayed development of ToM compared to typically developing hearing children; nevertheless Sundqvist et al. [679] found that—although the two groups of children did not differ on language and cognitive abilities at baseline—children with early cochlear implants solved ToM problems better than children with late implants.

It is worth pointing out, however, the significant outcome concerning the differences between deaf children with hearing parents and deaf children with deaf signing parents: the study conducted by Schick et al. [615], involving 176 children (from 4 to 8-year-old), in fact, confirms that the last group performed identically to same-aged hearing controls.

Assessment of play

The only play assessment tool that was found, specifically concerning the play of children with HI, is the *Play Assessment Questionnaire* (PAQ), proposed first by Yoshinaga-Itano in 1994 [774]. The PAQ is an adaptation of the observational tool named *Play Assessment Scale* (PAS; [250]), that consists of 45 developmentally sequenced items designed to elicit various play skills that typically appear before the third year of age [392]. Within PAQ, items appear in the form of a questionnaire and the respondents are parents and other non-professional caregivers. After validation with 170 deaf or hard of hearing infants and toddlers, the authors state that "the PAQ was found to be a useful nonverbal tool that assesses symbolic play behaviours and demonstrates a parallel development with specific language skill development of young children" [776]. The PAQ has been then used: to study language development in early versus later identified children with HI [775]; to evaluate language and play in students with multiple disabilities, visual impairment and deaf-blindness [554]; to carry out three case studies with young children who had both HI and ASD [390].

As it is clear, although the PAQ analyses also play, it is mainly used as a play-based assessment tool for study language development. Tools and scales clearly addressed to study the quality and the types of play of children with HI are not available, as far as it is possible to deduce from search in the databases of the field. In any case—whether play is assessed for itself or as a useful context—in order to give the child with HI the opportunity to show completely his/her skills, attention should be paid to the preparation of adequate settings, the availability of accessible materials, and the creation of dedicated test administration methods. There are many variables that must be considered, and that may interfere with the child's performance; just to give some examples: the communication methods adopted—spoken language or sign language—, the differences induced by the type of hearing technology worn, the quality of their attention capacity, etc.

Applying these considerations to the field of cognitive assessment of different populations of children with special needs, Schum's [621] study provides peculiar and insightful recommendations for adopting appropriate methods. Assessing the cognitive performance of children with HI is important, because a reliable prognosis is able to guarantee a more successful plan of intervention. But using standardized instruments to assess children with HI might be risky, since they are often hugely language dependent, thus possibly introduce a bias in the evaluation process; moreover, simply translating verbal tests and directions into sign language is risky, because sign language is iconic, and the posed question can result less complex.

Moreover, when non-standardized methods of estimating a child's abilities are used, they can be over or underestimated. The author proposes a team approach, where different professionals take charge of the assessment of different skills separately; tools that are not based mainly of language and that explore various mental functions—such as memory, processing skills, etc.—can be adopted. These reflections may suggest similar considerations regarding the play assessment of special populations, a research field yet to be developed.

3.6.3 Factors Affecting and Favouring the Play Activity[94]

Similarities and differences have been ascertained between the play behaviour of children with and without HI, and they were mainly associated with expressive language [344, 616, 661].

As universally recognized in the field literature, both play and the overall communicative functions are not compromised in the children who are exposed to sign language or in situations of bilingualism [304]. For instance, in 1990, Spencer et al. showed that deaf children with deaf parents, who use sign language as their first language to communicate, spent equivalent amount of time in pretend play and produced the same amount and level of pretend play as their peers without HI [660].

Furthermore, the assessment of the play difficulties of children with HI can in some cases be influenced by the quality of the language skills they are able to show. Working with videotaped play sessions and adjusting the audio volume, Short et al. [635] demonstrated that when the language was not audible, children with language difficulties were perceived to play better than when the language was audible. This did not happen in the case of children with ASD, whose play was interpreted as poor in both cases.

Types of play and their tools

Practice play

Spencer and Waxman [658] did not find any difference in engagement states in play between deaf and hearing children aged 9 to 18 months. There is a lack of specific

[94] This paragraph is also inspired by Andreeva et al. [17], and Périno and Besio [542].

research related to this particular type of play in children with HI. As for all children, also in the case of HI the interest towards toys for practice play comes from perceiving the effects of their actions: exploring, understanding cause-and-effect, discovering surprising effects. By using these tools, they also enjoy a sense of mastery, pleasure for internal control and social connection.

The need to recur to alternative sensorial channels suggests to propose toys with visual or tactile stimuli and/or effects. It is preferable that the feedback offered by the toy is immediate.

Symbolic play

According to Cejas et al. [165], young deaf children with hearing parents, compared to their hearing peers, have deficits in joint engagement, and spend more time in unengaged states. Due to their direct interrelation with language development, pretend and symbolic play have been widely and deeply studied in the area of HI. In what follows a short review of them is presented.

Some studies on pretend play did not report significant differences comparing typically developing children and children with HI. In another study, with a sample of mother-child dyads with and without hearing impairment, Spencer [659] found that children's play levels were not associated with the hearing status rather with the language competence. This was confirmed by Spencer and Deyo [657], who studied three groups: children with HI with their hearing parents, deaf children with deaf parents, and hearing children with hearing parents. Categorizing them by hearing status, no significant differences were found for time spent in sequenced, ordered sequenced, or substitute play, and pretend play overall. Frequency and length of play sequences were also not different. When categorized according to language level, however, differences emerged for time spent in ordered sequences, in substitute play, and for play diversity. These results suggest that language delay is associated with delayed pretend play, not HI. On a larger sample of children, Spencer [662] found that toddlers with HI spent more time in pretend play than hearing children and this might be due to the major time required by children with HI. Nevertheless, once she grouped children according to their language levels, she found that those with higher language levels produced more abstract behaviours and longer sequences while low language levels were associated with shorter and fewer ordered sequences.

The outcomes of Bornstein et al. [104] contradict the previous ones; in fact, the researchers found they did not find significant differences in amount of pretend play, highest level of pretend play, or number of object transformations, despite the hearing status of the children's parents. Thus, they did not find any association between pretend play and language except in the two groups of dyads in which the hearing status of child and mother were mismatched. Other studies (e.g., Brown et al. [124]) concerning children of various ages proved the otherwise, i.e., children with hearing loss engage in pretend play less often than hearing children, and their pretend play is delayed and less abstract. In 2001 another research group [126] carried out a complete experiment by classifying more in-depth the children's play behaviours in the various increasing levels of pretend play (decontextualization, decentration, sequencing, planning; the first three with 4 stages each and the fourth with 3 stages) in relation to their age. While pretend play scores of the hearing children were age-appropriate, the scores for the deaf children were overall lower, but the descriptions of the characteristics of pretend play in deaf children are even more interesting. As to the level of decontextualization, they used real objects as such, and they substituted objects more than their peers; they never invented new objects.

As to decentration, deaf children always produced actions on another recipient, and never through another identity. Sequencing was very poor in deaf children: almost all their actions were isolated, while those of their peers were classified as sequenced.[95] Finally, for what concerns planning, less of 30% of the actions of deaf children resulted as planned.

These children's difficulties in pretend play were then correlated with specific language delays; what is more interesting here, is that their modalities of pretending do not seem to be ready for higher and more complex levels of symbolic play, appear repetitive, are weak in fantasy, imagination and planning: all these characteristics are bad predictors of a balanced and coherent play development towards further types.

Another experimental study in symbolic play worth mentioning is presented by Quittner et al. [571], whose goal was to demonstrate that increase in auditory input via a CI would have led to improvements in various developmental areas. They proposed to the involved children two sets of toys different according to their age, and request to the dyads parent-child to play as at home, to be able to measure parent sensitivity and joint attention. The adopted methodology for what concerns play is here particularly interesting, since the researchers adopted both a method to select toys for symbolic play according to a procedure used by Hill and McCune-Nicolich [345] and then a classification of symbolic play, adapted from Belsky and Most [57], that is organized in 14 levels. In what follows, the authors' conclusion: "The deaf children's play levels ranged from simple manipulation of objects to a basic level of symbolic play involving the use of a meaningless object (e.g., wooden block) in a creative way (e.g., as a bed). In contrast, hearing children's play was concentrated in the 4 highest levels of symbolic play. The hearing children developed sequences of play with and without stories and were able to transform two meaningless objects into imaginative play [...] These results confirm our hypothesis that deaf children show cognitive deficits in their use of representational or symbolic play" [571]:551.

Constructive play

Apart from pretend and symbolic play, that gave rise to a substantial number of studies, mainly related to the related development of language, the other types of play are not significantly present in literature in the case of children with HI. This general lack of specific interest testifies also that constructive play of children with

---

[95] This is confirmed by a study of Gregory and Mogford [302], who, while demonstrating the ability to use the objects symbolically in six deaf children aged 1–3, found also that they did not enact imaginary play, nor sequences of similar length and complexity of their peers, without HI. The study is reported in Slade et al. [648].

HI does not require particular shrewdness. It demands concentration on an activity over time, while these children usually do not like to stand and prefer to move around. Choosing more attractive toys might be helpful, in this case, as well as supporting them to become concentrated and committed on the task. Quittner et al. [571] used different set of puzzles to study the parental sensitivity (facilitating problem-solving) at different child's ages, finding a correlation between more supportive mothers and children who were able to generate more solutions to the problem.

Rule-based play and games

Attention and concentration restriction can not only influence the quality of this type of play in the case of children with HI but also their willingness to participate. Due to their impairments in understanding language and in speaking fluently, they might find it difficult to enjoy games in which communication abilities are a substantial aspect of play, for example when discussions and debates are crucial, or where mediation is needed about rules or the ludic process.

As in the case of other types of play, these reflections may change if the child uses the sign language and can share this opportunity with other players (for example, when the sign language has been taught also to other children or if an interpreter is available). The cognitive challenge implied by the game might in some cases prevent sharing the game with peers unless appropriate adaptation and facilitation strategies are adopted. It is worth noting that the world of games and videogames is widely used to create playful environments, in order to propose to the child, in a fun and joyful way, activities that have didactic, learning, or rehabilitation purposes.

Physical and social environments

Deafness and HI are not problems per se, rather because they might provoke a severe failure of appropriate early communicative interactions between adults and the deaf child. A really fruitful relationship requires sharing of languages and communicative codes, as well as abilities to interpret and anticipate the needs, and to support growth in all the developmental areas. As known, play is not unrelated to this important exchange: it is contemporarily the drive and the outcome of it.

Evidence is available in research describing the interactions of mothers and children with HI during early play. Lyon [451] found that HI children with higher levels of pretend play were associated with mothers generous with suggestions and prompts, and not only using modelling strategies. In a subsequent study, Spencer and Meadow-Orlans [662] found that maternal responsiveness has significant influences also with older children. This suggestion is verified also as a negative feedback: Blum et al. [91] found that children with low quality of pretend play were associated with high level of maternal control. Interaction within the dyad mother-children with HI may show also difficulties in maintaining joint reference [214] with shorter, less complex play episodes. A study of Pratt [559] indicates that mothers of children with HI observed their child less and less elaborated on their own behaviours, while they were more directive, suggesting they regarded play interactions as instructional opportunities. According to Hartup [325] such directive style of interaction may create less secure attachment, and a sort of a dependence of these children on adults in early childhood settings.

Brown and Remine [125] underline that mothers of children with HI usually reduce the levels of abstract commentary during symbolic play; in some cases, their behaviour is so addressed to scaffold the child's initiative, that the interaction may result less playful and creative.

For all these reasons, it should be recommended that, in carrying out play situations and activities, the roles of adults, their place, and the distance from children are very carefully considered to facilitate the players' autonomy. For example, to sit face to face is required to show toys, invite to play as suitable partners, and promote visual or physical interactions. Above all, within a group of children, adults must not forget to ascertain that all verbal messages are understood by children with hearing impairments. However, when a play sequence between children is starting, adults should not interfere, leaving that communication between them develop as it is possible—through gestures, signs, or verbal cues—so that they can play freely.

Within the environment where the play activity occurs, toys are always in view, and they are grouped according to the type of play they favour. The areas devoted to pretend and symbolic play are the most important and critical ones, so the more well-ordered they are, the easier it is for the child to organize his/her play activity. This, in fact: (a) facilitates imitation between children and adult; (b) facilitates adults in handing toys, as well as gestural and verbal communication; (c) allows children with HI to observe the other players, to encourage social interactions and joyfulness; (d) allows sharing of complementary roles within the same scenario and the development of that scenario.

The child and his/her play companions

The peer play of children with HI has been more extensively studied, focusing on the amount, duration, and type of play, as well as on peer interactions. Nevertheless, these studies are strongly addressed to increase knowledge about language and skill development of these children and recovery of their impairments.

At the beginning, when the issues related to social participation and inclusive contexts were considered secondary to the achievement of rehabilitation results, research was strictly related to observe the social development of the single child. Thus, the preference of children with HI for solitary play, mainly in constructive activities, instead of that in pretend or dramatic play [237, 344] has been often underlined. Darbyshire [208] found that children with HI tended not to play with hearing peers.

Recently, more studies on groups of players and inclusive contexts have been produced, even if attention to the creation of inclusive play situation is still poor and occasional: the prevailing accent of research is still concentrated on recovery and psycho-physical outcomes. Brown et al. [122] discovered that both children with and without HI used language while pretending, and also that they talked about plans and the meaning of objects, although with different degrees of frequency, precision, and complexity in language.

Children with HI were found to produce fewer initiations and comments than their hearing peers in one-to-one play, although they took verbal and play turns [93]. In free play, there is evidence that preschoolers with and without HI are more likely to select play partners with the same hearing status as themselves [581] and that this affects subsequent levels of play [421]. But, very interestingly, when children with HI play together, they tend to choose constructive play, while they shift to dramatic play when playing with hearing peers. Pre-schoolers with HI are not willing to enter a peer play, and at the same time hearing children are not likely to initiate to children with HI and they tend to ignore initiations from them [215, 587].

The entry behaviours of children with CI seem to be more successful in one-to-one interactions, while the duration of the CI may be connected to improved social competence [462].

Wauters and Knoors [743] found that two groups of children with and without HI were similar with respect to peer acceptance and friendship, while they differed in social competence: this is another inspiring outcome from research, because—unlike the other two components which are more related to the individual's personal traits—it is possible to create social situations where this competence is expressly taught.

In summary, relationships with peers seem to be highly influenced by the language delays of children with HI and by their strong reliance on visual awareness of peers rather than the use of their hearing [123]. Anyway, although the research unambiguously and clearly indicates that the knowledge and early use of sign language favours a more coherent and consonant development of the deaf child, closer to that of their peers, on a linguistic, communicative, social, and even cognitive levels, a radical direction change at scientific and educational level is still to be implemented. In the cited studies there is no trace of play activities that include alternative modes of communication, which for example introduce the sign language as a communication code for all, thus favouring the creation of contexts able to welcome differences and considering this opportunity as an element of progress to all.

This is probably due—as in other cases that have been considered in this chapter—to the predominantly technical (if not medical) approach adopted to address the topic of disability. However, changes, novelties, and real achievements will only occur when the child, each child, will be observed within the contexts in which he/she lives, grows (and plays), and when the researcher, and the educator, despite being experts in disabilities, will first of all look at those contexts, to understand where, how, and why, they must change, to guarantee that child all the space he/she needs to become a competent, possibly happy, adult.

Part II
Playing Robots

This part introduces the technological aspects related to robots that could be used to play. Robots are devices that are physically interfaced with the real world through sensors and actuators, and may have some degree of autonomy. The physical and technological issues related to the development of robots able to play, the playing activities that could be implemented with these robots, and how they could be designed to cope with the need of generating inclusive playing experiences that exploit their possibilities are presented. All these aspects are organized in a framework that could be used to analyze and design such experiences.

Chapter 4
Playful Robots

Andrea Bonarini

Abstract What is a robot, how can it be designed considering sensor and actuator possibilities, materials, shape, and control? How can it operate in the unstructured world that it should face when interacting with people? The definitions of robot given by international agencies (ISO, IEEE) open a wide spectrum of possibilities for the implementation of robotic devices, that go beyond the classical mental images that we may have of robots, and get closer to what entertainment producers are proposing in the last seventy years, since electronics has reached the reliability and costs compatible with this mass market. What is important to consider in the design of a robot able to play with people with different abilities in an inclusive way? We discuss different aspects of the development of playing robots, from the ones related to physical aspects, such as shape, external appearance, dimension, material, to the ones enabling functionalities, such as sensors and actuators, and to the ones related to data elaboration and behaviour definition, including adaptation to the human player, a relevant aspect when interacting with people that may exhibit a wide range of possibly unexpected reactions. The final aim for a playing robot is to produce a feeling of animacy, which makes the robot a companion to play with. The goal of this chapter is to provide an insight about the set of tools that could be used to implement playful robots.

4.1 Definitions

Since few years major normative institutes such as the International Standards Organization (ISO) and the Institute of Electrical and Electronics Engineers (IEEE) decided to formalize a definition of the term "robot", to try to put order among the different meanings that different sources, including major dictionaries, attribute to the term. This is also needed to set up norms that cover and rule the use of robots not only in the controlled environment of production plants, where normative has already been defined, but in the free environment of everyday activities, play included.

According to ISO [363], the term "robot" denotes "a drive mechanism programmed in two or more axes, having a certain degree of autonomy, moving inside its operating environment and performing tasks for its intended purpose". The IEEE

A. Bonarini and S. Besio, *Robot Play for All*, Research for Development,
https://doi.org/10.1007/978-3-031-05042-8_4

definition [362] is not far: a robot is "an agentive device in a broad sense, purposed to act in the physical world in order to accomplish one or more tasks". These definitions share the main aspects of the robot: it is a physical device, able to move, with some autonomy and the ability to aim at fulfilling a task, i.e., trying to achieve a goal. These are the kind of devices we are considering in this book.

The IEEE ontology [362] also includes some specifications, which are useful to point out some features of robots that enable possibilities for their application in play activities. They are reported and commented here below.

- *automated robot*: "A role for a robot performing a given task in which the robot acts as an automaton, not adapting to changes in the environment and/or following scripted plans". This is a robot that is programmed to perform always the same activities, like an industrial robot. This could be used, for instance, to tell stories, or act following a script, but it is not intended to interact. Actually, it is not able to participate actively in playing activities, but it could be used as a mobile toy.
- *semi-autonomous robot*: "A role for a robot performing a given task in which the robot and a human operator plan and conduct the task, requiring various levels of human interaction". In this case, a person may play with the robot a collaborative game, each partner achieving partial goals, communicated, or perceived by the other.
- *fully autonomous robot*: "A role for a robot performing a given task in which the robot solves the task without human intervention while adapting to operational and environmental conditions". In this case, the robot can be a full companion of the player, able to follow rules, propose activities, actively pursuing personal goals.
- *tele-operated robot*: "A role for a robot performing a given task in which a human operator, using sensory feedback, either directly controls the actuators or assigns incremental goals on a continuous basis, from a location off the robot. A tele-operated robot will complete its last command after the operator stops sending commands, even if that command is complex or time-consuming". This kind of robot can be used as an avatar of a player to provide special abilities and functionalities, and to enable the development of abilities such as attention, movement control, strategy, and many others. The fact that the robot can be assigned an activity to perform may relieve the player from the full real-time control of the activity but can also be exploited in the play activity to drive the attention of the player to the way the robot is performing the action.
- *remote-controlled robot*: "A role for a robot performing a given task in which the human operator controls the robot on a continuous basis, from a location off the robot, via only her/his direct observation. In this mode, the robot takes no initiative and relies on continuous or nearly continuous input from the human operator". In this case, the robot is a manually controlled device, and becomes a tool enabling specific play modalities, to play with, like any other toy. Actually, this is one of the most appreciated kind of toys for some ages, since it provides the power of fully control on a device that is acting in the physical world. Also, this type of robot can become a sort of avatar. The need for continuous control from one side encourages

identification, on the other side, may require abilities of perception through the signals that the robot sends (or from the playground if the robot is in sight), and of actuation since the player should be able to control all the degrees of freedom of the robot.

We would like also to consider, and extend, the definitions given by Dautenhahn et al. [209], in order to provide a clearer framework to define robots that play. These robots are embodied in the sense of their definition of "embodiement": "A system S is embodied in an environment E if perturbatory channels exist between the two. That is, S is embodied in E if for every time t at which both S and E exist, some subset of E's possible states with respect to S have the capacity to perturb S's state, and some subset of S's possible states with respect to E have the capacity to perturb E's state". This definition puts in evidence the fact that the presence of a physical body is not enough, but the robot should be able to modify the state of the environment in which it operates, and be influenced by it. We consider in this book only robots that satisfy the definitions given above, which were defined after the mentioned paper, so excluding systems that do not have a physical body that can physically move. Notice that the definition in [209] calls also for the need to have open channels between the robot and the player for all the signals needed for the play activity, since we may consider that the player is part of the environment where the robot operates.

In principle, it is possible to define a function like:

$$DOM\{S, E\} = f(x, y, t)$$

that "expresses the degree of embodiment (DOM) of a system S with respect to an environment E as a function f of the vectors x and y, and time t. Vectors x and y are vectors of variables measuring the perturbation of S by E, and the perturbation of E by S, respectively" [209].

The critical issue for playing robots, and for social robots in general, is the definition of x and y. We may assume that they include a subset of the state variables of the robot (S) and of the environment (E), which, in turn, include the playground (P) (the limited space where we play) and the human player(s) (H). The state spaces which we are interested in are those that can be modified by the interaction channels open in the robot and the player(s), typically vision, hearing, and touch. We will analyze the possibilities to exploit these channels, but the relevant aspects are those that affect what is perceived as the "state space" of the play activity. We may envision at least two levels of state variables: the ones directly related to sensors and actuators (*basic variables*), and the ones (*cognitive variables*) that are related to play, or, in general, to the performance of the activity, which have to do with cognitive interpretations of the basic variables. Several issues may arise in this "signal to symbol" transfer, related to the abilities of the players (both human and robot) to perform it within the time needed to play, to their sensor and actuator possibilities, to the openness of the channels, and possibly other issues.

In the rest of this chapter, we will first explore the possibilities to implement the physical body, then the way we may activate the interaction channels and obtain the basic variables' values. We will see in the next chapters, how these features can be exploited to devise play activities with known characteristics, and how it is possible to cope with the just mentioned potential issues.

4.2 Body

A physical body enables interaction through the channels people normally use to live in the real world. It offers at the same time the possibility to act on the environment (so also on the human player), to influence it and be influenced by it establishing an interaction. The type of interaction strongly depends on all the features of the body, introduced in this section.

If we plan to have a robot that should e perceived as "intelligent", as possessing some "animacy", we may take also the statement by Dautenhahn et al. [209] to further support the need for a proper design of all the body features: "Intelligence cannot merely exist in the form of an abstract algorithm but requires a physical instantiation, a body".

4.2.1 Shape

The shape of a playing robot is important for its acceptance, the expectations it may raise [318, 546], and affordance [286], so the way in which it could be perceived to be used. The external appearance is related to the contest of the playful activity, and coherence should be granted.

A general consideration should be done about the so-called "Uncanny valley effect", proposed by Masahiro Mori in 1970 [489], according to which the affinity a person can feel with a robot increases with its similarity to the human shape, but drops suddenly when this similarity is high, but not enough to match humans well. This drop is even stronger when the robot is moving. This may have an even more negative effect on some subjects, especially those affected by neuro-developmental disorders, who may feel uncomfortable with people. Mori's considerations concerned the human appearance but could be extended to any bio-inspired appearance: a robot appearing like a fake animal may be less well accepted than a robot that may just suggest an animal shape, but is clearly different from the real one.

Many aspects could be put in evidence to classify robot embodiments (e.g., [47, 495]). We introduce here below a shape categorization functional to the role a robot may have in playful activities.

- *Human-like*: a robot with humanoid body, i.e. head, arms, and legs, can trigger different emotional responses. It could be perceived like a companion, with abilities similar to those of a person, and so raise expectations for a similar performance. Unfortunately, technology is still far away from a strong similarity with human movements, and human-like performance is hard and expensive to obtain, and always imperfect. For instance, most humanoid robots cannot now engage in games like hide-and-seek. A common solution to maintain both human-like shape and mobility is to put a human-like body over wheels, so adding to the expressive possibilities of head and arms, the ability to move even at a relatively high speed. Humanoid heads may have different shapes, inducing different expectations [222]. If the humanoid head includes a mouth, expectations about the ability to interact in natural language may arise, so humanoids are often used to engage in games that involve question-answering or storytelling. Unfortunately, natural language performance is still inadequate to fully cover the expectations and the requirements for a full, free natural language interaction, and it may be problematic to go over simple question-answering games. A shape more close to the imaginary of humanoid robot than to a human may reduce expectations and may allow to expose the actual abilities of the robot, as discussed in Chap. 5.

- *Animal*: an animal shape is often used to recall the sensation of a pet. The type of games it enables are often related to expected abilities of the specific animal, so a dog [380, 667] or a baby seal [739] can play the role of a pet, usually related more to touch than to sight. As for humanoids, some pet bodies have been mounted on wheels to gain mobility and add further play possibilities (e.g., Zoomer[1] [74, 727]). The implementation of pet robots often includes small movements of head and tail, the most expressive parts of an animal body, in reaction to some perception. A general consideration that holds for any robot that tries to resemble a biological being (either animal or person) should be done: as much similarity is attempted as much expectations that the actual ability of the biological being is implemented; this is a potential issue, since the present technology does not allow to obtain the expected results. As mentioned also in [572], the shape of non-familiar animals or fantasy creatures may be better accepted than more realistic shapes, because they leave open possibilities about the actual abilities the robot may have. In some situations, a robot with limited abilities, if properly contextualized, may trigger behaviours aimed at overcoming the limitations, which may be engaging (e.g., [409]), and interesting. However, a robot not able to reach the quality level needed to play will be soon left apart; therefore, known limitations should be presented to the players and integrated in a play context.
- *Cartoon*: Anything that has at least eyes or any element that may recall a cartoon-like aspect is often welcome, since it reminds positive experiences with cartoons, and may anticipate playful activities. Often, shapes explicitly recalling recognized, specific cartoon characters trigger positive emotions, and even just a detail like the shape or the colour is enough to remind a known cartoon and trigger attention, and positive engagement [114]. A cartoon character may do many different things, but there are no specific expectations about it: it is clearly a fantasy creature, so its abilities have to be discovered, and any ability or limitation could be expected. The same principles that are adopted to define emotionally engaging cartoon-like

[1] https://www.zoomerpup.com/.

movements in animation [374] could be considered also for robots to improve animacy, or illusion of life [583, 724].

- *Toy*: A reaction similar to that of cartoon-like robots may be triggered by robots that resemble usual toys, like a ball [479], enhanced with autonomous movement, vibration, lights, or sound, in other terms, animated. Autonomous movement and reactions may be exploited in playful activities, as discussed in Chap. 5.
- *Robotic arm*: this shape comes directly from traditional industrial robots. The ones used in playful activities usually can grasp (light) objects, are tele-controlled or tele-operated, possibly through appropriate interfaces, and used to provide capabilities not otherwise available. They are less expensive, less precise, less dangerous, and less performing, in general, than industrial robots.
- *Vehicles*: robotic vehicles used for play can bring the player on board, or be driven from outside. In the first category, we have both the same vehicles that support mobility of people with physical impairments (e.g., wheelchairs), or special toy vehicles [168]. In any case, they are equipped with sensors that provide some degree of autonomy to the vehicle, which can thus support safe mobility. They may be driven with assistive technology tools so to support a kind of shared autonomy [99] between the driving player and the vehicle. Vehicles that can be remotely driven can be small cars and trucks and can be used in multiple activities like bring or push objects, follow tracks defined on the playground, and many others. In most cases, the remote control is often implemented with the support of assistive technology.
- *Other*: Some robots have shapes that cannot be classified as any of the above mentioned, e.g., a cube or a stick, or a ring. In some cases, these shapes can be functional to a type of interaction, presenting an affordance that can be exploited to play. In other cases, they may trigger curiosity and attention because of the unexpected movement or expressions they may produce.

In general, simple shapes are preferred to more complex ones, especially by children with ASD [532].

4.2.2 Size

Another aspect of the robot that influences the possible play activities is its size.

- *Tiny robots*
  There are few notable examples of tiny robots, 2–3 cm long, that could be used for interesting activities. In general, they may not have computation on board, but may have reactive behaviours, or even behaviours that emerge from the body

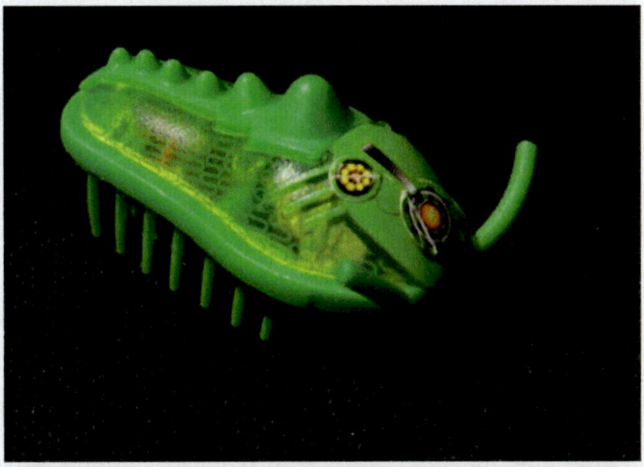

Fig. 4.1 HexBug, one of the many vibrating bugs on the market

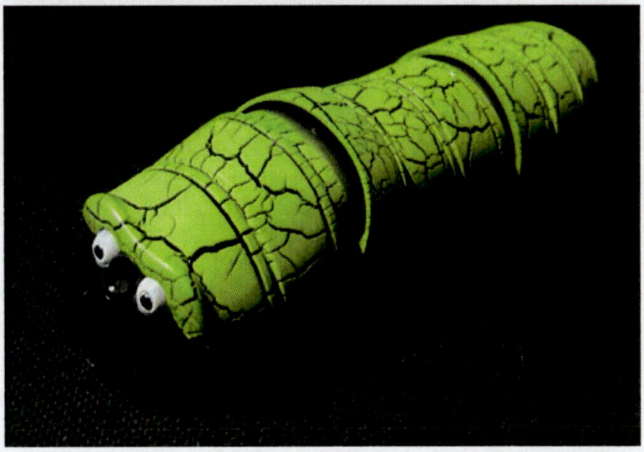

Fig. 4.2 GhostBug, the sensorized caterpillar

design. We mention here the vibrating bugs (like Hexbug,[2] see Fig. 4.1[3]) and the sensorized caterpillar GhostBug (see Fig. 4.2[4]).

The vibrating bugs move quite fast on any horizontal surface, almost straight, and, when they hit a non-horizontal surface, they continue moving, escaping from it by design. Given their speed, it is not too easy to catch them, even if they do not have any sensor to perceive anything of the external world. These bugs can be used just to try to reach them, and possibly to pay attention to where they could go, at the sound of their motor, plan how to catch them, improve the skill to reach them, and so on. They have also been integrated in a popular game (La Cucaracha) where they run in a labyrinth whose walls can be rotated by players,

[2] https://www.hexbug.com/nano.

[3] Picture by Andrea Bonarini. This work is licensed under a Creative Commons Attribution 4.0 International License (http://creativecommons.org/licenses/by/4.0/).

[4] Picture by Andrea Bonarini. This work is licensed under a Creative Commons Attribution 4.0 International License (http://creativecommons.org/licenses/by/4.0/).

one at his/her own turn, to try to drive the bug to the other's home. This game may need cognitive abilities to plan the proper movement and manual abilities to modify the wall position. Moreover, timing is important since the bugs are not waiting and continue running.
The sensorized caterpillar has an attractive, characteristic movement, and when it gets close to some obstacle it moves back rotating about 30°, then it starts again to go straight. This behaviour might be used to place a set of obstacles to make the caterpillar to reach a target. This requires some cognitive ability to forecast the possible behaviour and to estimate the correct placement of the obstacles as well as some manual ability. Although the caterpillar is slower than vibrating bugs, also this game requires a proper management of timing.

- *Manipulable robots*
Manipulable robots are sized between about 5 and 40 cm, a size that stimulates manipulation. Depending on size, external material, and affordance of the parts, the robot can be manipulated in many different ways. All may be grasped, the smaller ones may be thrown, as well as the ones with a tail or limbs. If the robot can sense, e.g., through an accelerometer, that an undesired behaviour is about to be activated [8, 9], it may react to try to prevent it, e.g., by emitting sounds. Manipulation may be integrated in free play, by associating to manipulation some reaction; moreover, it is one of the basic components of touch-based affective interaction, and can also be considered to implement games. For instance, they can be used to ask to be gently transported to another place, where they can be delivered to someone else, who can bring the robot in another place and so on. If the robot is moved too fast it may complain, if it reaches the target it may provide a positive feedback. Time could be also considered in this game, to provide a goal such as "deliver as fast as possible" and a winner may be identified by the robot itself when reaching the target.
Some of the robots of this size can also be mobile and can be used both on a table or on the floor, enabling play activities that involve reaching, avoiding, clearing, path finding and many others, as mentioned in Sect. 4.3.1. Usually, robots of this size are not too fast, and do not mount sophisticated sensors, although the technological advancements are starting to make accessible to the market solutions that can improve amount and quality of the information these robots could exploit with the limitations in power typical of this category.
- *Kid-size robots*
These robots, with a height in the range of about 50 to 120 cm, are intended to play on the floor, interacting with kids moving at their level. This is the main advantage for these robots, which could also mount bigger batteries, last longer than the previous ones, and have sensor and computational power on board adequate for a rich interaction. Most of the play activities in which they may be involved exploit movement of the robot.

Examples of these robots and their play potentialities are presented in detail in Chap. 8.

4.2.3 Color

Colours may activate reactions and moods. The choice of colours for the body of the robot may induce attitudes and ways of interacting. For instance, the white fur of Paro [739] is not only coherent with the representation of a baby seal, which, after the campaign of the years when it was first proposed to save baby seals from hunters, is associated with something to have care of, but also induces a neutral mood, and a sensation of cleanliness, and harmlessness, shared with most of the white, robot-shaped robots on the market (e.g., Pepper [518], Nao [486], MIPArcade®).

Pale colours are neutral, and, when not associated with any specific cultural meaning (e.g., pink for females and light blue for males, in some Western cultures), can be safely used for robots. Bright colours (e.g., red, orange, bright green) are often used in cartoons and may help to establish a link with pleasant experiences. However, they may also trigger negative reactions if they are exciting, or stimulate too much the sensor apparatus of the player. Black is usually associated to villains or Hi-Tech devices. The effect of colour, in general, has been widely studied in psychology and design, and colours have a lot of different association in different cultures [605].

4.2.4 Material

The material of the robot body is directly related to touch, and may induce different interaction modalities. Most of the robots have a plastic body. This has many positive aspects: it can be easily cleaned, it may be robust, it is cheap for mass production, it can be shaped in any way. However, plastic does not stimulate touch: it is rigid and cool, while people touching a companion would expect a warm and soft body that may be deformed under pressure. A first step in this direction is done with silicon covering many commercial toys, either flat like skin, or arranged as a kind of relatively hard or flexible hair. Silicon is easy to model and quite cleanable, like plastic, relatively cheap, and it can be used as a skin also on a deformable body. It is not so pleasant to caress, still cold, it has limited life time, and it is somehow prone to improper interaction, like stretching or punching.

Other solutions are textiles, both as fabric or as synthetic fur. Textiles are cheap, washable, warm and can be tailored to any body. In addition to traditional cotton or wool textiles, for robots, it is possible to consider also elastic textiles, like Lycra®, soft textiles, like fleece (pile), or semi-rigid textiles, like felt, each providing different possibilities to implement a skin pleasant to touch and enabling different movements. Synthetic fur is another option, widely used for pet-like robots, since it provides a nice touch feeling and may also have a look similar to the real animal fur. A textile skin makes it possible to implement soft bodies and certainly presents an affordance that calls for touch.

There are many other possibilities, not much explored, yet, including metal (the iconic material for robots, not much used for toy robots any longer, because of weight

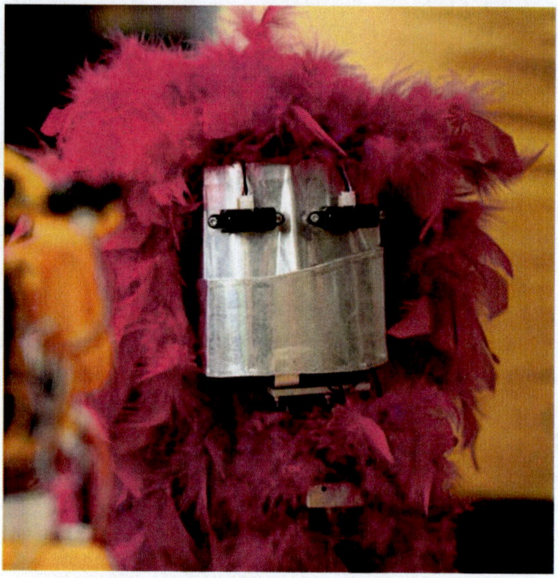

Fig. 4.3 Concierge, developed at AIRLab, Politecnico di Milano. It can follow with its eyes a person moving in its range. It can be used for attention and control play. Body in aluminium, hair in feathers

and production costs disadvantages with respect to plastic), up to leather and wood (e.g., the robots of Amit Drori[5]) as well as feathers. Feathers can be used for aesthetic purposes like in Tofu [758], and also to characterize the robot movement and enhance the emotion expression as in Concierge (Fig. 4.3[6]) and E-2? (Fig. 4.4[7]).

Figure 4.5 contains a visual summary of the considered robot body features. In the next chapters, we will see how these can be exploited to define play activities.

4.3 Actuators

In this section, we present the different ways a robot can generate signals that could be perceived by a human player. We consider all of them as actuators, in the sense that they enable the robot to act. They involve motion, sound, and light.

4.3.1 Motion

A robot may move in the space in different ways, listed here below.

[5] https://amitdrori.com/.

[6] Picture by Andrea Bonarini. This work is licensed under a Creative Commons Attribution 4.0 International License (http://creativecommons.org/licenses/by/4.0/).

[7] Copyright: ©Lab Immagine—Politecnico di Milano.

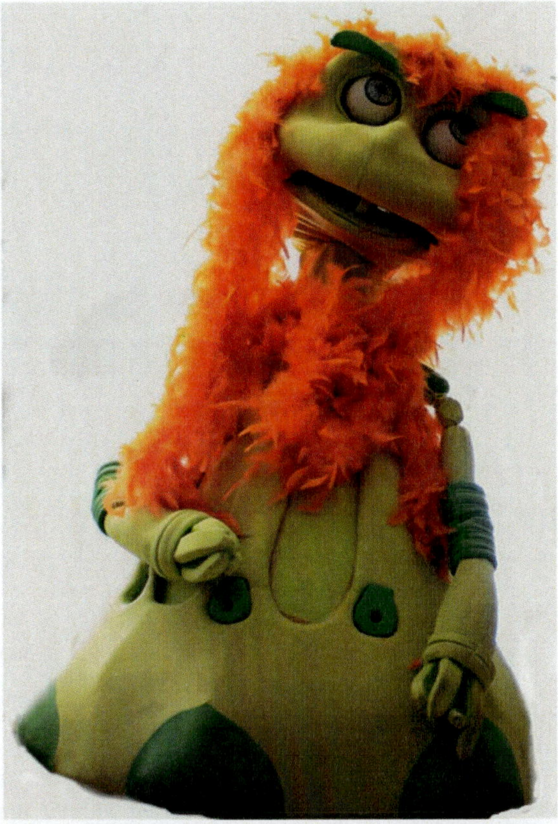

Fig. 4.4 E-2?, developed at AIRLab, Politecnico di Milano. It can navigate in indoor environments, and interact with people, capturing and showing emotional signal. Body in Ethylene-vinyl Acetate (EVA), skin in Lycra®, "hair" in feathers

- *On place robots*: these robots can only move parts of their body, but cannot move on the floor, on a table, in the space. They may be designed as pets, animals, robots, humans, or cartoon characters. Their movements are usually intended to express emotions in order to get engagement in interaction. The movement may involve head, chest, less frequently arms or legs; this last movement is more complex to be made realistic, and limbs have a potentially dangerous affordance that may induce to grasp them and to tear them off. Some of them can express emotions also through vibrations. Often, they have lights and the possibility to produce sounds, so to improve the communication. Notable examples on the market are Furby, My Real Pet, Minions. A special type of on place robot are robotic arms, a shape borrowed from industrial robots, which gives the possibility to grasp objects or to draw, according to the end effector mounted on the top of the arm. These are usually tele-controlled and may be used to provide manipulation abilities to people with physical impairments (e.g., [2]).

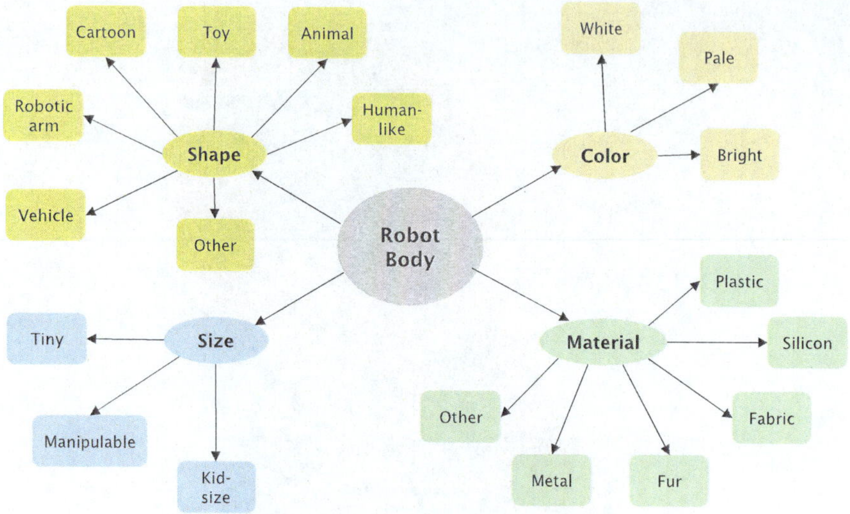

Fig. 4.5 Visual representation of the considered robot body features

- *Moving robots*: these robots, depending on the size and on the sensor abilities, can move on a table or on the floor. Mobility can be exploited for the play activity. A typical set of play activities may involve the fact that the robot should be reached and touched, or should follow or reach a target, or the player, as when playing fetch. In this, the robot needs to have sensors to recognize the elements of the game, and to be able to run at a speed that is coherent with the play activity and the player's abilities. Another set of possible games involve obstacle course, or labyrinth, where the robot should follow a path matching some elements of the environment with its sensors. This requires from the robot to be able to sense what is needed, and from the player either skill in controlling the robot or cognitive ability to set up the play setting. The movement can be obtained by wheels, mostly arranged in a dual-drive kinematics (with its typical constraints on turning), tracks, usually not fast and anyway constrained, omnidirectional wheels, which enable holonomic (i.e., free of constraints) movements, legs, usually slow and unstable, or directly by the spherical shape of the rolling robot.
  In the category of moving robots are also flying robots, like drones and blimps. Both are usually tele-controlled and can be employed in games of ability to drive them through 3-D obstacles. Drones are more suited to external environments and are often equipped by cameras that may allow real-time view from the drone. Blimps are slower, but bigger and less dangerous and scary, much easier to control than drones.
  It is also possible to express emotions through movement in space, even when no other parts of the body are moving (e.g., [18, 38]). Managing emotional expression while performing a task is a challenge worth to face, given the return that emotional expression can give on animacy.

Motion is a primary source of animacy, and can be perceived, depending on the situation, either by sight or touch. A robot may move parts, in a way functional to its role in the play activity, to manipulate objects, but this is often difficult and expensive since both dexterity and sophisticated sensing are required. It is much more common to see movements that give an expressive meaning to the robot's activity, and in particular that are designed to communicate with gestures or to convey emotions, which will be discussed in Sect. 4.8.

4.3.2 Sound

Sound is a natural complement of motion, may enforce attention and may be functional to the play activity. Robots playing sounds not associated to any proper motion are as expressive as loudspeakers and hardly can catch attention and involve players. Sound and motion should be matched in rhythm and expressiveness to provide a coherent behaviour. Even a speech not associated to movement give a fake impression, and reduces the possibility to establish a good quality relationship.

There are different options to use sounds.

- *Speech*: utterances are emitted by the robot in natural language, so that they could be understood by the player. These can be either pre-recorded and just selected among the available files, or generated by a natural language generation system. In the first case, a relatively simple dialogue manager may be enough to manage interaction, often based on a kind of state machine. When interacting in natural language, a drawback may arise if the interlocutor drives the dialogue far from expectations and there would be the need to manage difficult situations. Full natural language generation may require computational resources only accessible through the internet web, possibly introducing in the dialogue undesired delays that have to be managed. Failing the interaction with a fragile subject may be critical. The type of voice contributes to characterize the robot, both as gender, and as more or less human-like, cartoon-like, or robot-like.
- *Non-verbal sounds*: sounds without any explicit meaning can be used to express emotions and characterize situations, as we have been trained by science fiction movies like Star Wars or cartoons like Wall-E and Minions. They can also be interpreted as non-linguistic utterances [575], often expressing some emotional status. There are rules to be followed to design these sounds in order to obtain the desired effects, which consider pitch, dynamics, volume, rhythm, melody, and timbre [369, 462].
- *Motor sounds*: often disregarded, motor sound is usually perceived and may be integrated in the experience. It may be perceived as disturbing [713], because of pitch or volume, or as putting in evidence the mechanical nature of the robot, thus reducing animacy. It may be explicitly used to express emotions such as anger, fatigue, or frustration [272] and others. Of course, the possibility to express something with motors that have been designed to produce movement relies on the

specific motor, the resonance of the body and the control system. Some playing activities cannot be implemented because of motor noise. For instance, the robot cannot hide itself in a hide-and-seek game, since everybody would listen where it is going. Other activities may exploit motor noise to make the robot evident, for instance, to short-sighted players.

4.3.3 Light

Coloured LEDs can be used both as tools to express emotional status, as well as signal emitters functional to the play activity. Emotional expression is related both to colours and to the rhythm used to switch on and off LEDs. Again, colours may be associated with cultural meanings, some of which are being somehow "globalized" in these last years by mass market entertainment media (movies, books, cartoons), at least in Western countries.

Luminosity can be controlled to express different emotional status: a slow-fading light may express sadness, a fast rhythm excitation, and so on. Emotional rhythm is well perceived and interpreted by most of the players (e.g., [100, 114]. This may have a strong effect on the interaction: it contributes to provide a good feeling of animacy and may also become functional to the game mechanics. Rhythm and intensity should be carefully modulated when using a robot with people with special sensitivity, since they may suffer from convulsions [82].

Light is also the channel exploited by screens, often used to represent facial expressions. It is a solution that offers rich expressions, sometimes limited by the low luminosity of the screen (as in the last generation of Furby), mostly in conditions of strong illumination, such as natural light or spotlights.

4.4 Sensors

The robot needs to perceive what is needed to participate in the specific play activity. Typical sensors are listed here below, together with their main features that can be exploited in playing.

- *Buttons and switches*: these are the simpler sensors producing a digital signal (On or Off) when they are pressed. They can be used to accept answers to questions, to turn on or off some actuator, and, if properly placed on the body, to detect the presence of a material, for instance as bumpers or surface detection for mobile robots operating on suspended surfaces, like a table or a stairs-delimited room floor.
- *Presence sensors*: they detect the presence of anything in the range of the sensor. Movement detection sensors used in security (PIR—Passive Infra-Red sensors) can distinguish objects from persons and animals moving in their range, but need

to be mounted in a fixed position, not on the robot, if this is moving. Other active Infra-Red (IR) sensors may be set to trigger at a given distance, acting as proximity sensors. They are often used to avoid that a mobile robot run off the table, and to trigger actions at a given distance, such as avoiding obstacles or following a target.

- *Distance sensors*: implemented by different technologies (e.g., ultrasound, radar, or IR), they can provide a distance to the closer object that can enter in their conical range. By considering different ranges, it is possible to trigger different actions. By considering the time between readings it is possible to estimate the speed of a moving object in the range, and possibly trigger different actions, e.g., emotional expressions, according to the approaching or leaving speed. With an array of distance sensors, it is also possible to estimate the direction of the movement of the closer object in the range.
- *Ego-motion sensors*: accelerometers and gyroscopes provide, respectively, acceleration and rotational speed with respect to the three perpendicular axis relative to the sensor. They are usually integrated in a single chip, which in some cases hosts also a dedicated microcomputer that provides the quaternions, mathematical entities that characterize absolute displacement. They can be used to compute the different characteristics of movements, for instance, they can be used to identify how a robot is manipulated, to recognize gestures, to estimate vibrations. They are adopted in touch-based interactions and to monitor robot movements possibly induced by the player. A simpler version of motion sensor is the tilt sensor, able to detect whether it has been tilted or shaken over a fixed degree. This is usually a Boolean sensor, providing one of two possible values, like a switch.
- *Touch sensors*: resistive sensors can detect pressure by deformation, capacitance sensors can detect touch or the proximity of a hand or a body in a short range. They are mostly used for touch-based interactions, for instance to recognize gestures such as pat, caress, punch, and hug [114]. They may also be used in place of buttons to accept either answers to questions, or simple commands. Other robots integrate touch sensors to detect the level of stress. For instance, Therabot [76] is a dog-like robot equipped with touch sensors to detect the level of stress of people with mental health disorders, and eventually adapt the behaviour of the robot to it.
- *Light sensors*: Cameras provide either 2-D or 3-D images. In general, images are (possibly very large) matrices of numbers describing pixel's colours (or distance in case of 3-D cameras) organized in a bi-dimensional table. Understanding something from this bunch of numbers requires computationally demanding operations, nowadays often based on machine learning models. It is possible to identify objects and persons in the range, to identify the main joints of the person and, from this information, perform activity recognition, to recognize a person, to estimate the gaze direction, or to analyze the emotional expression from face and body gestures. These operations may require time, which may affect the quality of interaction and playfulness.

  Thermo-cameras are also available to exploit the thermal signature of a subject. For instance, with these, it is relatively easy to detect a person, her thermal shape, without being able to recognize her/him, which can be exploited when strong privacy constraints have to be considered.

Light sensors include also light detectors, implemented with different technologies, that act as a single pixel of a camera, providing the intensity of the light that reaches the sensor. These can be used to provide a guide to the robot, for instance by pointing a lamp in front of it, so that it can follow the light. There are also colour sensors that include three different light sensor each covered by a coloured filter so to detect only one of the three basic component of a colour: red, green, and blue. These are usually adopted to recognize colours at a close distance, since they need a quite uniform coloured area in a controlled light situation. A typical use of these sensors consists in putting them below the robot, pointing at the ground, to detect coloured lines or markers that could drive the robot.

- *Microphones*: these provide the sound input to the robot. At a low level, it can be used to trigger activities when the signal trespasses a threshold. A more intensive elaboration may provide frequency analysis and filtering, improving the amount of information that could be exploited. For instance, the whistle of a referee can be distinguished from background noise [101]. It is also possible to analyze the sound signal to interpret possibly emitted Natural Language (NL) utterances. We cannot list here the many techniques that could be used to interpret NL, but we would like to comment about services offered by different companies to obtain at least a good quality transcript of what has been told by a person. In most cases, they work very well in controlled environments, and, anyway, they may often take few seconds to provide a transcript. This should then be interpreted, and finally associated to one of the reactions that the robot could exhibit in similar situations. The importance of a fluent and correct interaction cannot be enough stressed. Delays in the flow, improper utterances, mismatch between sound and motion may reduce animacy, as well as confidence. Full natural language interaction is still an open problem, mostly when interacting with persons affected by communication and interaction issues. Multiple microphones can also provide the direction of sound.
- *Tag detectors*: either RFID, NFT or vision-based (e.g., reading bar codes, or QR-codes), they can detect a tagged object with a very low computational cost. Tagged objects can be parts of the environment (e.g., used to localize a mobile robot, or to make it doing some movement), or elements presented to the robot (e.g., cards, or buttons embedded in some plastic object). Magnetic field detectors can be considered in this category, as they are often used in commercial products to detect objects containing a magnet in their proximity (the magnetic field decreases with the cube of the distance), such as pretended food for animal pets.

Figure 4.6 contains a visual representation of the considered categories of sensors and actuators, i.e., the tools to open communication channels for the robots. In the next chapters, we will see how it is possible to exploit them to implement playful activities.

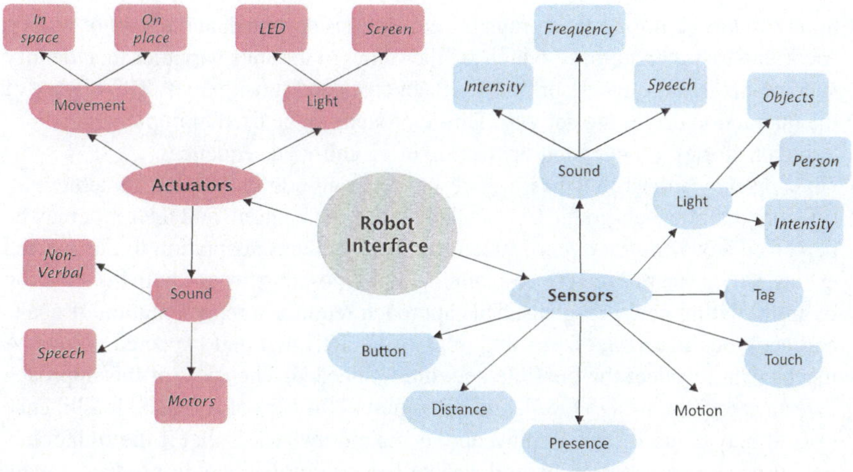

Fig. 4.6 Visual representation of the considered sensors and actuators

4.5 Behaviour and Play

The robot abilities needed to play depend on the type of play and on the reliability that is required. About this last, often when playing we expect that the other players have their own degree of ability to participate to the game: it is part of the playing contract, and a functional play community works to integrate the players in the activity, as long as they reach a commonly agreed ability level [213]. This holds for human players, but also for robots; so, it may be accepted that a robot could not play in a perfect way. However, the behaviour of the robot should be coherent with the aim of the activity; the robot should be able to show what is needed to understand that it is purposely playing, following the rules and aiming at the play goals.

Issues may arise from poor sensors or inadequate sensor interpretation, from inappropriate actuators and actuation, and from behaviour design. Any issue should be solved before delivering the robot, possibly by defining a play activity or a game coherent with the possibilities of the robot. All the players should be integrated in the play activity, to let engagement, pleasure and fun develop freely, without worries.

The behaviour of the robot can be designed according to different paradigms, shortly introduced here below.

- *Reactive behaviour*: according to a given perception, the robot reacts in a given way. Reactions can be independent from each other, and no relationship with the past events is considered. This type of behaviour can be exploited to implement free play, where the relevant aspect is to offer the same reaction to the same input, in order to be perceived as consistent, and develop self-confidence, trust, and control. Depending on the number of reactions, the playing activity may be too simple and boring, so abandoned once discovered the few possible relationships, or too complex and difficult to manage and even to understand.

- *State machine*: a pre-defined graph of sequences is designed, and the robot visits it according to its perceptions, which are the values of the state variables that identify states. This is the typical control of videogames and most games. The history of the interaction drives the activity. This approach can be used to implement games based on stories, on question-answering or on sub-goal sequences.
- *Goal oriented*: the robot has a goal and can autonomously plan to achieve it, possibly defining sub-goals. Classical planning can be used, and the robot may be perceived as a *rational agent* [502, 728]. This includes adaptation to unexpected events, which can be faced by re-planning, if it is possible to cope with the situation by instantiating new sub-goals. This approach requires a representation of goals, and activities in terms of preconditions to be activated and expected effects. A mechanism to select the possible activities is needed. The roots of this approach date back to 50 years ago [252], and it was part of the core of Artificial Intelligence (AI). It may be used for free play, and its main drawback is that if the situation is not covered by any action, then the robot has no rational way to produce a plan, but it should produce anyway an action (inactivity is also an action in interaction), which may be inappropriate.
- *Black box, learned model*: building on experience, it may be possible, in principle, to learn how to do in any situation, adopting a Machine Learning (ML) approach. Although possible, this approach requires to collect enough samples of any possible situation and apply the preferred ML algorithm to the data. This may be foreseen, but it would require many data from situations that may be very different from each other and complex to describe, therefore cannot be considered for our purposes. Moreover, being a black box approach, it would not comply to the principles of transparency that have now to be implemented in any autonomous device, as discussed in Chap. 9.

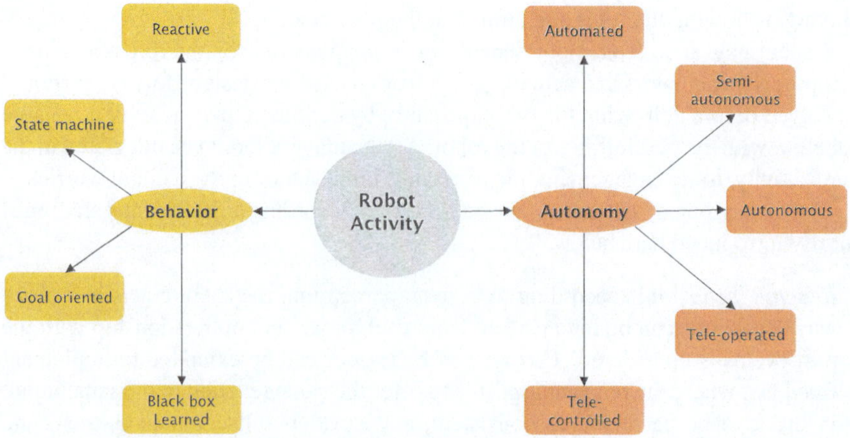

Fig. 4.7 Visual representation of the ways a robot can be controlled and how behaviours can be implemented

The just listed basic activity paradigms can also be adopted in tele-operated or remote-controlled robots, where a player, an operator, or a play companion is in charge of controlling the robot. The way they do so is characterizing the activity. If they are just reacting, the initiative is mainly left to the human player, if they have a plan, or goals, they may participate actively in the play activity driving their avatar, if they use their knowledge about the situation and the specific player(s), the interaction would be similar to the last one, non-transparent to the player, but this is typical and expected in traditional play.

Figure 4.7 contains a visual representation of how the robot can be controlled, as reported in Sect. 4.1, and how behaviours can be implemented.

4.6 Playground

We have seen in Chap. 2 that the playground plays a fundamental role for the playing activity. When a robot is involved, we may have different scenarios, depending on the size of the robot and its capabilities.

If the robot is only moving on place, it is often placed on a table and the playground is limited to the table, the chair where the human player is sitting, if any, and the things that may be nearby. Rarely the robot used for these activities can autonomously manipulate objects, so the interaction is mostly verbal and gestural. If the robot is intended to be manipulated, it may be possible to leave the table, with the robot, for a chair, or a sofa, or even the floor; in this case, sensors and actuators are mostly dedicated to close and touch interaction, possibly including sound and lights. In this situation, a camera is of little help, since it would be often pointed to some irrelevant direction, or too close to be able to understand anything from the image.

If the robot can move in space, the playground can be a table, the floor, or a 3-D space, if the robot can fly. When moving on the table, the robot should be equipped with sensors that guarantee that it cannot drop from the table. The table is a quite limited environment, but, still, there may be a part of the table that a person sitting on a side can reach, and a part where only the robot can go: this may enable reaching and escaping games. The table may be equipped with frames to keep the robot in, and it is possible to put objects on the table, which may become part of the play activity. For instance, one may put juice bricks that may be considered as targets, and may be also pushed by controlling a robot to clean up the table or to collect them in a place. Another robot running on the table may enable a social interaction in a limited space. Many games may be implemented, sharing the constraint that the player has to stay at the table, possibly moving around it.

If the playground is the floor, it may be limited to a room, or extend to a set of rooms, a whole apartment or care centre. This is the space where also the human players usually move, and also in this case they can actually move while playing. Here, games involving fetching, reaching and escaping, dancing, taking positions can also be envisioned. It is also possible to introduce elements in the environment, such as obstacles and targets, as well as other toys to interact with, such as balls.

The robot should be designed to be safe, since in this setting, it has often a size comparable with that of a kid. Safety can be intrinsically guaranteed, by having the robot moving slowly, and not weighting much, or should be guaranteed by reliable sensors and control software, which may be available only on quite expensive robots (see Sect. 4.9).

4.7 Animacy

Moving objects may be perceived as having some animacy [557], and animacy perception may influence perception of intelligence in robots [46]. Theory of mind refers to those social skills that allow humans to correctly attribute beliefs, goals, perceptions, feelings, and desires to themselves and others [782]. The presence of a theory of mind in people facing a robot enables the attribution of animacy. Robots that induce the perception of animacy are usually engaging people, and can take a richer and more engaging role in playful activities.

Animacy is related to different elements that should coherently work to be believable. Any action of the robot, including movement, sound, and light should be integrated to produce the desired effect.

A first aspect concerns movement. Biological movement is different from "robotic movement" because muscles' physiology and arrangements are different from motors and robot links. It is possible to control movements of a robot by implementing proper control systems. The typical control systems used in industrial robotics are aimed at obtaining the best performance in terms of speed and repeatability, so they are often actuated with high acceleration, which produce fast movements and abrupt stops. This is also what is obtained when controlling motors without a proper control software, just opening or closing a power circuit on the motor. Physiological movements, instead, are characterized by smooth changes, and high accelerations are only used to express specific emotions, like anger, for instance. In the last years, a lot of efforts have been done to include also in commercial products movements that could be assimilated to physiological movements, so becoming expressive. They can exploit different speed and acceleration profiles to match the different ways biological beings are moving.

The possibility to modify the signal in the quest of expressivity is also shared by the other output signals, being them sound or light. For all the signals, different dimensions can be considered like: intensity, frequency, rhythm, dynamics.

With the possibility to modify parameters of the signals, it becomes possible to implement expressive robots [691].

Principles of cartoon animation [374, 414] have been considered to design robot movements that can convey animacy. These are based on dimensions characteristic of movement, well summarized in [583]. Of the 12 principles reported there, and taken from expert animators [374], we present and discuss here only the ones that may be considered for playful robots and that are not covered in other parts of this chapter.

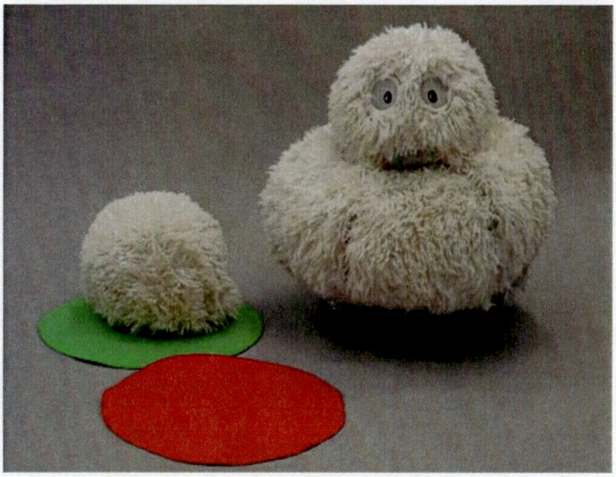

Fig. 4.8 Yeti, a robot developed at Politecnico di Milano—AIRLab, can express emotions through movement, body deformation, sound, and eyes shape and colour. Yeti is a mobile robot, whose body is made of metal nets covered by polystyrene foam and cotton fur

- *Squash and Stretch*: body deformation is a cue for animacy, not easy to obtain with robots, usually made in hard materials. Some effect may be obtained by connecting parts with elastic elements, as commonly done in toy plushes to prevent breaking: this also gives the possibility to have parts vibrating or floating even if not directly actuated, and this contributes to represent a sense of animacy. Another possibility consists in using materials that naturally move with the general body movement, such as feathers, thin polyethylene, or voile. A solution adopted in few notable cases is the use of deformable materials and proper design to have a fully deformable body, such as polypropylene foam for Keepon [401], Tofu [758], and Yeti (see Fig. 4.8[8]) and knitted wool yarn for Blossom [678].
- *Staging*: This principle is related to the creation of a context for the action. In our case, this is done by inserting the play action in a narrative that can both explain and justify it [131], as well as setting the proper playground.
- *Straight Ahead and Pose-to-Pose*: These are two techniques in animation, the first used to develop the ideas of the animator directly, the second to accurately define the single steps of the animation. These could be mapped into basic interaction movements, and specific expressive sequences, respectively. Designing expressive sequences is a commonly adopted solution to implement expressions possibly proved as effective that require a sequence to be implemented; most emotional expressions require at least few seconds to be expressed and interpreted. This may pose limitations to the interaction, since the sequence, once started, should be completed to be effective, and in that time lapse the robot should not react to what may happen. This issue should be limited by designing relatively short sequences that block other robot activities for a short time.

[8] Picture by Andrea Bonarini. This work is licensed under a Creative Commons Attribution 4.0 International License (http://creativecommons.org/licenses/by/4.0/).

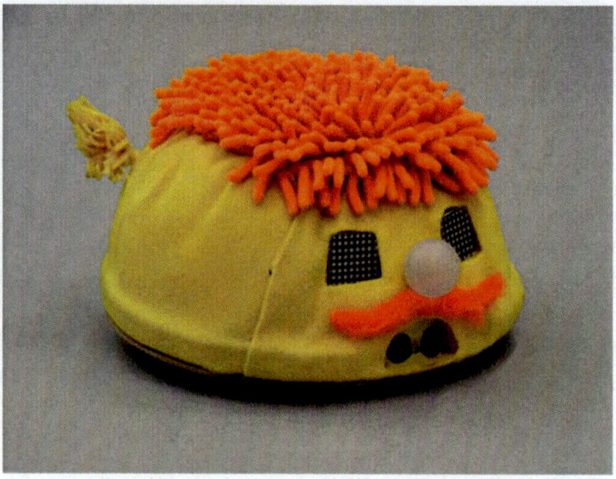

Fig. 4.9 ElRizo, a mobile robot developed at Politecnico di Milano—AIRLab, can express emotions through movement, sound, eyes shape and the movement of the tail,in reaction to relative movements, caresses, and light. ElRizo's body is made of a plastic colander covered by felt and a mop for hair

- *Slow In and Slow Out*: as mentioned before, physiological movements are not impulsive, and a smooth passage from one status to another one is coherent with animacy expression.
- *Secondary Action*: an action accompanying the principal one improves animacy, for instance, moving the head while speaking, or "breathing" while moving, or having a tail moving while playing a sound or going around. This is also a way to convey emotion while reacting to an external stimulus, as done by ElRizo, depicted in Fig. 4.9.[9]
- *Timing*: timing is an important element for expression. Both the duration of an action, the timing between an action and the respective reaction, the timing determining the rhythm of an action are critical to make the interaction effective. There are situations when the robot cannot answer in due time because, for instance, time is required to elaborate signals and produce the proper answer. In this case, it is possible to perform secondary, coherent actions, while the main action is to be defined, so to give the impression that the robot is present, and not just a dull prop blocked on some mysterious issue.
- *Exaggeration*: animation characters have exaggerated body features (e.g., big eyes and mouth, large head, ...) and make exaggerated movements, which make them more ridiculous and give them the possibility to express in a clear way what they have to. This would also be interesting for robots, in the direction opposite to trying to be similar to biological beings. However, some persons with disabilities may be disturbed by excesses, since they cannot easily manage them, or even understand the situation when trying to match their play experience with what they are used to experience. So, exaggeration, although potentially engaging, and triggering the pleasurable similitude with cartoons, should be considered with care.

[9] Picture by Andrea Bonarini. This work is licensed under a Creative Commons Attribution 4.0 International License (http://creativecommons.org/licenses/by/4.0/).

A laying robot should be always ready to be adapted, both in body features and in behaviour to the player's needs.

- *Solid Drawing*: we agree with [583] that an extremely regular body is less interesting than an irregular one. This principle is not considered in most products, nor in most research robots, since symmetry is a proxy for quality in commercial products. However, many robots, including all the ones depicted in this book, exploit the fact that they have been handcrafted, or they have been designed in the effort of giving them some personality.

4.8 Emotion

Emotion expression in robots has been studied since many years, initially focusing mainly on facial expressions [112, 716], for which have been obtained results comparable with human expressions [52], then trying to extend emotional expression to gestures and body movements, as well as to speech and sound.

Emotional expression depends on possibly slight, still precise signals similar to those that we can recognize as emotional expressions in humans and animals. These may be associated to the movement of bio-inspired parts (head, mouth, eyes, arms, chest, body) that mimick human emotional expressions, but also to characteristics of the movement itself of non-bioinspired body parts. The same holds for sounds, where efforts have been done both to replicate emotional expression in speech, and to generate non-verbal expressive sounds.

The research on emotions has produced a large number of models that try to capture different aspects of this phenomenon, so important for social life. One of the most adopted in Robotics is the circumplex model [598] according to which emotions can be distributed along two quantitative axis: arousal and pleasure/displeasure (valence). While arousal has been associated to acceleration (e.g., [604]), it is more difficult to associate the valence axis to parameters that could be directly implemented in robots without adding some contextual knowledge [18] or other emotional cues, such as direction of eyebrows, the shape of eyes, or an emotionally loaded sound.

Other models, directly related to movement, have been considered, coming from observation (e.g., [157, 399]), from the dance tradition (e.g., Laban [408]) and from animation principles (e.g., [374, 414]). There is no full concordance among the different elements that may characterize an emotional expression, but this also depends on the different interpretations that are given to the words labelling emotional expressions, on cultural background, and on the expression possibilities of the robot's body.

Promising approaches follow the model that Rudolf Laban defined to describe movement for choreography [408]. Among the qualities he defined, two are useful to describe emotional aspects: *Effort*, which depicts how the body concentrates its effort to perform the movement and deals with expressivity, and *Shape*, which describes how the subject modifies the shape of his body. Unfortunately, a precise definition of the components of these two dimensions was not in the aims of Laban, but roboticists

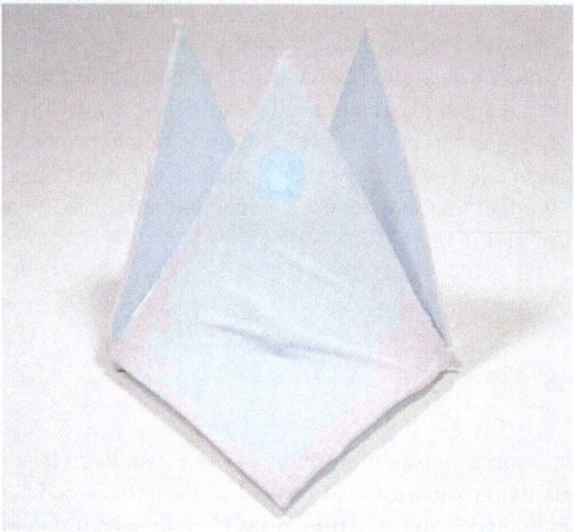

Fig. 4.10 The robot EDRO developed at Politecnico di Milano—AIRLab. It can express emotions with displacement, movement of the doubled triangles that compose the tetrahedron and LED colour and rhythm. EDRO is a mobile robot, made of wood frames covered by Lycra® and reacting to the perceived ways to approach it, detected by a sonar sensor embedded in the body

have tried to put them in relationship with movement parameters that could be mapped on robots (e.g., [38, 714]).

A lot of robots with a bio-inspired form rely on facial expressions to show emotions, either mechanically implemented (e.g., [52, 113, 583]), or shown on a display as on the last version of Furby. Other robots, like Nao [486] and Pepper [518], rely on movement of head, arms and chest for emotion expression, but have a fixed face.

The same basic movement principles can be applied to any part of a robot, as well as to the whole body, also when it has no bio-inspired appearance as is the case EDRO, shown in Fig. 4.10[10] and Theatrebot [18] (see Fig. 4.11[11]) expressly developed to identify what are the basic characteristics of movement needed to express emotion, depurated from bio-inspired elements.

Saerbeck et al. [604] state that the perceived affective state of a robot is independent of the embodiment, suggesting that we can use motion design tools across different embodiments. In our experience, we verified that many different embodiments can express emotions, provided that motion and the other signals are properly designed. Based on observations and on theatrical representation background, we experienced that, if there is the possibility to have joints in the body, whatever the shape of the body, at about 60% of the height (corresponding to the human waist) or at about 80% of the height (corresponding to the human neck), it is possible to exploit inclinations of the body sections to support emotional expression.

[10] Picture by Andrea Bonarini. This work is licensed under a Creative Commons Attribution 4.0 International License (http://creativecommons.org/licenses/by/4.0/).

[11] Picture by Andrea Bonarini. This work is licensed under a Creative Commons Attribution 4.0 International License (http://creativecommons.org/licenses/by/4.0/).

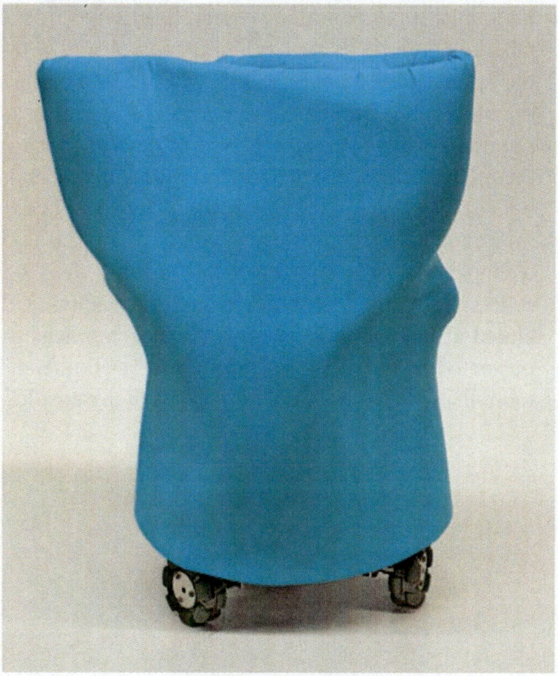

Fig. 4.11 Theatrebot, developed at Politecnico di Milano—AIRLab. It can express emotions only with displacement. It has been used to study how to express emotions on stage

4.9 Cost Considerations

We would like to close this chapter with some considerations about the cost of robots that could be used to play, which is important for their diffusion. Both families and care centres can rarely afford expenses of thousands of Euros for a single device, so the development of play activities and of playing robots should consider also the abilities that cheap devices may be able to exploit.

As it could be imagined, complexity is associated with costs in materials, sensors, computation power, programming, maintenance. In the chapters of Part III, we will present many playing robots and how they implement the features they need to play. The present situation is articulated in different possible categories of solutions, discussed here below.

- *Toys*: the (robot) toy market is very competitive, and products should target the whole population. The cost for a toy rarely goes over 199 Euro, since the product should be accessible by a mass of customers, in the order of hundreds of thousands, so to cover the production and distribution costs. As we will see, also with low-cost products (in the order of tens Euros), it is possible to devise interesting play activities involving autonomous robots.
- *Professional robots*: professional robots, like industrial arms, social robots like Nao and Pepper, and even Paro, have a relatively small market and a lot of features, so the cost goes well beyond 1,000 Euro, and a careful cost-effect analysis is required.

- *Self-made robots*: in many research activities, robots have been developed in the labs, and their plans are beginning to be shared with the community in the spirit of the makers movement (e.g., [35, 371, 413]). For the shared projects, the possibility of autonomous implementation by care centres or families is open and may be an important way to spread this type of devices among people interested to play with them. This brings also the possibility to improve or adapt the robot to special needs, which is a common request from many specific situations. The cost of materials may range from tens to few hundreds of Euros, depending on the amount of technology that is embedded in the robot. It is possible to develop very cheap robots that can support interesting play activities. We will see many examples aimed at providing inspiration for development in Part III. None of the robots presented in this book and developed at Politecnico di Milano—AIRLab costs more than 300 Euros in material, and many cost less than 100 Euros.

Chapter 5
Robots and Play Activities

Andrea Bonarini

Abstract How play activities could be structured when a robot is involved and why? What is working and what it is not in a robotic playing activity, not only for persons with disabilities but also for normally developed people? The accent is on physical games, where autonomous robots can move, act autonomously, and become effective game companions. We present issues related to the type of movement, and in general the use of actuators, which should be carefully designed to engage the specific player in an interesting activity. In free play, the robot should be interesting and propose activities that could match the abilities of the player, while in structured games, it should also be able to comply with the game rules, and to adapt abilities to produce behaviours that could keep any player in the state of *flow*. We analyze the role of robots in the type of play and the contexts related to the different disabilities introduced in Chap. 3, providing a conceptual framework that could be used to analyze the examples that will be presented in the third part of this book. We discuss how it is possible to obtain a playful robot at a cost compatible with the market, overcoming the intrinsic limitations that may come from imperfect sensors and actuators. Robot and game design should interact to originate play situations that can be perceived as appropriate and engaging, also when the available technology cannot achieve the performance that we may like to have.

5.1 The Role of Robots in Play

Play can be supported by two main drivers, common to all the players, since they are intrinsic to human (and animal) nature and deeply rooted in primitive needs: *curiosity* and *challenge*. Both are functional to a very basic need: survival. Curiosity is triggered by anything that we do not know, or master, yet. The need to be in control in any situation that may occur pushes in the direction of exploring new situations, in a broad sense, as soon as we may perceive them. Challenge is a consequence: once we face a (new) situation, we would like to acquire the competence to face it, so that we may control it and feel safe. Facing a challenge requires confidence in the own possibilities, so the challenge should not be too complex, otherwise the player may feel to be stressed and possibly leave the play situation. Since the challenge is posed

A. Bonarini and S. Besio, *Robot Play for All*, Research for Development,
https://doi.org/10.1007/978-3-031-05042-8_5

by a play activity, in which the player voluntary decided to be involved, as by the definition given in Chap. 2, he/she has all the right to leave it when it is no longer enjoyable [213]. At the same time, a too simple challenge is not worth the energy to be spent to face it, since the player is already able to manage it. These are the basic mechanisms behind the application of the *flow* theory to play [199]. Moreover, this theory states that when people are in the flow state, they are completely absorbed in their activity, engaged with all the senses to enjoy it, and that this is also the best way to exploit it. Therefore, the aim of the design of play experiences with robots should bring the players in their *flow* state, considering all that may be relevant for this. In the rest of this chapter, we will analyze the different aspects that may be considered to achieve this goal.

As we have seen in Chap. 4, a robot may be able to react to signals perceived by its sensors and to propose actions. In both cases, some animacy is attributed to the device, which is not an inert object, but shows some intentionality and can play an active role in the interaction, whatever the channels it could exploit. This strongly modifies the traditional way of playing with toys, where the player decides what to do with the toy and how to play. With a robot, this responsibility is shared. From one side, this may be interesting for subjects that cannot easily decide what to do with a toy: a robot can stimulate reactions, or respond to even simple interactions, enhancing the sense of control of the situation. From the other side, the autonomy of the robot may stimulate attention, memorization, planning, possibly negotiation: most of the abilities needed to play (and interact in general) with people. This is one of the original aims of playing.

A robot can be designed to engage a person in one-to-one playing activities, thus enabling situations where persons with disabilities may decide to play even if nobody else is assisting them, so improving their autonomy and, at the same time, relieving care-givers and families from the burden of continuously assisting a person.

A robot can also be a motivation to interact with others, to show how to play with it, or to play all together. This can be a way to foster inclusion. The game should be designed to exploit the abilities of all the players, possibly requiring also to people with no disability to use some reduced ability, as part of the play contract.

A tele-operated or tele-controlled robot can be used as an avatar, to play without being involved in presence. Controlling a robot may be satisfactory per se, and this is already a good motivation for this setting. An avatar can do things that a person cannot do (e.g., seeing, or moving in a controlled way) so it may empower a person with disabilities. A robot has its own limitations, so, used in a game by a person with other abilities, may make available only some possibilities to interact with the world; a relevant aspect of play is related to the decision to cope with difficulties, for fun. It has been said that playing consists in putting ourselves in a challenging situation just for the fun to cope with it.

Finally, what it is possible to do with an avatar is different from what it is possible to do with a person. We have seen in play for the sake of play interactions that subjects decided to hit the robot, or to tear it down, or to kiss it. This might not have been done with a person, being this a therapist or a companion: the robot can open new expression possibilities.

Another motivation to have a robot involved in play activities is that it may be equipped by sensors that could record data useful both for the progress of the play, and for objective evaluation of the performance, which could be used to plan new activities and possibly assess progress in skill acquisition.

5.2 Aims and Issues

The main goal for a robot to play is to engage the other (human) player(s), since this is the aim for any player, and the robot should be perceived as a play companion. When the players play for the sake of play they are continually defining and redefining rules of playing, rules that actually define the fact that they are playing. If they are playing a game, rules are defined a priori and shared by the players. In both cases, the presence of rules and a setting define the fact that there is a play activity in act. As mentioned by De Koven [213], when we play, we are building a *community* that agrees to play in such a way that all players are enjoying the activity. To achieve this goal, the robot should comply to some general standpoints.

- The robot should have the *ability* to play, to understand and follow the play rules, to aim at the goal coherently with its role in the specific play activity: a robot perceived as not able to play is not a player. If there is no possibility to obtain the needed abilities with a robot, the game should be changed, either by design, or online by a supervisor (if any) or by the robot itself, or by the human player that should have been made aware of this possibility [213]. In play for the sake of play, this should happen dynamically and both the human player and the robot should be able to understand the possibilities of the other.
- The actions and reactions of the robot should be understandable by the human player. In particular, when playing for the sake of play it should be clear what is the signal that triggered an action, so that the play rules could be dynamically set. In most situations, also the goal of an action should be clear, from both sides, to assign a degree of rationality to the other player. Sharing, or discovering, causes and expected effects of actions is part of the play mechanism.
- The robot should not show to be too skilled for the game; if it is a competitive game, it should not show to be able to win all the time, otherwise the human player may get frustrated and lose engagement. In principle, the player should reach and maintain the state of *flow* [200] as long as possible, fully enjoying to play. This can be obtained only if the activity is easy enough to be manageable, and difficult enough to be a challenge. Of course, this may not be easy with players belonging from diverse populations, having different skills and attitudes. This issue puts in evidence the need for some adaptation capability in the robot and/or in its driver, if any.
- The robot should be able to exploit the possible disability of the player(s) in order to make them enjoying the game and feel to be included among the other players, if any.

In this book, we focus on playing activities where the robot fully exploits its physical being, so it moves, perceives, acts. Other types of technological games may be considered, most of which share some of the principles we are mentioning here, but we strongly believe that the physical interaction that is possible with a robot offers a large amount of possibilities that is worth to explore and exploit.

We have mentioned different categories of games in Chap. 2, and we discuss here the role a robot may have in each of them.

- *Practice play* includes simple body actions and visual and tactile experimentation of objects. The robot here may offer a set of reactions to its sensor perceptions that may enable free exploration of the relationship. This may develop confidence in controlling the situation, stimulate attention and engagement, support the formation of cause-effect relationships. The type of reactions should be compatible with the abilities and attitudes of the human player. Reactions should be clear and clearly related to the action the player can do. Discovering what are these actions, and how to perform them is part of the activity, triggered by curiosity. This means that the set of reactions should be rich, possibly matching the quality of actions that the player can perform. For instance, if the player can only perform rough movements, with strong acceleration, a robot to be manipulated should not be designed to react to precise movements, but should be able to recognize general features of the movement, such as a qualitative direction, or average acceleration, or composite movements like shaking. A reaction compatible with the recognized movement (e.g., a cry when shaken too strongly, or a pleasure sound and a smooth vibration when moved slowly) is possibly getting to the goal.
- *Symbolic play* involves giving a different meaning to objects, persons, actions, or events. Here, the robot can take a role, impersonate a character, behaving accordingly, participating in a story, not necessarily exploiting natural language, but behaving coherently with the assigned role. Sometimes, it may be enough a simple characterization, and leave the players to complete it in their mind.
- *Constructive play* consists of building or assembling something. Physical construction needs good manipulation, which is usually not available for the category of autonomous robots we are considering. However, it is possible to explore constructive play by driving a robot, like a robotic arm to build simple structures (e.g., with wooden bricks), or a vehicle to push bricks to build a wall. We may extend the principle of "building" and consider building a story, or setting a path to make the robot reaching a goal by following a line traced on the floor, or by avoiding obstacles it can find along a path.
- *Play with rules* encompasses all those play activities that have rules accepted and followed by the players, i.e., games. In this case, we need to have defined and shared the rules of a proper game. The robot should be able to follow the rules, and there should be someone, the players (robot included), or someone of the public that plays the referee role, in charge of checking that rules are followed. Rules may be designed or adapted to exploit the abilities of all the players in the way that implements a fair game.

5.3 The Player

The players, both human and robot, may have different characteristics, abilities, engagement attitudes, and mood. The designer of the play activity should consider all these aspects and devise a setting where all can play and enter the flow condition. This requires a clear identification of the functionalities needed to play, which have to be recognized and declared before playing. When we start playing, a kind of silent contract is virtually signed among the players, to behave as the activity requires, and to be free to change the game or leave whenever the activity becomes no longer interesting [127].

Achieving engagement is a task to be seriously considered. This requires to keep the play at the correct challenge level, and, at the same time, to satisfy the primary play stimuli: curiosity, and mastering. Animacy tends to support this aim: an object that is behaving in a way similar to a biological being rises expectations and curiosity. As this object is far from a bio-inspired aspect and possibilities in sensors and actuators, as much curiosity rises and expectations lower. Therefore, a trade-off between bio-inspiration and abstraction is to be targeted. The right proportion may be different for different players, and, since the robot body cannot be much modified, most of adaptation should be obtained by motion, sound, lights and behaviour.

Issues may arise when there are more players playing with the robot. In single-player activities, the robot is interacting only with one player and it could adapt to the player's needs. In parallel play, either the players interact independently with their own robot, or alternate on the same robot, while the others are playing with something else in the same environment. In this last case, the shift in the possibility to directly interact with the robot should be managed smoothly, to avoid to originate a cause for conflict that should be then managed. In cooperative play, the robot is a tool to play with, the players may interact with it all together, but this will reduce the possibility for the robot to effectively participate in the interaction. The best situation is when the play community agree to interact at turn with the robot, possibly aiming at achieving the same goal. Turn-taking is one of the abilities that should be developed in kids, particularly in children with intellectual disabilities.

5.4 The Design of Play Activities with Robots

We list here some notes to drive the design play activities with robots.

- *The play activity should be designed so that robot and players can effectively play.* Abilities of all the players should be taken into account and matched by the definition of the play activity. Moreover, the possibilities of all the players should be declared at the beginning so that everybody is aware of what is the play situation, and act accordingly.
- *The play activity should not require special attention other than what it is needed to play.* The robot should be able to play, so there should be no need to pay special attention to make it playing, if this alters the spirit of the activity. All the attention should be dedicated to play, not to take care of the possibly poor performance of the

robot. The play activity should be defined such that the robot, as well as any other admitted player, could play. In particular, if the robot has not enough capabilities, the play activity should be re-designed to make it exploit its possibilities to play.
- *The play activity should be engaging for the players.* In particular, the players should be motivated to play, by curiosity and/or challenge, so that they may autonomously decide to participate to the game. As we will see in the next chapters, in most cases play activities are proposed to the player as part of a therapy session and may be taken more as an exercise, something that "should be done" instead than a play activity. One of the roles of the robot should be to transform this situation in a play situation, triggering interest that may lead to fun.
- *The play activity should adapt to the player mood and abilities.* Adaptation is important since everybody has particular needs, interests, and also moods that affect the participation to the play activity. The robot should try to match them. This can be made offline, by setting parameters of the robot and of the play activity, or also online, if the robot has the ability to detect what is needed from the analysis of the available signals.

5.5 Robot and Game Design for the Market

An important issue arises when we decide to consider the market. As we will see in Chaps. 7 and 8, play experiences can be designed either with robots that reached the market or with prototypes that still have not left the research labs.

As known, to reach the market there are cost-effectiveness issues to be considered. The regular toy market is highly competitive and tends to offer products at a low price, in many cases not customizable, except for the toys aimed at customizing the body to program the build robot exploring different configurations. With this type of robots, the design of the play activity should exploit the available possibilities, and usually develops around the elements that could be added to the robot or the playground to make playing interesting and accessible to the players. Examples are provided in Chap. 7.

On the other side, experiments are done in research labs and care centres with prototypes or with robots that hardly could directly reach the mass market because of their cost or of their relatively low reliability (see Chap. 8). In most of these cases, the play experience is aimed at some sort of therapeutic session, and it is used to understand what may be the relevant aspects of such kind of intervention, leaving to somebody else the role of making it a possible product for the benefit of a large number of people. These experiences, usually done in a context of research and exploration of features and possibilities, may provide useful insights about what could be done to obtain interesting play activities.

We will see that, in both cases, the type of play activity may be analyzed within the so far presented framework, so that it would be possible to select or produce the robot that best matches the needs.

Chapter 6
The Role of Robots in Play Activities for Persons with Disabilities

Andrea Bonarini

Abstract How could robots play in inclusive, physical games? Issues and opportunities are introduced in this chapter. A robot is different from a simple toy, since it can produce its own reactions, and, possibly, take initiatives. This ability provides a new dimension to the use of the play instrument, which does not require the creative act of inventing a kind of pretended interaction, or the cognitive load of following game rules, but enables the engagement in a relationship with an active object. This may be easier than playing with inanimate toys, and reassuring, for instance, for people affected by neuro-developmental disorders. Moreover, it gives the possibility to play autonomously, without the need for assistance, and, possibly, to play with companions. Independent play is an important achievement for persons with disabilities. It may be also possible to provide the robot with sensors that can collect data about play that may be used to objectively assess the progress of the players. We discuss in this chapter what can be the role of a robot in inclusive play, and what are the requirements to obtain a successful experience.

6.1 Play and Disability

Different types of disabilities may enable different types of play. The aim of studying inclusive robotic play is not to provide tools that could be used by everyone, but to develop devices and experiences that can match specific needs. As we will see, it is possible to develop devices that could be accessible by people with different disabilities, as well as play experiences playable by many, but the goal of full coverage of all cases with a single robot cannot be achieved, while nice, inclusive experiences may be designed also to match specific disabilities.

In the next section are listed categories of disabilities, as described in Chap. 3 and the corresponding accessibility and playability conditions that may enable a satisfactory playing activity. In Part III, examples of some of the systems that implement some of the presented possibilities are presented, while we have preferred to present in this chapter only general suggestions that may stimulate the development of new play activities.

A. Bonarini and S. Besio, *Robot Play for All*, Research for Development,
https://doi.org/10.1007/978-3-031-05042-8_6

6.1.1 Physical Impairments

People with physical impairments are not only limited in movements, but may have also perceptive, attentional, motivational, cognitive, and emotional-affective limitations, that should be taken into account to design the play activity. Practice play may be oriented to manipulation of robotic objects that may produce movements, light or sounds when manipulated in a certain way. The robot should consider that the player cannot produce precise movements, so the trigger to obtain some effect should come from gross movements, possibly detected by accelerometers embedded in the body, which has to offer handles (e.g., arms, legs, big nose) designed to enable sure grasping. The cause-effect relationship should be evident, so that even an imprecise movement should trigger an easily identifiable effect. If sound can be produced, in any way, as vocalization or through an instrument, the robot may react to sound intensity, or even frequency. For instance, it may move ("dance") or make sounds ("sing") answering to notes played on a keyboard, possibly adapted to be used. Timing is essential to make it possible to understand the cause-effect relationship between stimulus and action.

Another explored possibility consists in providing the access, through augmentative technology (AT), to the control of a robot, either an arm or a vehicle. These may be used both also for construction play and for symbolic play, where the robots may play roles in a story.

Once the robot can be used to provide operational abilities needed for a game, it is also possible to play rule-based games, provided that the required ability be compatible with what the robot can express when driven by the person.

Another interesting possibility involves mobility. Often, people with physical impairments use electric wheelchairs to move, and they acquire good skills in operating them, which may be challenged and improved. Play activities may be defined where the wheelchair becomes a tool to move around and interact with the robot, in a game that involves reaching a goal whose complexity is compatible with the abilities of the player. In other play activities, the wheelchair itself may be the robot to interact with, if equipped with sensors and play enabling software.

When these people can actively participate to the game, they enjoy interacting with others. It is thus possible to implement social game situations where different people with the same disabilities interact, e.g., through robots that they drive to achieve a competitive (e.g., sumo, race, hit-the-skittle) or a collaborative goal (e.g., clean the playground from big boxes). The game should be even, otherwise the player with a poor performance may abandon; to achieve this goal, the robots may also be tweaked to obtain similar performances when driven by people with different abilities. This would enable the inclusion of people with physical abilities in play activities with normally developed people.

6.1.2 Intellectual Disabilities and Autism

The term "intellectual disabilities" covers a really wide range of situations, and the characteristic of each one should be considered to design a successful robotic play experience. We may have high level subjects with ASD, who may show some social issues, but can participate actively to most play activities (and many of the experiences reported in literature are done with this type of people), or we may have people that have difficulties to associate symbols to colours, or to keep attention for more than a short time on some object or activity. Each one needs to put attention on different aspects to design the play activity.

As discussed in Chap. 2, among the most common issues, we may have verbal comprehension, working memory, attention, perceptual reasoning, quantitative reasoning, abstract thought, and cognitive efficacy. Problems in verbal comprehension reflect on verbal expression and social relationships. Verbal interaction is difficult and should be guided. Natural language effective dialogue management is still problematic also from the robot side, so play activities based on natural language exchanges may not be easy to implement.

These subjects show, in general, a strong interest for technology, mostly when it refers to known elements such as everyday situations, or cartoons. The shape of robots may recall something known so to make these players at easy, and feel safe, in a comfortable situation. Many of them, especially people with ASD, may be sensible to specific things or features. Some of them may be extremely reactive to some specific colour, strong sounds, or elements such as a face; therefore, even the body of the robot should be ready to be adapted, and, actually, many of the robots used with subjects with ASD are designed to make it possible to eliminate the face, or reduce the sound intensity or the rhythm of lights.

Difficulties in remembering may reflect on difficulty in participating to games with complex rules, so, even when rule play is possible, rules should be very simple and the effects of the actions of all the players should be clear and immediate to be connected to the stimulus that has generated it. Cause-effect relationships can be well accepted if clear; exploring the reactions of a robot may be interesting, if these reactions are not disturbing. There may be a tendency, mostly in people with ASD, to repeat actions that provoke a known reaction, as a kind of confirmation of the ability to obtain it. The robot itself or an adult may help the children to explore something different to disengage her/him from a too stereotypical behaviour.

People with ASD are attracted by details that come unfiltered to their perceptual systems. This brings them a lack of attention that reflects on some play abilities. A robot may try to attract attention with smooth and nice movements, which may not be perceived as disturbing, and gradually gain attention and induce the exploration in free play. Many interesting and sometimes unexpected reactions may happen in free play, when the robot can match the needs of the specific children. The interest in details may also be considered to capture attention. If details are interesting for a specific person, for instance details on the body of the robot, the robot can interact in a way that exploits this interest to capture attention and engage the children in further activities, such as being followed, or try to catch the interesting spot.

Poor movement control, mostly in people with Down syndrome, may lead to actions that may harm the e-robot or the co-player. The robot should react to these possibly violent actions, so to induce a sort of social containment not imposed by an adult, but directly coming from the tool used to play; the play contract may have a role in making the containment understandable and acceptable.

Self-regulation is another issue that may be educated, for instance with play activities that require turn-taking, where the interaction with other human players, or even the robot itself, is subject to the simple rule that an action can be done only by the agent that is in charge to do it in the current turn.

There are many robotic activities that are aimed at making the children imitate the robot's gestures. We consider this activity more a kind of exercise than a play activity, but if done in a non-prescriptive way, involving robot and players in a play activity that naturally requires gestural expression, this may become a kind of play.

Role-playing is often difficult because it requires a good cognitive status, but simple roles may be taken in a well-defined context, possibly integrated with the reality of the life of the subject, and a kind of pretend play may emerge.

Attention is a critical issue: any activity should be short and interesting enough to keep the attention. Play for the sake of play with an autonomous robot may have this characteristic since activities are short cause-effect exchanges and develop naturally from the interaction, so also preventing the negative surprise effect that sudden changes may induce. Certainly, the robot's actions should be smooth enough to avoid to be scary; it should be possible to predict them (this may be supported by announcing them or providing explicit cues), and they should be clearly related to activities of the player. For instance, sophisticated relationships between relative positions of the robot and the player may not be understood, and induce insecurity, while a natural, simple interaction (such as keeping a distance, or getting slowly closer), may be better accepted.

Joint attention could be obtained with robots that may act as companions, which is possible to trust once they have gained confidence. The robot may share attention with the player on something interesting, for instance a toy to play with, and the next activity may be to play together with that toy (e.g., making the plush riding the robot, or throwing a ball to the robot).

Social play can be played by a robot that may become the centre of attraction for the activity done by different players: to satisfy its "needs" the players may do something that may involve physical activity, possibly integrated with some simple cognitive activity. Physical activity is needed to engage the players, cognitive activity may be a plus that adds interesting possibilities to the basic play situation.

6.1.3 Sensor Disabilities

The role of robots in play activities with people with sensor disabilities is to enable them to participate to an engaging and playful experience. This means to use robots to exploit the present abilities. Literature is not rich about robots playing with people with this type of disability.

Visual Impairment

For people with visual impairment, one of the known issues is the lack of physical activity. Many sports have been modified to be accessed by these people [426] and technology has also been used for this purpose, e.g., using vibro-tactile sensors to enable the participation to exergames [487]. There are also proposals to use robots to enable physical activity, e.g., to guide them running with a robot drone [258], or to support in assembling a Tangram puzzle, by physically guiding the selection and the placement of pieces with an industrial robot, remotely driven by an operator [97]. However, none of these activities can be properly considered as play.

What a robot could do to support blind people in playing, in particular, physical games? As we have seen in Sect. 3.5, many issues may arise if visual impairment affects children from the beginning of their life. The lack of visual comparison may delay the development of associations between concepts and terms, which are one of the bases for cognition. The lack of orientation may develop a general sense of uncertainty and insecurity. The development of play activities with robots should consider these aspects.

For instance, it would be possible to use the motor sound as a way to signal where the robot is and where it is going, so that, in an open space without any other obstacle, a kid-size, soft robot may try to escape, in a tag game. If equipped with a human detection system, it may also try to catch the player, or to throw balls to her/him. All these play activities should be done in free, delimited, safe space, and the robot itself should have a soft body and move so to prevent actions dangerous for the player(s). As done already with blind football (a paralympic game) it is also possible to ask all the players to wear a blinding mask so that also people without visual impairment can participate in the game sharing the same disability.

A free play activity may involve reactions of the robot to sound or touch. For instance, the robot can take a direction according to the frequency of the voice or an instrument like a flute or a whistle (a note), and may react with interesting sounds. If the robot can declare what it is doing, and maybe what it is perceiving (e.g., "I'm detecting an obstacle at 40 cm"), it is also possible to drive it to a target that is making a possibly interesting and contextualized sound.

Tools such as ReCog [3] and the others developed by the same group at IBM use AI to recognize objects and elements of the environment and describe them so that people that cannot see them may become aware of what is around. These are available on mobile phones, so they may be easily integrated in game systems that can interact also with robots.

For younger children, a manipulable robot providing sound and vibration reactions to different types and positions of touch may also be interesting to be explored.

Auditory Impairment

People with auditory impairments can actually participate to activities that do not involve the hearing channel, like most of the possible activities, including those presented in this book. For them, we should consider that no auditory feedback can be perceived, so all kind of feedback should be provided along the other channels, e.g., through movement or light, including visualization of signals on screen. Another critical issue concerns possible rules for a game, which have to be presented by a text or sign language, if there is enough competence to understand any of these, or by examples. In general, complex rules may be difficult to be remembered and organized, so simple games should be devised.

6.2 Inclusion

We interpret inclusive play as the possibility of a person with disability to play together with other persons, both normally developed and persons with disability: all should enjoy playing.

Both device and experience design affect inclusion, and it is often enough to consider inclusion in the design process to implement a play experience that may really be inclusive, even with devices not explicitly designed for this.

Play can be inclusive if the conditions for playing are satisfied for all the players, i.e., if they have similar possibilities to play also in non-competitive games. Competition is often a motivation for playing, but it may not be relevant or effective with many kinds of disability, in particular where cognitive abilities are compromised. However, the self-satisfaction for being able to achieve a goal is present in most players. If the possibilities of participation are not equally distributed among the players, it is possible to intervene either on the robot, on its interface (for instance the interface to control it), on the settings (the playground, how to access the game elements, ...), and, not less relevant, the structure of the play activity itself. For instance, it may be interesting to have a buddy flanking the player with disabilities, possibly suggesting what to do, but always leaving space for a full expression of the abilities and the decisions of the main player.

6.3 Data Collection

An important aspect of the presence of a robot in a play activity is related to the fact that it can collect data by its sensors to enable objective evaluation of the activity and the analysis of possible progress in a series of play sessions.

For instance, we have implemented at AIRLab–POLIMI a game where a person receives a ball that embeds an accelerometer and a gyroscope. The person has to launch the ball against a target placed either on the floor or on the wall. The target

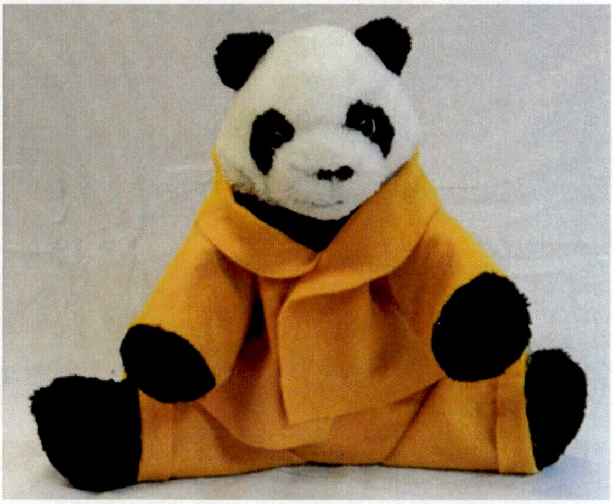

Fig. 6.1 Kung, a panda plush developed in different instances at AIRLab-POLIMI. It has been used as a plush for free play, and as a doll for a dressing game

can sense touch. Both ball and target are wireless connected to a ground station, to provide data about the performance. These data can then be analyzed to evaluate objectively the kind of movement the subject had performed, how much time the subject had taken to decide to launch, how was the trajectory of the ball, whether the target was reached or not. The system can provide both sound and movement as feedback, which is often perceived as the game target, and motivates to play and aim at a good performance.

In another setting, accelerometer and gyroscope sensors embedded in a panda plush are used to monitor the manipulation of the object, to provide feedback about different recognized gestures (hit, shake, throw, pickup, drop, idle), to record how the object has been manipulated, e.g., by people with movement impairments, and to monitor whether the plush is used in a violent and potentially dangerous way, possibly stimulated by the affordance provided by arms and legs, or protruding body elements; in this case, the panda reacts with sounds trying to prevent the dangerous situation [8, 771].

Another instance of the same panda (Kung, Fig. 6.1) has been equipped also by sensors able to detect whether the right cloth has been put on in the right way. This was requested by a psychologist operating in a care centre to stimulate attention, manipulation and identification of the right pieces. There are jacket and trousers and the panda gives a feedback when it perceives that the right one is on (it is not possible to put on the wrong one), or when too much time has passed since the beginning. Again, data about manipulation modalities and time can be recorded and then analyzed.

A more recent version of Teo [114],[1] Oimi (Fig. 6.2), has been equipped with a camera and Deep Learning devices (Google Coral, and Intel Movidius2) to detect objects, the subject's skeleton and direction of sight (Fig. 6.3), so making it possible

[1] A description of Teo is provided in Sect. 8.2.

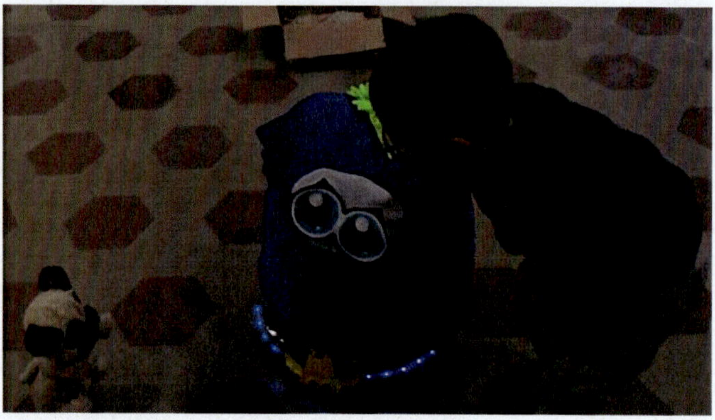

Fig. 6.2 Oimi, an omnidirectional robot developed in different instances at AIRLab-POLIMI, in action to bring the attention on the puppy dog plush

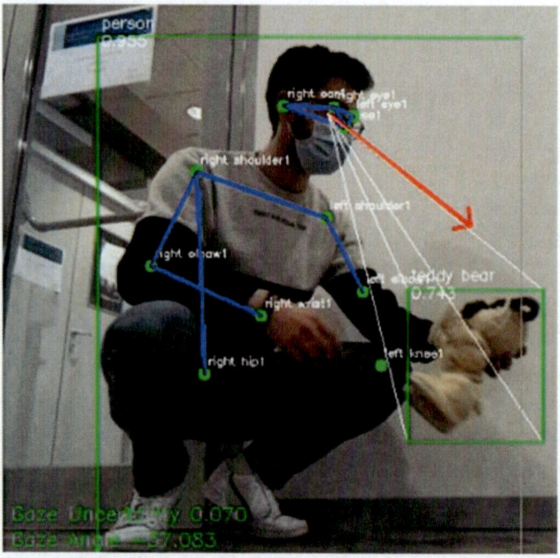

Fig. 6.3 The recognition of a plush and some subject's skeleton points. From these data, it is possible to compute their position, as well as the direction of sight of the subject

to have in real-time data about joint attention that the robot tries to induce in subjects with autism, or attention deficits, in general. Automatic computation of eye contact and attention can be performed without the need of any manual tagging of the acquired movies.

A detailed log of all the activities, including timing, attention shift, and whatever could be deduced from the robot's sensors can be recorded and analyzed to produce an objective report about what happened in the session. The intrinsic limits of the sensory apparatus and of the interpretation system should be considered when using these data for assessment and may be integrated by data observed by the care-giver to obtain a complete and still objective set of data to be analyzed.

6.4 Usability and Accessibility

Both usability and accessibility play a relevant role for the acceptance of a robot in a play activity with people with impairments. A general set of considerations about usability and accessibility for toys has been already presented in Sect. 2.9.2. We recall here the basic principles and definitions as well as the structure of a set of guidelines that we have defined to evaluate and consider them in the design of technological toys, including robots.

Usability is defined as "the extent to which a product can be used by specified users to achieve specified goals with effectiveness, efficiency and satisfaction in a specified context of use" (ISO 9241-11:2018 [364]).

Accessibility is defined as "the extent to which products, systems, services, environments and facilities can be used by people from a population with the widest range of characteristics and capabilities to achieve a specified goal in a specified context of use" (ISO 9241-11:2018 [364]). Accessibility involves both ease of use and success of use (ISO/IEC Guide 71:2014 [365]). It is clear that the two concepts in our case merge in the call for robots that could effectively participate in the specified play activity enabling the specific users to play their role and to enjoy the full richness of the play activity.

It is not possible to assume that everybody can have a specific play experience with a robot, since this would limit the number of possibilities to develop play experiences targeted to specific players. However, in the definition of a play activity and of a robot player, we need to know what are the abilities required to have access to the game. An analysis of the game and of the players may also bring to different versions of a robot or a play experience that can match different specific needs.

In [368], we have reviewed some of the guidelines and tools available to design technological objects that may be used to play by considering accessibility and usability. In [367], we have proposed some guidelines for such development, whose structure is summarized in the rest of this section. This work has been developed within the COST EU Network "LUDI: play for children with disabilities" in collaboration with care givers, therapists, persons with disabilities, and engineers.

These guidelines consider different figures that may need support in the development or selection of a technological device for a play activity, namely: parents, professionals, designers, makers, and researchers. Each one has different needs, in particular: parents would like to identify the proper tool and play activity for their children, professionals would like to design a play activity and select a tool to achieve a therapeutic goal, designers should design the technological device and the play activity so that they can be accessible and usable, makers may need to understand also how to hack existing devices to make them accessible and usable, and researchers are aimed to develop research and trials to improve knowledge.

For each figure, reflective questions are first proposed to frame the situation and make all the relevant aspects emerging. Then a guided track drives the user through evaluation steps to consider the different aspects involved in accessibility and usability. The tracks are different for each figure, since the needs of each one are different.[2]

[2] We leave the interested reader to the original paper [367] available open source from https://sciendo.com/chapter/9788395669613/10.1515/9788395669613-008.

Part III
Experiences with Playing Robots

This part is dedicated to present playing experiences designed to include technological toys, commercial and experimental robots, to discuss ethical issues related to robotic play, as well as to identify and frame the possible activities that have not yet implemented, but could be designed and foreseen in a next future.

Chapter 7
Existing Robotic Toys

Andrea Bonarini

Abstract In this chapter, we present some of the categories of robots that the market is presently offering to play with, and what it is possible to do with commercial robotic toys, including the toys that are not presented as robots, but actually comply with the definitions given in Chap. 4. Millions of robotic toys reach our homes every year. The framework defined in Chap. 4 drives the analysis of categories of robotic toys, their features, and their possible limitations to be used for inclusive play.

7.1 Toy Categories

Robots have triggered imagination and expectations for centuries and have been implemented as toys well before technological advancements could make them available to the large public. We are considering here only toys that match the robot definitions given in Chap. 4. They started to reach the mass market when technology had become mature enough to make it possible to implement at a relatively low cost enough reliable devices that could be attractive as toys.

In the analysis, we consider the main categories introduced here below. In Sect. 7.2 we will mention how it is possible to play with robots belonging to each of them.

- *Pets*. In this category are included robots imitating pets (e.g., FurReal,[1] Joy for all,[2] Therabot [76]), but also robots that may substantially react to caresses and food, either with animal-like body (e.g., Moflin[3] Paro [632], Qoobo,[4]) or cartoon-like body. Some of them are relatively rich in sensors, like Furby,[5] which can react to sounds and shake, and Pleo,[6] which has also touch, distance, and food sensors. They are usually non-programmable, and have pre-defined reactions implemented both

[1] https://furreal.hasbro.com/.

[2] https://joyforall.com/.

[3] https://www.indiegogo.com/projects/moflin-an-ai-pet-with-emotional-capabilities#/.

[4] https://qoobo.info/.

[5] https://furby.hasbro.com/en-us.

[6] https://www.pleoworld.com/pleo_rb/eng/products.php.

A. Bonarini and S. Besio, *Robot Play for All*, Research for Development,
https://doi.org/10.1007/978-3-031-05042-8_7

by moving parts of the body, by emitting sounds, or sometimes, when compatible with the character and market price, by using lights and facial expressions.

- *Tele-controlled and tele-operated robots*. From the old wire-controlled cars, to the new robot-shaped devices and flying robots, controlled by joy stick or smartphone, tele-controlled robots may be either vehicles or arms. Most of them are dummy: direct commands can drive them around, and, sometimes, can make them emit sounds or light signals. They are suitable to impersonate driven characters.
  Tele-operated robots can be remotely controlled not only in their low-level movements, but also to activate behaviours either through remote control or through voice and gestures (e.g., Zoomer[7]). Sometimes, tele-operated robots can be programmed at least in easy ways to select pre-defined behaviours corresponding to high-level commands, or facing situations possibly detected by sensors.
- *Programmable robots*. These have sensors, usually can move around and produce sounds and light. They may be shaped as vehicles (e.g., Edison,[8] Pixy,[9] Dash and Dot[10]), or even balls (e.g, Sphero[11]). Also LEGO Mindstorms®,[12] can be considered in this category, since it adds to the traditional LEGO possibility to make objects by bricks the possibility to integrate sensors and actuators connected to a computing brick that can be programmed.
  They can be programmed either by graphic languages like Scratch [582] or Blockly [268, 529], or common, general programming languages, such as C, C++, or Python.
  Often, programming (and building in the case of LEGO Mindstorms®) are done by persons without impairments to produce in a short time adapted robots that could be used also to play.
- *Button-operated robots*. These robots have coloured buttons that trigger actions. In some cases, the possible actions are limited to simple movements associated to music (e.g., dance or sing), in other cases, the robot may ask questions that are answered by pressing buttons. Usually, their body is implemented in robust plastic materials, often robot-shaped but also having a shape coherent with a context (e.g., a school-board or a farm with animals), and they cannot be programmed. One of these robots is depicted in Fig. 7.1.
- *Robotic assembly*. These are robots that can be assembled in many different ways and then programmed. The first commercial success was LEGO Mindstorms® [249, 445, 721], which adds a programmable controller, motors, and sensors to the classical LEGO construction possibilities. ClicBot[13] and EZ-Bot[14] make it possible to

---

[7] https://www.zoomerpup.com.

[8] https://meetedison.com/.

[9] https://it.clementoni.com/products/pixy.

[10] https://www.makewonder.com/.

[11] https://sphero.com.

[12] https://www.lego.com/en-us/themes/mindstorms.

[13] https://keyirobot.com/.

[14] https://www.ez-robot.com/.

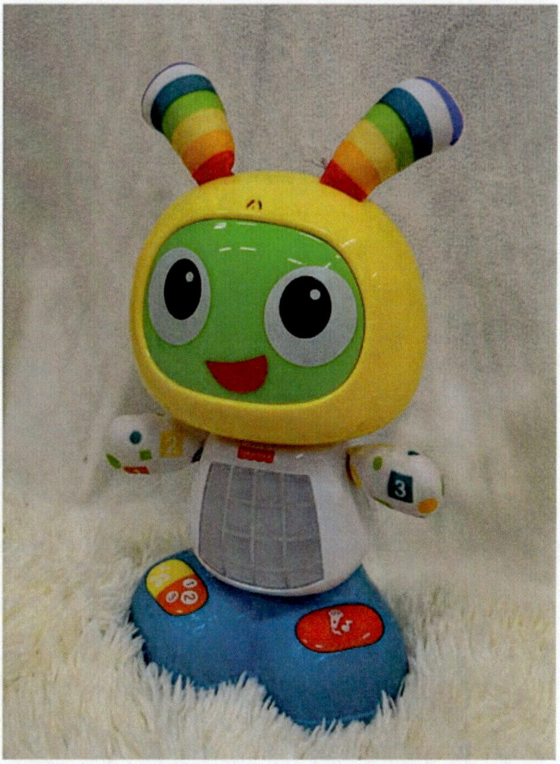

Fig. 7.1 A commercial button-operated robot. Buttons on the feet activate different modalities. This robot can dance, sing, and show coloured lights

assembly and control both arms and mobile robots, with few modules. Cubelets™[15] provide a set of cubes with different functionalities (sensors, motors, power) that can be magnetically assembled to build a robot with simple functionalities interacting with the external world according to the way it is assembled, without the need of being programmed with any programming language, in a kind of "programming-by-assembly" way.

- *Autonomous robots*. In this category are robots that can act autonomously in the world using sensors and actuators.
  Many autonomous robots are complex devices, usually implemented with a plastic body, whose size is between 50 and 130 cm, quite expensive, intended to be programmable and to be considered as social robots to be used in interactive applications, including playing. Examples are the small humanoid Nao [296], the child-sized half humanoid Pepper [518], and the animal-humanoid robot Sanbot.[16] An interesting autonomous robot for which a wide set of pre-programmed activities have been implemented explicitly to interact with persons with disabilities

[15] https://modrobotics.com/.

[16] https://www.sanbot.co.uk.

is Leka[17] a commercial evolution of Roball [480]. It is a rolling, transparent ball including a screen and interaction capabilities. The ball shape reminds one of the basic toys, and autonomous movement and expression trigger curiosity and engage the player.
Although we tend to consider autonomous robots as very complex machines, actually there are robots in this category that show relatively simple behaviours, but are fully autonomous, like HexBug Nano®[18], and the Ghostbug Caterpillar, already presented in Chap. 4.

7.2 Playing with Robots Available on the Market

Having defined the main categories of robots that can be found on the market, we report for each of them some of the play activities that have been or could be implemented considering people with special needs. Let us remember that there are a lot of ways to use any object (including a robot) to play, and we can list here only some of them, with the aim to inspire applications and further exploration.

7.2.1 Pets

The main activities that could be done with robots belonging to this category are based on the kind of interaction that they may enable. With respect to a traditional teddy bear-like plush, these robots can react to sensor stimuli, thus enabling the implementation of a cause-effect mechanism that could be recognized, and also searched for confirmation. Robots like the Paro baby seal have been used both with elderly affected by dementia (e.g., [601]), and with autistic children (e.g., [65]). These people obtain a feedback from caressing, or from giving "food", or from a limited number of other actions. The motion and sensor richness is mostly constrained by market motivations like cost: there is a difference of two orders of magnitude between the cost of Paro and that of a commercial toy with similar appearance, with the expected repercussions on reliability and the complexity of the interaction. However, limited interaction possibilities may be acceptable and beneficial for people with limited cognitive or sensory capacities, since they can usually manage only a small number of alternatives, and too many possibilities may create confusion and disaffection. The same holds for people with motor control issues: although these robots may be used to recover raw and fine motor control, e.g., by triggering reactions to some of them, a high number of gestures obtaining different reactions from the robot may be confusing and difficult to distinguish from each other.

---

[17] https://leka.io.

[18] https://www.hexbug.com/nano.

Among the sensors we may find on robotic pets, a common one is a magnetic sensor, typically used to detect "food" consisting in a magnet embedded in some plastic-made food appearance. The robot may react to the presence of food in the mouth, but usually it is not designed to actually eat the food. This means that it may not be suitable for children not able to perform pretend play, which requires imagination: the action "provide food" may be effective to obtain a feedback, so to activate the cause-effect relationship, but may not hold the cognitive effect of "providing food", which has consequences on the sense of taking care, one of the possible targets for this play activity.

Other sensors are adopted to detect gestures like caresses or hugs. These are mostly implemented by capacitive sensors and are designed to detect proximity of a part of the human body to the sensor, usually embedded below the skin/fur. Although affordance of the robot body calls for the expected gestures, it is possible that these sensors trigger pleasure reactions from the robot also as a consequence of different ways to get close to the sensor, like a smash, or sitting over. The body design here plays a relevant role, providing, such as in the baby seal, a clear suggestion about the way to interact with the robot, as well as about the sensible parts. The skin of the robot has also its relevance in this kind of activities. Pleo, the baby dinosaur, has a plastic skin, coherent with the character, since a dinosaur is expected to have a hard skin. However, this does not naturally invite to caress, although it has been designed so that a caress triggers a well-designed behaviour to show pleasure. On the other side, the affordance provided by the long neck of Pleo, just close to the caress sensor placed on the head, may induce dangerous behaviours, since it calls to be taken in hand and to be shaken or even to throw the whole robot.

Another sensor that may be embedded in a robot pet is an accelerometer/gyroscope, used to detect how it is moved and manipulated. This may trigger reactions, but a proper detection of the movement is not easy to obtain reliably at a low cost and this possibility is not much explored in toys. A simpler sensor that detects shaking and reversing was implemented in Furby both to detect general activity, intended to promote the improvement of the robot's language from Furbish to English depending on the amount of activity, and, in the more recent versions, to enable a change of character of the toy, which becomes rude when agitated and reversed for a time long enough. These effects are quite long term, require continuous coherent actions, and usually cannot be perceived by people with cognitive disabilities, while people with other disabilities may understand the mechanism although the direct relationship with movement is not evident (except for the character shift), and may require good control of movement. Therefore, this is a not much effective mechanism to involve people playing. The other, more direct reactions of Furby may be more interesting.

7.2.2 Tele-Controlled and Tele-Operated Robots

These robots come mainly in the shape of vehicles, with a solid plastic body, or robotic arms, and can be controlled either by a dedicated remote control, or by a joystick or through an app running on smartphones and tablets. Vehicles can be controlled to move on the floor or on a table, thus enabling play activities related to spatial relations, while arms can be used to facilitate the interaction with objects.

Vehicles may be just driven around, exploiting the fine control abilities of the human players, but leaving them free to explore the play possibilities. Often, without a clear goal, this type of entertainment runs out quickly. It is possible to define targets to reach, or paths to follow, which may provide a goal to be achieved, and stimulate both fine motion abilities and cognitive abilities at different levels, depending on the complexity of the defined task. Unfortunately, these toys are usually not designed to be able to identify these goals, so the design and check of the play activity is on the assistant or the players themselves.

Arms may be used to move objects, grasp, pick and place. They are usually complex to operate at single joint level, but may be provided with pre-programmed routines that enable to perform basic actions on the simple push of a button, so they may be interesting for persons with disabilities.

These robots may become avatars to explore a world of possibilities, even when these are not accessible by their human controllers, due to their disabilities. For instance, we have tried to explore the possibility to control a fish-shaped blimp by subjects with motor disabilities, which gave them the possibility to virtually move and interact by flying around [74, 727]. In this specific case, we had to face a typical problem of toys not designed to be inclusive, i.e., the standard joystick was difficult to operate by these subjects and they had to be supported by the assistants to enjoy the experience, which was anyway much appreciated.

In another setting, we have sometimes observed in children affected by mild ASD, the use of the vehicle as a sort of avatar to try to interact both with the therapist or with a companion. We have also observed some competition between subjects in trying to get control of the robot, promptly exploited by the assistant to start a turn-taking game setting.

It is possible to define tasks (e.g., clean an area from bricks, or search for a ball and push it in a target), which provide further motivation to achieve a performance that may require to exploit and develop abilities.

In play for the sake of play, the players usually explore the way they can control the robot and soon come to face challenges like pushing heavy objects, disentangling the robot from obstacles and so on. As we already said, challenges are essential parts of play.

Tele-controlled robots can be used to implement social games, either competitive, like the classical sumo wrestling (push the opponent robot out a circular ring) or cooperative, like pushing together a brick to a target. The robot gives to the players the same body with the same possibilities, although differences may be present in the control abilities. Usually, commercial toys do not provide possibilities to adapt the controllers to match the uncommon abilities, but some systems may accept different types of controllers, often interfaced through standard protocols such as USB or Bluetooth, possibly designed just to match special abilities.

Tele-operated robots may have some sensors, mostly to detect obstacles (typically infrared sensors) and possibly to detect noise or speech; this gives them some extrapossibilities, automatically activated by sensor readings, like avoiding obstacles or reacting to sensor data (e.g., emitting a sound when getting close to an obstacle, or activating a pre-programmed behaviour in response to a vocal command). These may be used to implement cause-effect relationships that increase the engagement and the desire to play. In some of these robots, e.g., Zoomer, the activated behaviours are so engaging and well-designed that subjects aimed at activating them just for fun. Unfortunately, the quality of sensors does not always support a reliable interaction, possibly also due to the expression possibilities of the player, and this may induce frustration [74, 727]. Hence, the importance of identifying toys that could reliably support the declared features, or to set up a play activity where possible faults could be integrated in acceptable situations. For instance, if the game is based on score, this should not depend on sensor reliability. If there is a story that should go on, this should not depend on sensor reliability or there should be an escape possibility.

7.2.3 Programmable Robots

Programmable robots are proposed to players to program behaviours. This requires some cognitive and motion abilities not available to everybody, so this feature is not much directly exploited by persons with disabilities. However, the possibility to program behaviours of the robots, establishing a relationship between sensor readings and activity, is completely in the hands of the caregiver that could personalize the behaviour of the robot to the specific abilities and interests of the subject. This opens a full range of possibilities to implement games and playful activities, both based on more or less direct cause-effect relationship between the subject actions and the robot's response, or based on more complex activities such as question-answering games, theatrical interactions (e.g., [111]), pretend play, motion challenging games, and much more.

For instance, we have explored the possibilities given by Cubelets™ to program-by-assembly a robot that could implement many cause-effect relationships, for instance, it could escape when the player approaches with the hand the sensor on the top cube. This was implemented by simply putting the light sensor on top of the robot and arranging the Cubelets™ so that when there is a reduction of light on the sensor the robot runs away. This was tested with people with physical and cognitive impairments in a game where they had to "capture" the robot by taking care of not covering the sensor, so by controlling their movement [74, 727]. Even if magnetic connection makes the assembly of the robot simpler, they could not manage to do this autonomously, and also the basic behaviour of the robot was not easy to explore for these specific subjects.

7.2.4 Button-Operated Robots

These are very simple devices, aimed mainly at young kids, and the activity is based on simple action-reaction turns, either promoted by the robot or activated by the subject. Each turn requires a simple exchange and runs out with that. The type of activities that can be done here is based on the recognition of the button to operate and on the actual action to perform, which could be challenging for people with motor disability or visual impairments, but also for some people with cognitive impairments. The reward provided by the toy is often enough to engage the subject at least for a short sequence of activities.

7.2.5 Robotic Assembly

The robots belonging to this category are aimed at developing imagination and manual capabilities. The principal system belonging to this category is LEGO Mindstorms™, where the traditional possibilities to put together parts typical for LEGO are enhanced by a control brick that can be programmed either with a visual or textual language. Sensors and actuators can be connected to the control brick and it is possible to explore a wide range of possibilities building a body around them. People with cognitive disabilities may have problems to understand what to do to assemble a robot, and how to program it, while assembling may be challenging also for people with motion disabilities. However, as already seen for programmable robots, the subject may become the director of activities performed by assistants and companions, and contribute to build a robot that may reach a target, such as navigating in a maze, or collecting boxes, or turning down a paper tower. The assistants and partners could always set up a play setting appropriate for the subjects, where all can play with satisfaction, by following the basic principles mentioned in the previous chapters.

Other experiences have been done with Cubelets™ and people with physical and cognitive disabilities [74, 727]. Construction of the robot was too difficult, despite the well-designed magnetic connection among cubelets, because it requires fine motion control, anyway. Moreover, the function of each cubelet had to be experienced, or explained, in advance so that the assembly could be planned to obtain a behaviour. This requires cognitive abilities to imagine the possibilities offered by the cubelet, and short-term memory to remember them till the moment to assembly the robot. The task may be challenging even for normally developed young children.

7.2.6 Autonomous Robots

Autonomous robots do not need human intervention to operate. They may be pre-programmed, even with quite complex behaviours, or may implement simple behaviours that could be exploited anyway to implement interesting games.

It is interesting to consider what could be obtained by very simple autonomous robots such as HexBug, shown in Fig. 4.1, in Chap. 4. This is a vibrating robot that simply starts running on its vibrating rubber legs when turned on. The shape is designed so that when it encounters an obstacle simply bounces on it and continues running. It is possible to set up different games with it either by building race fields, where these robots should compete, or by building a closed environment with only a small opening to be reached to escape, or by participating in a more complex game (commercially available) where two bugs should reach the opposite exit, but the players may turn rotating elements on the field at each turn, to try to address their robot in the right direction and the opponent one in the wrong one. This is a strategic game, but strategy is often forgiven due to the short time to take decisions and can be used to stimulate both fine control of movements and turn-taking. A possible drawback is given by the relatively high speed of these robots that may prevent the generation of a proper action in people with some cognitive or physical impairments.

A different setting can involve the GhostBug caterpillar shown in Fig. 4.2 in Chap. 4, which has a distance sensor on the head so that, when it gets close to an obstacle it can turn back by a random angle and then start to go forward again. This can be used to try to address the robot to a target by putting in front of it an obstacle, or a hand. This stimulates strategy and fine control to position obstacles. Again, with two or more caterpillars it would be possible to implement also competitive games, or even cooperative ones, such as coordinated dancing. Since the speed is slow, the interaction with this robot is easier than with HexBug.

With the more complex autonomous robots any kind of play activity can be designed, exploiting the sensors that most of them have to detect obstacles, sounds, and in some cases also shape and pose of people. Many of them have also the possibility to self-localize, so they can offer a very wide range of possibilities, generally at a high cost. Given that most of these activities are performed in experimental settings, and that most of these robots cannot really be considered as toys, but rather expensive devices, we will present some of them in the next chapter, dedicated to research experiences.

Chapter 8
Experimental Robots

Andrea Bonarini

Abstract This chapter analyses, according to the presented framework, playful robots developed in research labs in the world and at Politecnico di Milano AI and Robotics Lab. In most cases, these have not reached the market nor development levels that could bring them to the real users in a real setting without the presence of the developers, but they have been used in experiments limited to labs or few, selected care centres or schools. However, it is interesting to analyse these experiences to understand what kind of playful activities have been explored, how these have been evaluated, what kind of outcomes have been obtained, and what kind of technologies have been used, since they trace the directions that are bringing to the next future products. At the end of the chapter, the scenarios to bring these innovative products to the market are analysed. These include the evaluation of effectiveness of this technology, and of the different characteristics that should be taken into account, such as playability, playfulness, accessibility, and usability.

8.1 Introduction to Experimental Robots

There is a vast literature about the use of robots by persons with disabilities (e.g., [1, 148, 210, 261, 340, 608]), and in many cases the reported activities are referred to as playful interventions, although often they do not fully satisfy the main characteristics of play experiences that we have introduced in Chaps. 2, 3, and 5. In the following, we will report many of these experiences, as examples of what could be done and has been tried. We have excluded all experiences with robots that do not exploit their physical body, but act only as tablet holders or speakers, since these types of playful activities are not designed as playful robot interactions. We have also excluded the play experiences where the robot plays a secondary role (e.g., of commentator) for a game to which it does not directly participate (e.g., [511, 539]), since we are focusing on playful robots and not on general social robot interaction. The focus is thus on robots directly involved in playful activities exploiting their physical body to play.

In most of the cases reported in this chapter, either the robots or the play activity, or both, are prototypes, sometimes tested with real users in a real setting, but not having reached a mass market, yet, as mentioned also in [340]. There may be many reasons

A. Bonarini and S. Besio, *Robot Play for All*, Research for Development,
https://doi.org/10.1007/978-3-031-05042-8_8

for this: either the prototype was designed to test an approach, but still needs further improvements, or the market is not the goal of the researchers that developed these robots and play activities, or the steps to reach the market have not been taken (yet) due to the need of resources to complete all the steps required to obtain a product from a prototype. In any case, research results continue to be collected and it is possible to foresee the time for commercialization of these results as it would be beneficial for a large set of potential users, when cost-effectiveness could be obtained.

This chapter is organized per type of playful activity, according to the categorization presented in Chap. 2.

8.2 Play for the Sake of Play

In play for the sake of play, the robot and the player interact freely without any predefined goal. To consider an activity as a play for the sake of play, the rules defining what is play should be satisfied. This requires that the players share the playing context and interact to set the interaction rules and possibly evolve them. Play for the sake of play may make emerging relationships that are enabled by the fact that the robot is either reacting to what it can perceive, or take the initiative to propose activities, so that it can have an active role in play development. The quality of the robot's actions is extremely relevant to trigger interesting behaviours and to engage the player. In particular, perceived *animacy* plays a relevant role in trusting the robot and recognizing it as a companion and able to participate in this type of play activity. The perception of animacy is enabled also by the robot's physical aspect, but, it is in large part related to the ability of the robot to interact, so to perceive inputs from the human player and to select an action that should be considered as related to the perception and play goals, as noticed also in [572].

For instance, in [667] is reported a comparison between the experience made with a toy dog, able to move but not to sense, and with AIBO, a robot dog that could react to actions perceived by a camera, a microphone, and touch sensors on the body. Eleven children with ASD were introduced one at the time to one of the two devices, and then to the other, and left interacting with it. The toy pet was quite similar to a small dog, the body covered by fur, while AIBO showed its robotic, plastic body. Despite the less pleasant touch experience, the fact that AIBO could react, and even show some patterned autonomous behaviours, made most of the subjects detect animacy in it, and start rich and natural interactions, while the pet toy elicited some interaction that was soon left for activities more related to the traditional toy nature of the object.

Teo [100, 114] was originally developed as a tool to be integrated with an external depth camera and projections on a big screen, to play a role in structured games, but a set of capabilities were also implemented to enable a free play activity, intended to be played as familiarization with the robot at the beginning of a session. The robot (see Fig. 8.1) has a 60 cm high soft body that offers an area where patches with Velcro™ on their back can be attached to compose a face with different expressions of eyes and mouth. It can run on omni wheels, freely in any direction, at a speed

Fig. 8.1 TeoG, a soft, omnidirectional robot developed in different instances at Politecnico di Milano—AIRLab

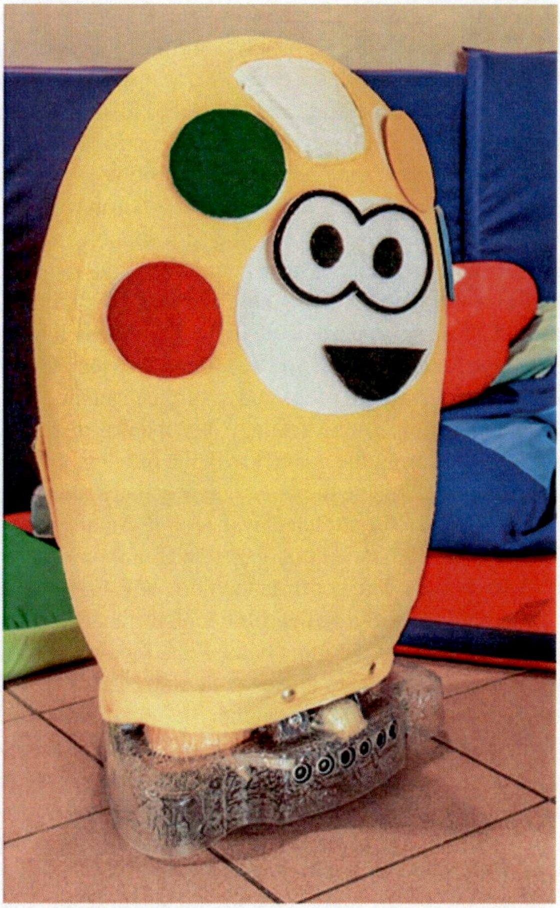

in the range of human speed (1.4 m/s). It can sense distance, movement (through an accelerometer), and localized touch on patches and on body parts like the back and the sides. It could also be remotely driven by joystick.

It turned out that many unexpected and interesting situations occurred during the play for the sake of play activity, more than in structured play. The free play activity usually started with the robot turned off, present in the room with the subject(s), ready to be explored. After a first familiarization with this static "big plush", the robot is turned on and starts gently to look for interaction.

At this point, in a case, a kid with ASD was surprised by the movement of the robot and then run against it, tearing it down. The reaction of the robot was to start crying. The child, surprised, turned it back standing, then went to look for a piece of yellow cloth, the same colour of the robot body, offering it to the robot in reparation.

In another case, again in the familiarization activity, one of the two involved kids with mild ASD, independently working around the robot, without interacting with each other, noticed that the robot was tele-controlled by the operator, and asked to have the remote control. Once become the robot controller, one kid used Teo to search for an interaction with the other kid, as it was freed from direct personal interaction. This trial was successful, and the other kid started to interact with the robot, finally going to the first one to ask for the controller. So, interaction was obtained first through the robot, then because of the robot.

In a third case, a person with Down syndrome was introduced to a structured game where a remotely driven Teo played a support role to induce associations between colours and positions. After having overcome the initial fear of getting close to the robot (at the time not being able to control the quite high and scaring acceleration), the kid accepted to participate in the game, which was possibly too easy for her, and went touching the robot. She was asked to associate a colour selected among the ones of the patches on the robot body with the same colour on one of the patches on the floor, and to help Teo to get there, but she was distracted by the presence of the robot and was exploring the contact with the moving, soft body. Finally, she answered the question asked by the therapist in a way that showed how she considered it as trivial, and continued to be attracted by the robot. At this point she take the initiative, escaped from the boring association game and autonomously started a free play activity for the sake of play. She got from the floor a tie, originally part of Teo's dressing kit, and the operator controlling the robot took the chance to move the robot as it was able to perceive the tie in the kid's hands. The kid, in turn, suddenly perceived animacy in the robot and started to move the tie in front of the robot to stimulate it to follow the tie, in a kind of keep-away game. The operator could drive the robot to participate in the game and the kid was fully involved up to the moment when the robot rushed too fast in her direction, stopping very close to her, although without contact. This was enough to scare her again: she rushed to a corner of the room and kept the distance, although maintaining interested attention to the robot's movements. Notice that this type of activity couldn't be implemented so easily by a human player, nor by an autonomous robot, which, in general, is not able to discover autonomously a play possibility, or even to perceive the tie in the player's hand. Notice also that the ability of the operator was here in selecting the proper timing for Teo's actions. The unexpected outcome of this activity was that the kid then tried to explain to other kids, later introduced in the room, how to play with the robot; before this experience, she didn't interact with any others.

In [379] are reported other studies where robots are left with children free to interact with them (e.g., [198, 438, 500]), obtaining interesting and sometimes unexpected behaviours.

In [198] children singularly underwent a standardized stress situation and then members of one group freely interacted with the robot Paro for 15 min, while the others interacted with the same robot turned off, i.e., reduced to a common plush. The goal was to evaluate the use of a social robot to alleviate anxiety and mood symptoms in children. Participants who interacted with the robot after the stressful task showed significantly higher levels of positive affect than participants in the control group, possibly due to the type of interaction they could experience with the robot. Novelty to face a reactive robot may also have played a relevant role, and 15 min are enough to explore Paro's capabilities, possibly less than what is needed to become acquainted with it and start to consider the interaction as no longer stimulating the curiosity needed for play.

In [438], three groups of hospitalized children could freely interact, respectively, either with the robotized teddy bear Huggable [370], with a computer animation avatar of the same robot, or with a traditional teddy bear. Children exposed to the robot reported more positive affect than those who received a plush animal and the interactions with the robot were more joyful than in the other two situations.

In [500], the robot Paro was left in a psychiatric ward where it could be freely accessed by inpatients with ASD, after obtaining permission from the staff. For some subjects the interaction turned out to be useful to develop good communication and reduce anxiety. Other patients didn't like the aspect (in particular the big eyes) and the motor noise. The authors conclude that the use of robots with patients with ASD should be carefully evaluated considering the many potential issues.

In [284] a simple wheeled, tele-controlled robot was used for free play with autistic children and the authors conclude that "the mobile toy robot in an ecological situation such as free, spontaneous gameplay could be used as a mediator of social stimuli in order to reduce the impairment of autistic children skills related to social information understanding and interaction".

At Politecnico di Milano—AIRLab, we have implemented Skunky (see Fig. 8.2), a skunk-like plush, able to move on a flat surface, like a table; it is intended to interact with people with motor or cognitive disabilities. It can be called by emitting sounds or knocking on the table, it can be "fed" with magnetic food as many commercial toys, so triggering a pleasure movement, it can be caressed on the head, which triggers a different pleasure movement and sound, it can sense a caress close to the back, just at the tail connection with the body, which triggers a short escape movement, simulating nuisance. Discovering these reactions and acting to trigger them stimulate a free play activity intended for people with limited physical and cognitive abilities. The number of possible reactions to discover is small, and the type of actions to

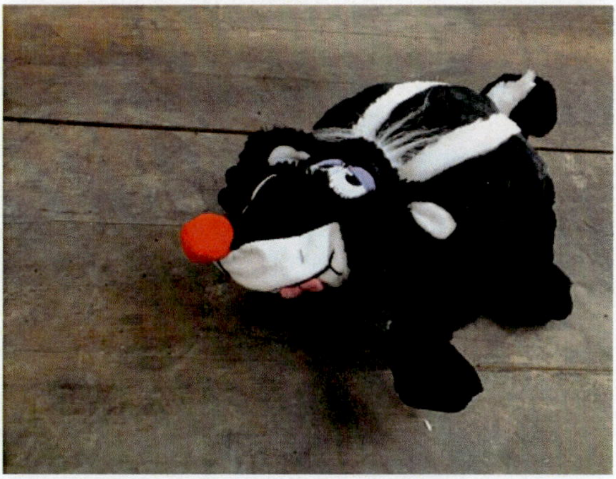

Fig. 8.2 The Skunky robot developed at Politecnico di Milano—AIRLab

trigger it enough challenging to be faced more times, to be sure to have understood the cause-effect relationship. The feedback is clear enough to be perceived by most of the subjects.

8.3 Structured Play

In structured play, a play setting is defined explicitly, rules of the game are declared, and all players should understand them and be able to play according to them, which may raise issues both for the robot and the human players with special needs. As we will see also in some of the examples, this does not mean that there is no room for play for the sake of play, if the player likes. In many cases, the structure that has been presented is explored and it may be modified in different ways, since an engaged player may always decide to change the rules of play, in search of fun and enjoyment.

We have seen that we may have *solitary* games, where a single human player is involved and where a robot usually becomes a (robotic) companion, or *multi-player* games where different players, possibly with different abilities, play with the robot, sharing the interaction with it. Another classification regards the goal of the game: the players can *collaborate* to achieve a common objective, or *compete* to achieve contrasting objectives. Finally, we can distinguish situations where the robot is either fully involved in the game as an active player, or it is tele-controlled, or it can stimulate the game without being directly involved [495]. In this book we are not considering this last category, since these robots are not playing, nor fully exploiting their physical abilities in the game, such as robots that play games by talking, controlling a board, or making expressions (e.g., [511, 539]).

In the following we mention as examples of structured play some of the robotic games developed at Politecnico di Milano—AIRLab. All these robots are based on the Arduino[1]-related technology, so they can be easily replicated at a relatively low cost, to make them available to the largest public.

8.3.1 Solitary Games

In this section, we present some games that can be played by single players. Usually, this implies a direct physical interaction with the robot, and the game mechanism should be designed to provide engagement for the different kinds of players the robot may encounter.

[1] https://www.arduino.cc/.

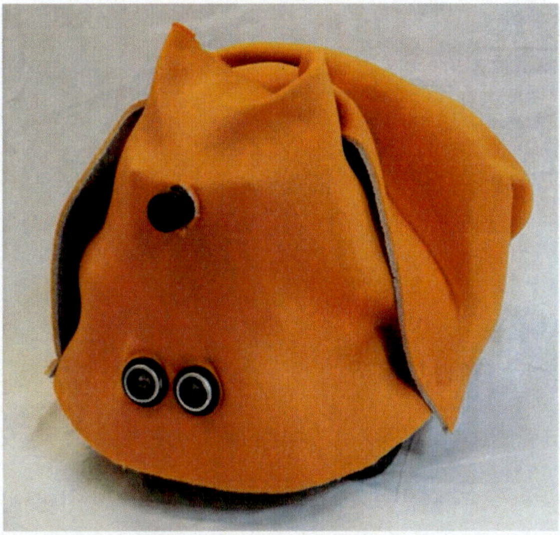

Fig. 8.3 Fixy, a mobile robot developed at Politecnico di Milano—AIRLab to play a game that may develop strategical abilities, associative memory, and motion skills

Fixy

Fixy is a small, mobile robot (see Fig. 8.3) able to detect obstacles using its sonar sensor, and to detect objects of three different colours (yellow, red, and blue) with its smart camera.[2]

The human player should place a pyramid with yellow or red sides in front of the robot, which will react by turning respectively left or right, then continuing to move forward as it was doing since the beginning of the game. The pyramid has also a third, white face, which will not activate any specific behaviour, but could be perceived as an obstacle. This enables the exploration of cause-effect relationships, as well as an associative memory (to associate colours and direction of movement) and coordination skills. The aim of the game is to bring the robot in view of the blue target (see Fig. 8.4). This goal is aimed at exploiting strategical skills to plan a sequence of diverting actions (colour presentations) that could bring the robot to the target. When reaching the target, Fixy performs a short ballet on a happy score that it can produce, in order to provide a positive feedback that could stimulate the repetition of the game.

When perceiving an obstacle, Fixy moves back and rotates to take a direction away from the obstacle, then starts to move forward again. The playground can be either left free of objects, so leaving to the human player only the goal of putting the right colour at the right moment in front of the robot, or it can be cluttered with objects. If the objects are either red or yellow, they can play their role of addressing the robot to the right or left. All other colours (except blue, which has to be avoided) are not recognized, so the object is detected as an obstacle, triggering the obstacle avoidance behaviour. In this case, the game would not require motion skills, but a

[2] https://pixycam.com/.

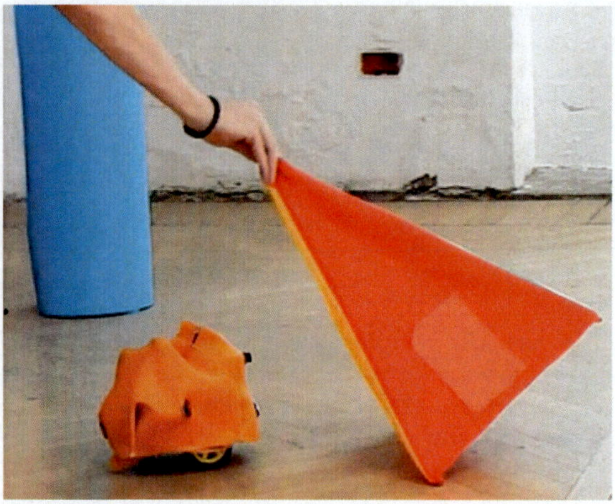

Fig. 8.4 The final phase of the game with Fixy. The player is putting the yellow face of the pyramid in front of the robot so to make it turning left and perceiving the blue target

higher level of strategical skills, since the position of the possibly coloured objects should be planned in advance, remembering the reactions of the robot.

This game is a typical cooperative game, where the player collaborates with the robot to make it reaching its goal.

The same setting, once being told or having discovered the relationships between environment and robot behaviour, could be used for play for the sake of play, where the player can exploit these relationships to make the robot acting as desired. Depending on the cognitive level of the player this may lead to more or less complex performances.

Chiappalo

Chiappalo is a mobile robot designed for two single-user competitive games (see Fig. 8.5). It can run at up to 1.4 m/s, avoiding obstacles and perceiving colours thanks to its Pixy smartcam.

The first game where it has been adopted is a kind of tag (or catch) game. The "UFO" robot runs away with random movements and the player should catch it by squeezing the extraterrestrial puppet that sits on its top. Sound is associated to the action. The robot can only detect entities from frontal sensors, and it is very fast in avoiding obstacles, so that chasing it from the side or from back would be the best effective strategy. The random movement has been studied to appear as a "realistic" escape strategy, so not too random, but also not straightforward. It is expected to be engaging and actually it has been in the trials. This game stimulates movement control, both in space and for squeezing the puppet. The speed could be tuned on the speed of the player. This play activity may stimulate a development of strategic thinking, although it can be played also as a simple reactive game.

When the first game finishes, it is the turn of the robot to become catcher. This game exploits the smart cam to detect green elements in the surroundings of the robot. A light cone is produced by a lamp to show the visual orientation of the camera. In the environment, the only green elements should be worn by the player,

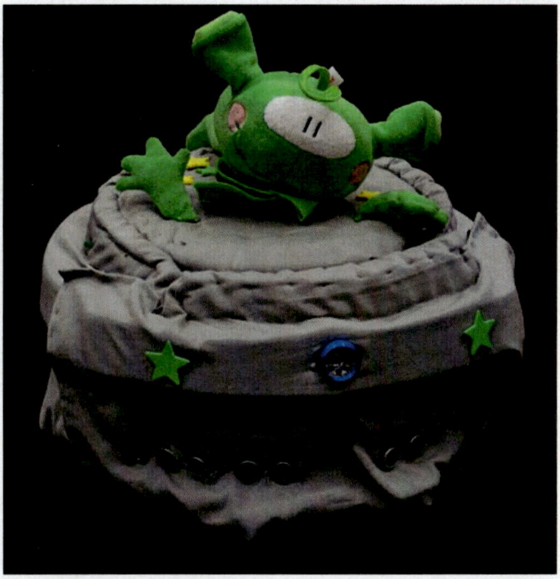

Fig. 8.5 Chiappalo, a mobile robot that could play

typically a green strip on the ankle. When the robot detects a green blob, it considers to have "caught" the opponent and starts a dance with a triumphal music. In the first version of this game, since this robot cannot manage the navigation in an unknown space, the robot was only rotating in place, starting suddenly after a short initial advice. Rotation in place is much more effective than running and it was difficult for the human players to avoid to be detected. We decided to give a rationale to the movement, as if the robot was looking for the player(s). This game has to be played in a closed environment, where there may be boxes that could be used to hide the detectable patches worn by the players from the camera, so that the players can just find a "safe" place behind a box, once they have understood that this may save them to be caught. Another alternative strategy would be to jump when the robot points in the player's direction. The first version of the game was too fast to allow most people to understand what was happening and to develop a strategy, so it was decided to reduce the rotation speed and to make the robot moving with an apparent intention. This made it possible to play in an acceptable way to most of the players that tried it, although it requires a certain motor ability to enjoy the experience and face the challenge. Actions to be taken were also suggested so that the players only had to perform them without the possibly frustrating attempt to develop a strategy.

The only other robotic tag (or catch) game we could retrieve in literature is described in [468]. This involved a human-sized, wheeled robot that implements the animal metaphor by projecting the head of an animal on the floor in the frontal direction, and a tail on the backward direction. The robot can implement three different movements, associated to different animals: dog, cat, and pig. The tail is moving left and right. The player should aim at jumping on the tail, in which case, the animal

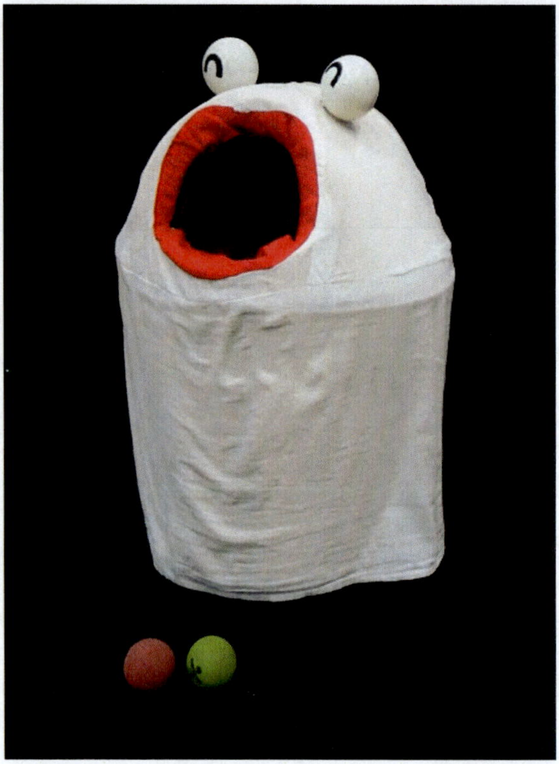

Fig. 8.6 ROB-E, a mobile, ghost-like robot that should be fed with coloured balls

screams both visually and with appropriate sound. In the paper are reported generically "successful" public demonstrations, but no results are available with physically impaired players, which were the declared target of the device. The robot is quite slow (22 cm/s), possibly too slow to really engage an able player, but appropriate for people with relevant motion impairments. Sound, movement, and projected elements have been designed to provide a realistic representation of the playing animal.

ROB-E
ROB-E is a mobile robot designed to develop motion skills in people with motion impairments, sitting on a wheelchair (see Fig. 8.6).

ROB-E can either move autonomously while avoiding obstacles (thanks to frontal sonars) or be remotely controlled by an operator, whose aim is to move the robot to match the ability of the player, so making the task more or less difficult and stimulating. This kind of adaptation would be difficult to obtain with such a low-level technology, but leaving this power to the caregiver may provide both a fine control of the session, and a deep involvement of the caregiver, who is actually playing in this activity by driving its avatar. The goal of the game is to put coloured balls in the mouth of the ghost robot. Balls are either blue, red, or green. Depending on the colour (detected by a colour sensor in the throat), a set of LEDs of the same

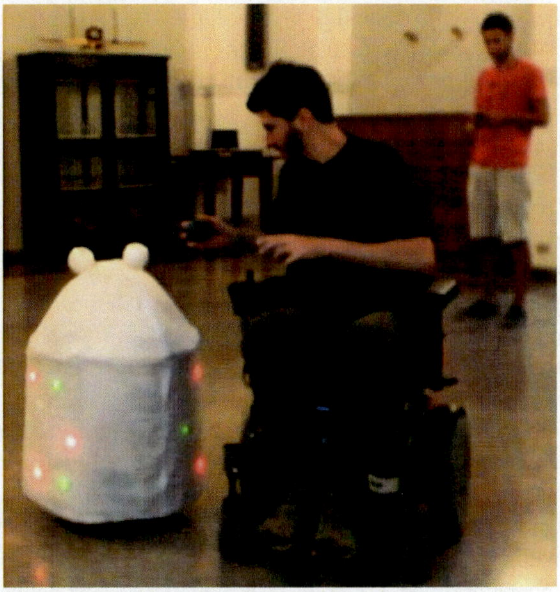

Fig. 8.7 A player inserting the last ball in ROB-E's mouth. On the background, it is possible to see the operator driving the robot with a joypad

colour of the ball and distributed on the whole body of the robot turns on, and a short jingle is played, thus providing a positive feedback at each achievement (see Fig. 8.7). When balls of all the three colours have been inserted in the mouth, the robot flashes all LEDs and performs a short dance. The behaviour of the robot, both when autonomous and when driven by the caregiver, is intended to be challenging to stimulate playing. This makes this game a competitive game, where the robot is acting in opposition to the player's will.

It is also possible to give the player more balls of the same colour; in this case, a selection has to be performed to obtain the partial feedback and to reach the final goal. This would stimulate an association between balls and missing LED colours. Moreover, depending on how the balls are made available to player, it is also possible to stimulate motion control to keep the balls and prevent them rolling down to the floor.

The same robot has been used in another setting, with people able to walk and run, leaving the back output of the balls open, so that when a ball is put in the mouth, in few seconds it rolls out from the back of the robot. Kids enjoyed the idea and started to play a game, where they were trying to get the balls expelled by the robot, which were rolling away on the floor, and then feed again the robot, to obtain the feedback and the final dance. This developed a kind of self-organization of the activity where kids were looking for the balls, run after them by exploiting motion abilities, and keep their turn to feed the robot. The presence of an assistant could also enforce a turn in getting the balls, so giving to everybody the right to participate to the game. This game may also be played by a person in a wheelchair and others feeding her/him with the balls retrieved once expelled. These two last versions of the game may suffer from slow timing and relatively long waiting time to be involved in the game; this issue may be mitigated by fillers produced by the robot, or by "easy" movements of the robot. In summary, also with such a simple mechanism, it is possible to devise many different play activities, and even restructure them on the fly as it happened sometimes.

The design of this robot considered different aspects, essential for its success. The height (about 70 cm) was defined to match the possibilities of users of common wheelchairs and was also compatible with standing kids. The width (about 60 cm) could provide good stability and is comparable with that of a person, so to provide similar mobility possibilities (made possible also by omni-wheels), which contribute to attribute animacy to the robot. The shape of the base is cylindrical, so to avoid as much as possible entanglement with the wheelchair. The body is soft to reduce issues due to possible collisions; it is made of a metallic network to provide robustness to the structure and non-deformability, covered by a 5 cm thick expanded polyurethane foam. The dimension of the mouth was intended to make feeding with the polyurethane balls (selected from the market, and easy to manipulate) not too easy, but at the same time not too difficult for a person in the wheelchair, possibly with other motion impairments. The speed of the robot was limited to the speed of a relatively slow wheelchair (50 cm/s) to make the game fair and give both the players similar abilities. The cheap white fabric was ideal to diffuse the LED light, and at the same time easy to be removed and washed.

Games with tele-controlled robots

In the following, we present some games where robots are tele-controlled by the players, so to become a sort of physical avatars that enable the players to play even if for any impairment they cannot directly perform the required actions. They enable a kind of transfer of abilities; for instance, the robot can implement moving abilities that the player does not possess. In most cases, an appropriate interface has to be defined and implemented to give the person with impairments access to the control of the robot.

Among the games exploiting tele-controlled robots, we present some developed at Politecnico di Milano—AIRLab.

Flipperbot

Another single-user, controlled robot game was FlipperBot (see Fig. 8.8). In this case, the robot is only 6 cm high, and operates on a table where a set of pillars are placed. Pillars have LED lights that are turned on one at a time by the game controller included in the table. The aim of the robot is to hit the switches that are around the pillar that has the light on. The players can control the robot remotely, with different devices, all connected via Bluetooth to the game controller embedded in the board. The robot is based on ESP32, a simple micro-controller that can be connected via WI-FI to the game controller.

This is a quite straightforward game, whose main issue was due to the speed of the robot, often too fast to allow a fine control of its movement. The playground was quite cluttered with the pillars, and its dimension had to be compatible with a regular table. Even if the dimension of the robot was reduced to a minimum compatible with

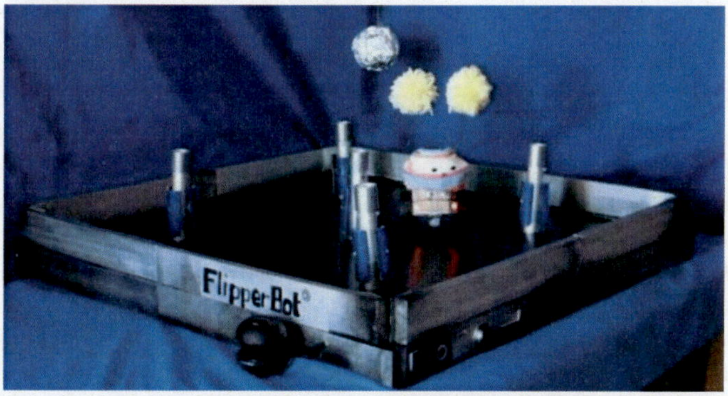

Fig. 8.8 FlipperBot, a remotely controlled robot working on a play table

Fig. 8.9 Mouse and cheese: a movement-controlled robot

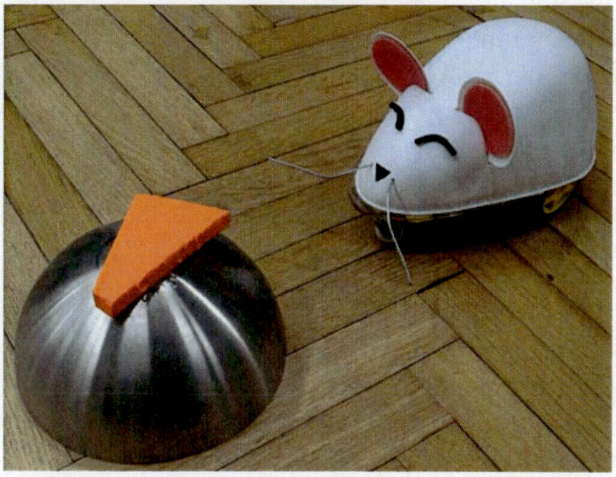

the available technology, it was not easy to make it move properly. The two big pom-poms at the top of the robot's antennas have the role to provide a way to bring the robot vertical again when it lays down: it is enough to push the pom-poms against any obstacle to make it arise and reach again the vertical position. This solution made the robot always visible and this arrangement to take the upright position was appreciated by the players. Despite the difficulty of movement, players were engaged and liked to play. The difficulty of the game could be adapted, by arranging the time the pillar light stay on. The usual arrangement on the control device had to be done to make it suitable to the players, since a traditional joystick was not adequate.

Mouse & Cheese

Mouse & Cheese (see Fig. 8.9) is a game implemented at Politecnico di Milano—AIRLab for people with motor impairments. It was intended for people in a wheelchair but could be used also for any people that could move in the space or that could move a part of the body.

It consists of a mouse-shaped robot that should be driven to a bowl containing cheese. Movement of the player is detected by an accelerometer and translated to the robot: moving forward moves the robot forward, turning makes the robot turning, and so on. Proper translation of player's movements to robot's movements should be tuned on the player. If the player is sitting in a wheelchair, the kinematics of movement is the same of that of the robot. If the player is standing, lateral movements cannot be realized with the devised robot kinematics, but it would be possible to implement a robot based on omni wheels that would not have the constraints of a differential drive, being fully holonomic, as people when walking.

This game is quite challenging and we noticed that it would be interesting to have a "free-me" button that can decouple the player's movement from the robot's, so to give the possibility to recover from possibly critical situations, as we usually do when rising the computer mouse to move the cursor over a position non-reachable with the limited operational space of the mouse.

Other games

Many other single-player games have been implemented. We only mention here imitation games (e.g., [225, 402, 553]), where a robot (usually an humanoid-like Nao or Kaspar [588]) shows some postures that have to be imitated by the player. All the literature reports positive effects of this use of the robots, also with respect to the imitation of humans, possibly due to the interaction with a toy-like robot. We do not consider this type of activity a play activity, even if it can be performed in a way that may make the player enjoying the activity, but more as a rehabilitation session.

Other games, addressing people with motion impairments, are based on robotic vehicles or arms that can be driven with appropriate interfaces to achieve some goal. Here the robot has the role, already cited, to provide the players with missing motion capabilities through the translation of motion (or vocal, breath, and others) possibilities to the robot's movements.

8.3.2 Multiplayer Games

In multi-player games, the players may participate either by waiting for their turn to take a role in the game, or by cooperating or competing to interact with the robot.

Turn-taking management is one of the goals in classical interventions with people with cognitive disabilities, like autism. Among the multi-player games that we have developed at Politecnico di Milano—AIRLab, we present here Yeti, DragonFlu, and Rosie.

Yeti

Yeti (see Figs. 4.8 and 8.10) is inspired to ToFu [758] and Keepon [401] for its body expressions, based on a vertical and asymmetrical deformation of an elastic body made of strips of polystyrene foam and metallic network, covered by artificial fur, and actuated by internal motors. It is 45 cm high, it can move on the floor, and it has very visible eyes, implemented by LED matrices, able to clearly show

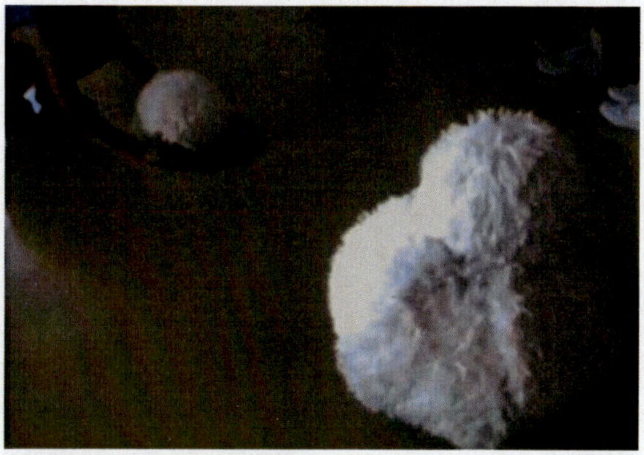

Fig. 8.10 Yeti during the play, showing an expression coherent with the player's action

expressions synchronously to the body deformation. It can move on the floor and acts as a stimulus and feedback relative to the achievement of the game goal. It has a companion, Snowy, similar in aspect, but smaller, without eyes and manipulable. This is perceived as a prop, while to Yeti was easily attributed some animacy by the players. Snowy's body is made by a transparent PVC shell, covered by the same fur of Yeti, which makes it possible to see the lights produced inside the body by LED strips. The human player holds Snowy, and has to place it on a patch of the same colour of the light that turns on in its body. The player should put Snowy on the right patch within 15". If he or she succeeds, Yeti shows to be happy both with body movements and with proper eye expression, otherwise it gets sad. After few seconds a new colour is produced by Snowy and another player may take the turn. In the meanwhile, Yeti goes around on the playground ready to provide its feedback.

Playing with a group of children with ASD, each one could take the right turn, and, while waiting, someone was also actively participating to the action by cheering the player urging to "make the robot happy", and suggesting what to do. In a session, after a while, some players, deeply engaged in the game, also discovered that it was possible to put Snowy on the T-shirt of another one, with the proper colour, instead of on the patches provided with the robot and laying on the floor. This started a new way of playing where kids were also offering (or asked to offer) their clothes to obtain a positive feedback. An important role was taken by timing, properly selected to give enough time to search for the right colour, but not too much, since this would require boring waiting time. The desire to take their turn was a stimulus to make the others participating also when not directly involved.

DragonFlu

DragonFlu is a mobile robot able to throw table tennis balls (see Fig. 8.11). It is controlled by the movement of a mobile phone, as detected by its accelerometers.

The player holds the phone and inclines it in the direction he or she want to drive the robot. The robot has a simple differential drive, that gives some constraints to the movement, functional to the game. By pushing a virtual button on the control screen the robot can shoot a table tennis ball from the mouth. The speed of the ball has been

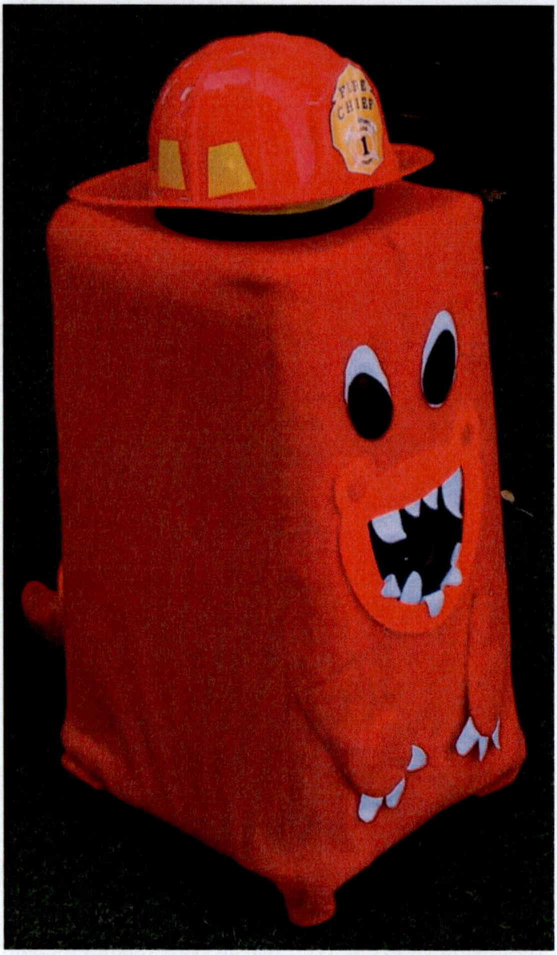

Fig. 8.11 DragonFlu, a remotely controlled robot able to throw table tennis balls

selected to be perceived as a shooting, but not to hurt when hitting a person. This game was designed for children with cerebral palsy, experiencing movement issues and possible cognitive disorders.

Two multi-player, inclusive games were implemented with DragonFlu. In both, a player takes the control of the robot, driving it by the phone and shooting the balls. The other players in the first game should avoid the balls, making this a competitive game between the controlling player (conceptually flanked by the robot avatar) and the others. This requires motion control from both sides. Moreover, the thrown balls must be retrieved from the floor. DragonFlu has a repository of balls below its cask. When all the balls have been thrown, the game ends, and the turn to control the robot may go to another player. If needed, a reward can be given to the controller for having hit with a ball someone, and to the other players according to the number of

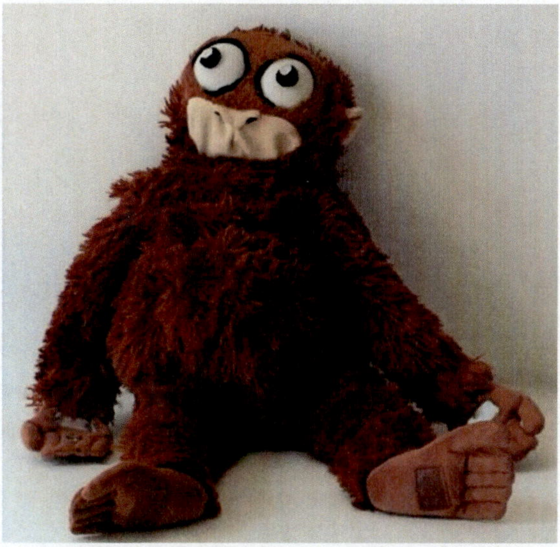

Fig. 8.12 Rosie, a robot able to play round-around-the-rosey and to react to manipulation

retrieved balls. Often, in practical cases, the game is engaging enough that rewards are not needed to motivate play. We observed that running after balls to retrieve them is appreciated and naturally accepted as a stimulus to play in most situations.

The other developed game is a cooperative game between the driven robot and the other players, which compete against each other. They stay behind a line and they have to catch balls on the fly. This is more difficult for these people, since fast reflexes and good control are required, but could be played by a person with motor disabilities and a set of normally developed companions.

DragonFlu was successfully tested in a camp dedicated to kids with cerebral palsy. Not all the players were able to manage the phone in a proper way, so a better handle was suggested and is being implemented. Moreover, children expected that the robot could speak and answer them. This would not be part of the game, but it would improve the attribution of animacy that was in the expectations.

Rosie

Rosie born upon the suggestion of a caregiver to whom was presented a gadget coming from the shop of a science museum. This was a small robot that, when hold by its hands, was producing sounds and lights. We decided to use the same principle (closing an electric circuit through human body) to make a robotic puppet that could play ring-around-the-rosey with a group of people with behavioural and mental issues, including ASD. The developed robot is a monkey plush, about 60 cm long, obtained by robotizing a commercial one, adding two metallic contacts in the hands, LEDs in the eyes, vibration motors, accelerometer and the possibility to reproduce pre-recorded sound (Fig. 8.12).

Rosie was used in a care centre mostly with adult people affected by intellectual disabilities. In a first phase, it was presented to the group and each one could singularly

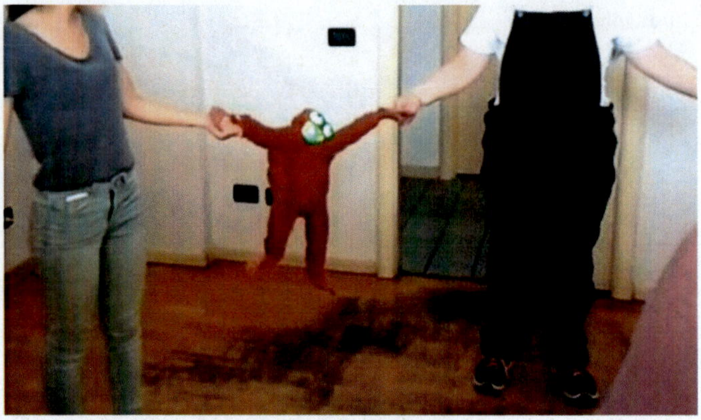

Fig. 8.13 Scimmiottondo in the round-around-the-Rosey circle

explore its expression possibilities: when shaken too hardly, the eyes become red and the robot vibrates and roars angrily, when caressed on the head, the eyes turn blue and emits a pleasure sound and a soft vibration, when both hands are taken by a person the eyes turn green and Rosie starts to sing the typical song for round-around-the-rosey. As soon as a hand is left, the circuit opens, the song stops. After the familiarization phase a group activity could be started, including both the robot, caregivers and persons with disabilities in a circle, hand in hand (see Fig. 8.13).

When the circle is closed, Rosie starts singing and everybody can dance in a circle with the song. Of course, closing the circle is not easy at the beginning, but as soon as everybody can understand that it is possible to start singing and moving when the robot sings, they usually collaborate to keep the contact, or start playing a game where anyone can take the turn to open and close the circle, in order to cause the production of the feedback from the robot, perceived by everybody in the group. At the same time, if the robot, which is held by its hands but cannot touch ground, is shaken too much, it stops singing and stars roaring; this may reduce disordered movements, since it is taken as signal of a behaviour which goes against the rules of the game. This is a case where one of the principles of play (satisfy the rules of a social pact) combines with the other one (face the challenge, here moving with care), to enforce engagement in addition to feedback.

8.4 Evaluation of Outcomes and Play Activity

The evaluation of the experimental activity concerns both the clinical outcomes obtained by introducing robots in interventions on persons with disability and the playfulness of the activity. We briefly discuss these two topics in the next sections.

8.4.1 Outcome Evaluation

The objective evaluation of the outcome of robotic interventions on persons with disabilities is the subject of contrasting positions. From one side, the majority of papers presents results on a relatively small set of subjects which cannot be considered as a representative sample of a population, although they are treated with statistically sound methods. This is even more true for impairments like ASD that have been recognized as a "spectrum" of disabilities, for which therapists know very well that treatments should be designed and fine-tuned on the needs of each specific subject. Most of the robots used in this type of interventions are designed by roboticists, often interacting with therapists, but a clinically sound assessment of the results is rare, and the need for evaluation procedures closer to clinical practices is becoming more and more evident [623], although not easy to implement, both because the population for diversified clinical trials could hardly be considered as uniform, and because clinical protocols are not easy to be defined in the conditions the trials are usually performed. On the other side, case studies are reported that present outcomes of real trials, specifying the experimental setting, and shed a light on the possibilities of these interventions.

Stanton [667] mentions two approaches to evaluate the outcome of the research with autistic children; since people with ASD have each different characteristics, as any people, including those with other disabilities, we may consider the trials, usually done with a limited number of subjects, either as case studies, which provide specific evidence and may be considered to design interventions, or as pieces of evidence to support a theory, but without any possible claim of generality.

Kahn et al. [381] propose a third approach based on the definition of benchmarks for the assessment of properties of social robots in general. Some of them have been proposed in [246]. Benchmarks would enable an objective and sound evaluation, although the open question concerns the proper definition of benchmarks. In many research fields, including Robotics and Machine Learning, benchmarks have been defined and research focused in facing benchmarks and confronting performance obtained on them, only. While benchmarks support research focusing, they also tend to bias research in the direction of the issues covered by benchmarks, often not even fully identified, sometimes forgetting the need to go forward, getting a step over the specificity of the benchmark and exploring new directions. Efforts are being done to face the definition and the selection of benchmarks in a scientific way, so to reduce undesired effects and at least make researchers aware of the benchmark characteristics (e.g., [161, 366, 699]). This requires a sound analysis of the benchmark elements so to precisely characterize it. This task is even more difficult when people are involved in the benchmark as in the case of robotic games, and human-robot interaction in general, but it is clear that this is the direction to be taken if benchmarks are considered.

Kabacinska et al. [379] list a set of specific, validated outcome measures for interventions with autistic children. Moreover, they report a set of recommendations to obtain a good quality study design, most of which are common to any sound study. We summarize and comment on them in the next paragraphs.

Any study should start with a sound definition of the goal of the intervention, in particular, what specific aspects are addressed. Then the outcome measure should be selected to be appropriate to assess the goal, and to provide the possibility to compare with other results aimed at the same goal. Possibly, the outcome measure should have been already validated. This recommendation goes in a direction similar to the one that could be taken when aiming at a recognized benchmark, with the same possible drawback of limiting the exploration dimension of the research. The set of subjects should be large enough and representative of the population, which is an open problem but also an issue that should be addressed at best. Appropriate control trials should be defined. For instance, as we have seen in this chapter, performing trials with the robot turned on, and the control trials with the same robot turned off, so to evaluate the effect of the robot behaviour separately from the effect of shape, material, colour, etc. Novelty effect may influence the effectiveness of the intervention, so it would be relevant to perform longitudinal trials that could wash out the effect of interacting with a new device. When possible, it is recommended to use blinded or automated scoring procedures to reduce biases that experimenters or caregivers directly involved in the trial may induce. Limitations and negative results should be put in evidence and reported.

Kabacinska et al. [379] provide also recommendations about the robot to be used. The robot should be safe and treated appropriately for the safety of the subjects; for instance, it has to be considered to be cleaned and sanitized before using it with different subjects. Since the robot may malfunction or even break, this situation should be considered in advance and mitigation actions should be considered to reduce the possibly induced stress in the subjects. Moreover, in planning trials, cost and availability of (enough copies of) the robot should be considered. The impact of taking the robot away from the subject at the end of the trial should also be considered.

The possible impact of the presence of the robot on the other actors involved in the intervention (e.g., caregivers, parents) should be considered. In particular, the robot should be presented as a further tool to be used to improve the status of the subjects, not as a substitution for the role of others or of other tools.

In the design of the study, the socio-cultural background of the subjects should be considered, in particular for what concerns robots and technology. Validated tests of attitude w.r.t. robots, such as Negative Attitude Towards Robots Scale (NARS [507]) and Robot Anxiety Scale (RAS [506]) are widely used, but cannot be used with subjects that cannot answer their questions. These scales assess the extent to which people feel unwilling to interact with a robot due to arousal of negative emotions or anxiety. They are largely used, although critiqued because they only investigate about negative aspects and do not consider motivations for this attitude, which may be deeply rooted or possibly due to unfamiliarity.

Another more general test to evaluate attitude towards technology is the Technology Readiness Index (TRI [523]), which investigates "motivating" and "inhibiting" dimensions with respect to the adoption of innovative technology. TRI is widely used, although it is not specific for robots.

A general issue against this kind of explicit expressions about attitudes has been raised in [606], where the adoption of implicit attitude tests, like IAT [301], is suggested to extract the deep attitude that may be different from the expressed one. The reported findings concerning the general attitude towards robots were matching what was obtained by explicit attitude tests in the considered sample.

Together with the presentation of some of the above mentioned critical issues, in [54] many different aspects related to the acceptability of a robot are discussed, namely: functionality, social ability, shape and appearance; however, no assessed measurement scales are proposed for them. An even more articulated set of these aspects has already been presented in Chap. 4.

The robots we are considering are interacting with people, so aspects related to Human-Robot Interaction should be evaluated. A widely used tool for this is the Godspeed questionnaire series [45], which has been defined to evaluate anthropomorphism, animacy, likeability, perceived intelligence, and perceived safety of a robot to interact with. Although still quite popular, improvements have been suggested from different researchers (e.g., [448, 746]) and a formal, widely accepted validation does not seem to have been obtained, yet.

Most of these tools are based on questionnaires that cannot be answered by people with cognitive impairments, but possibly by their caregivers and relatives.

8.4.2 Evaluation of Robotic Play Activities

Some aspects specific to robot involved in play activities can also be assessed. A large list of tests for playability and playfulness for play activities has been already presented in Sect. 2.10, and they could be adopted to evaluate also play activities including robots. Unfortunately, most of the roboticists' teams seem to be unaware of this possibility and in literature their application to robotic games is not reported.

An aspect that should be evaluated is playfulness Anita Bundy defined a test of playfulness for games [137], widely used to assess this characteristic especially critical when players have disabilities [139, 319, 497]. The test is aimed at evaluating intrinsic motivation, suspension of reality, internal locus of control, and framing, intended as the ability to frame the play activity by giving and reading social cues [49]. It is based on observation of the free play activity, usually done on video records. The test has been experimentally validated [139], although its clinical usefulness has still to be assessed [152].

Other aspects related to play and disability concern usability and accessibility as discussed in Chap. 3. For what concerns games, the evaluation of accessibility and usability have been developed mostly for computer games[3] (e.g., [263]), but issues related to the physical aspects of the game require the definition of specific procedures. We propose here a framework for this evaluation that includes elements

[3] http://gameaccessibilityguidelines.com/and http://www.includification.com/provide rich lists of guidelines for computer games.

from the methodologies used for objects and those used for games. In both the definitions of accessibility and usability, the user plays the main role, and guidelines for their evaluation always refer to the specific user that is targeted.

All these guidelines, and the ones proposed here below, are presented as lists of recommendations that can be used as a checklist for a posteriori evaluation, but also to design play activities and devices.

- *Introduction to the activity*
  At the beginning of the activity, the robot should be presented, together with its abilities, limitations and behaviours. The subjects should be aware of what may happen. Moreover, if the activity is a structured game, this should be described in a way that can be understood by the player, since in the game contract is included rule accomplishment by all the players.
- *Storytelling*
  It is often useful to give a context to the play activity, possibly inserting it in a storytelling that may motivate to play and becomes an integral part of the play activity.
- *Interface*
  The quality of the interface should match the abilities of both the human and the robot player. In particular, depending on the special needs, access can be provided thanks to careful design of the interaction devices and their use in the game. We have already presented examples where the interface was problematic for certain users and required a redesign. Sometimes, the game itself should be redesigned to be played with the interfaces more appropriate for a subject. Also from the robot side the reliability of the signal detection needed to play should be checked. It is not possible to have proper playing activities with robots that fail too often to play their role. It is better to design a reliable and simple play experience than one relying on sophisticated sensors that cannot provide reliable signals.
- *Start and stop*
  When the play activity starts the involved entities enter in a special situation that characterizes play (see Chap. 2). It is important that both robot and human players are aware that they are starting to play. In particular, if autonomous play is the target, it is important that the human player starts the robot, and this can only be obtained if the activation procedure is compatible with the specific abilities. The same holds for the end of the play activity. In a game, it is often proposed to play another game, or stop. This choice should be accessible to the player, or it would require the intervention of the assistant. The decision to stop or continue playing is always up to the human player, by the implicit contract underlying the play activity. It should also be possible to stop at any time, possibly avoiding traumatic actions such as turning off a lively robot.
- *Pre-game trial*
  Before actually start playing, it is suggested to give the possibility to explore the interaction possibilities and, in case of games, to perform a pre-trial of the game. This makes the subject more confident about the experience and at the same time makes it possible to tune the robot's abilities to match the ones of the player.

- *Adaptation*
  The performance of the robot should be adaptable to the special needs of the player, and possibly to her/his evolution in time. A typical solution may be to give the caregiver the possibility to tune parameters to match the subject's abilities. A simplified possibility consists in defining a priori difficulty levels as usually done in video games, although this does not allow a fine tuning of the parameters. A more interesting possibility would be to make the robot able to automatically detect the need to self-tune parameters, so that the game could be dynamically adapted, as done, for instance, in the games described in [98].
- *Signal intensity*
  The intensity of the signals used to interact with the player should be adapted both to the player's needs that may possibly be either the need for an intensity loud enough to be perceived, or the need of a low, gentle intensity to reduce anxiety and rejection. Moreover, the signal should be perceivable in the environment where the playing activity is held. For instance, a low volume may be critical in a large room where others are participating to the experience possibly by screaming, as well as a low intensity light, or low screen illumination to show expressions, may be wiped off in a sunny room or in outside settings, so cutting interaction possibilities that may be essential for the game functionality and appreciation.
- *Feedback*
  During the interaction, a perceivable feedback to any significant action of the player should be provided, both when this is functional to the experience (e.g., cause-effect evidence in free play, or question-answering in a game) or when it is just desirable (e.g., the score change in a game in response to some action).
- *Timing*
  Actions while playing should be done at a proper time, both for the game purpose, e.g., a prompt reaction to a stimulus, and to keep the rhythm of the play activity. Response timing is also critical to support animacy. Robot limitations due, for instance, to the time needed to elaborate a signal should be integrated in the character representation or in the robot's behaviour. It is not acceptable in a play activity that a robot requires the player to wait or to pay attention to timing, if not explicitly justified, since this may reduce the quality of the play experience and the player engagement. Timing should also be designed to match the timing needs of the player to perceive, understand, and react to the robot's signals.
- *Behaviour and game design* The design of the robot's behaviour should keep into account the specific impairments of the involved player. Parametrization may support the adaptation of a behaviour to special needs, but may not be enough, and the behaviour should be designed a priori to match them. If the robot is involved in a game, the game itself should be designed to consider the players' abilities so that they can enjoy the experience.

Chapter 9
Ethical, Social, and Psychological Issues

Andrea Bonarini

Abstract In this chapter, we discuss the ethical, social, and psychological implications of playing with a robot, in the physical world. Issues like attachment, bullying, and improper use of the device to which some animacy is attributed are reported in literature and in the authors' experience: they give the opportunity to reflect about social, psychological, and ethical consequences of this new play setting. Measures to limit undesired issues are discussed, together with their implications on design and readiness for the market.

9.1 Ethical Issues

Ethical issues related to the introduction of autonomous robots in the society have been raised since many years. The term "roboethics" born in 2004 [729] and the corresponding discipline cover different aspects, related both to the use and the design of robots and to the relationships between people and robots. Ethical issues arise when we have to evaluate what is good and what is bad in a behaviour. The general issues treated by roboethics extend much further than what is needed for the applications covered in this book, and we mention here only the aspects that are strictly related to our topic. Many concerns may drop when we consider that playing with robots in most cases does not imply to have the robot connected to Internet (so all data stay local to the robot and may not need to be recorded), nor to have the robot, at least the type of robot we are considering in this book, interacting through a screen, so that issues about de-physicalization of the interaction do not hold.

When ethical criteria are clearly established it is also possible to define rules and laws aimed at enforcing and assessing them, establishing what should be done to guarantee that they are matched. When available, we will mention them, but regulatory principles are based on the possibility to perform a kind of evaluation that, as discussed in Chap. 8, requires the definition of evaluation tools, not yet available. Many ethical principles are being stated both at the institutional level (e.g., the European Parliament Resolution on AI systems, the ISO 13482:2014 Standard for safety requirements for personal care robots, the BS 8611:2016 Guide to the ethical design and application of robots and robotic systems, and the IEEE Ethically Aligned

A. Bonarini and S. Besio, *Robot Play for All*, Research for Development,
https://doi.org/10.1007/978-3-031-05042-8_9

Design Standard 2017 from the IEEE Global Initiative and Standard Association), and at research level (e.g., [264]), but only limited official regulations have been issued, so the application of general principles is still left to designers, engineers, caregivers, stakeholders, and players themselves. In this, the development and adoption of robots for play follow the same process and rules that are taken for similar products like toys, video games, ad even apps.

When robots are used as tools for a therapy, they may be considered as medical devices, and so should comply to the (strict) regulations that rule the design and use of medical devices. However, they are not yet officially recognized as medical devices (with few notable exceptions like Paro, in USA), so they should comply to the same regulations of other tools commonly used for playing (e.g., toys and apps).

A last distinction should be done between "ethics by design", so producing a robot that has the capability to show an ethical behaviour, and "ethics in design", that is applying ethical principles to evaluate the consequences of a robot in its operational context, including potential replacement of humans, or changes in the usual procedures that may be detrimental [220]. Since we are in a play context, the ethical behaviour of the robot is subsumed by what is mentioned in the following sections, in particular by the need of acceptance of the robot in the play context, which is in contrast with non-ethical behaviour of the robot. We have already mentioned that the robot in this contest is just another tool to play with, so the consequences of its introduction in the practice have to be evaluated as for the other tools.

In the next sections we will discuss how specific risks can be faced.

9.2 Physical Safety

A first aspect concerns physical safety. Robotic devices should be guaranteed not to harm people. In most cases, robots used in play activities are intrinsically safe, in the sense that they are designed to have features that cannot harm people. For instance, they are small, lightweight, not too strong, without cutting edges, not too fast, and so on. In other words, they should comply to the rules common to all toys, as defined in each country.

When used by people with impairments, robots should also be designed considering their misuse, always possible if left free to interact with these players. In more than one session we have seen children jumping over Teo (described in Chap. 4) or riding it, without any harm, since it was designed to have a soft body and a robust, yet elastic, PET shell to protect wheels and sensors. In the specific case depicted in Fig. 9.1, the child with ASD was facing for the first time an active Teo, after having been in the room with the robot turned off for a while. The free play activity started with Teo moving slowly and dimming the lights to attract attention. Suddenly, the kid moved on Teo, and threw it down. The robot detected the situation by the accelerometer signal, stopped the motors and started to cry with a sad light flashing. The kid was surprised, raised the robot, and went looking for a piece of fabric of the same colour of Teo's skin, then handling it to the robot like he was asking to be forgiven. A proper

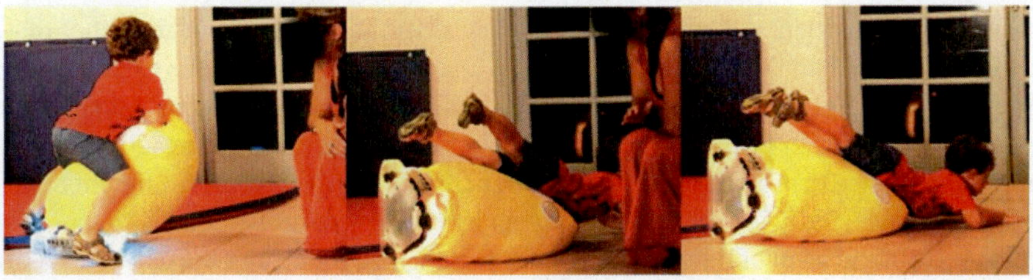

Fig. 9.1 A sequence from a session where a children jumped on TeoG

design made it possible to have this interesting, unexpected behaviour emerging. A fragile, or expensive robot may have led to a different behaviour, possibly requiring also a different setting and a different reaction by the caregiver, who would have tried to "save the robot", as we have seen in a movie involving Nao, presented at a congress. The caregiver in this session with Teo just left the child to manage the situation, having seen that no critical behaviour had been triggered.

We also worked to evaluate the risk of throwing a toy against a companion's head [10], a potential harm due to the misuse of the robot. After a careful analysis, it was possible to provide suggestions about the shape of a toy to reduce this specific harm. As a follow-up we developed a system to understand when a robotic toy is about to be thrown, by analysing with a machine learning model running on board (on a Raspberry PI) the signal of the embedded accelerometer [8], so to make it possible the implementation of some reaction from the robot itself to prevent the risky situation. This is another type of amendment to reduce the effect of misuse of a robot. Making the robot aware of a dangerous situation may also be used in the case of harassment, when subjects intend to damage the robot or make it fool. If it can detect the situation, the robot may be reactive and activate behaviours to try to bring the situation to a safe state.

9.3 Cognitive Safety and Social Issues

Cognitive issues may be related to acceptability, trust, dehumanization, or attachment [185, 265], and they may be connected to social issues.

Acceptability of the playing robot depends on many factors, including shape, behaviour, the play experience and how the robot is introduced. If the subjects cannot accept something of the robot (maybe the humanoid aspect, or the level of sound, or the light rhythms, etc.), they will not engage in the play activity, and the proposer should refrain to insist in the proposal. As mentioned in Chap. 4, a friendly shape (possibly reminding cartoon characters), the possibility to adapt robot features to the specific needs, a proper design of the play activity may raise acceptability to the proper level.

Trust strongly depends on the appropriateness of the behaviour of the robot that should participate in the play activities according to the rules and to the expectations for a companion's behaviour. A low reliability, difficulty in understanding the purpose of actions or even to perceive the relationship between actions and reactions, may bring to a lower trust, with the consequent decrease of engagement till the moment when the play activity is left. A related aspect is "perceived safety", that is "the user's perception of the level of danger when interacting with a robot, and the user's level of comfort during the interaction [45]". This requires a careful design of behaviours and of the robot itself. For instance, in the first version of Teo, the movements were always made at the same, sustained speed, which was appropriate for certain interactions, but not for others. When trying to engage a child the robot cannot go towards her/him at a high speed, since this may trigger fear, and the subject may no longer feel safe enough to play. The following version of Teo had the possibility to control the speed, so to move at the right speed for any different situation.

In another game that we developed, not intended for persons with disabilities, there was a drone flying around the player at a given distance. The game implemented a sort of Jedi training as seen in the Star Wars movies: the drone, from time to time made a sound like a laser blast, and the player had to "parry" it by rising his/her "light saber" in front of the chest [463]. Since the drone may be perceived as dangerous if it moves too fast and too close to the player, we devised a way to keep it active and safely out of the range of the laser saber (implemented by a coloured foam stick), while showing to be looking for the right moment to blast. This was not enough to eliminate fear, and we had to smooth the movements so to give the impression that they were under control. Since movements depended on the robot's perception of the shape of the player, it turned out also that the drone was moving with a style similar to the style of the player: either nervous, calm, or resolute. Matching the kind of movement expression of the player was also a way to improve acceptability and trust, as well-known from psychology [37]. If the player perceives that the robot is in control and can act as expected in the specific play situation, then he/she can be engaged and fully participate to the experience. Jedi Trainer was played with success by hundreds of players, none of which showed to be scared to confront a 50 cm wide drone operating four 10 cm blades at 10,000 RPM to generate a quite significant air flow.

Another issue related to trust is deception. In many play activities, a certain kind of deception is part of the game. For instance, when playing football or hide-and-seek or many other games, feints are expected as legal ways to reach a goal, and coherent with the play contract. As any other aspect related to performance, this kind of deception shouldn't make the play participation of the other players too difficult or prevent them to contribute to the activity at the level they can play. We have included deception among the possibilities to make the game interesting in another game experience not designed for persons with disabilities [510].

Another cognitive issue is related to the possible dehumanization of the experience. These robots are used as tools to improve the play experience, so they should be considered as any other tool by the players and possibly by their caregivers, who usually attend the sessions and may also participate to the playing experience. As mentioned in Chap. 4, one of the goals is to induce the subjects to interact with the robot, but the play situation makes evident that the robot is just a tool, even when animacy is attributed. A playful robot can enhance a play moment that would be otherwise managed using another tool, possibly a traditional toy. In most of the playful experiences that we have presented the robot does not substitute a person, but plays a role in support of an engaging play experience, possibly together with others, and most often at least together with an assistant.

A lack of longitudinal studies and of objective and quantitative evaluation of the activity does not allow us to understand what may be long-term effects of the interaction with robots [461], whether habituation will influence future interactions, or whether any form of attachment may arise, under what conditions and settings. The reported experiences are usually positive and effective, but more thorough analysis have still to be done, subject to the definition of proper evaluation tools (see Chap. 8). In our experience, we have seen in many situations that returning the robot where it was already used to play triggered a positive memory also in cognitively impaired subjects, in a way similar to what could happen with a toy that was used in a positive experience, but no specific attachment.

Attachment may be possible in situations where a robot is intensively used like a reactive pet. In this case, the robot may induce a stronger dependency than a traditional plush, and the prevention of excessive attachment is up to the caregiver.

Another aspect related to animacy concerns "life" of the robot and malfunctioning. The need for power, in many cases, when batteries are needed, brings to situations where the robot requires to be recharged. If this is managed directly by the robot, possibly asking to be recharged before "dying", a possibly stressful situation may be prevented. Being a (more or less) complex device a robot may always incur in malfunctioning. This cannot be foreseen and should be managed by the assistant. Minor malfunctioning may affect the ability to play, which may be acceptable until the play contract expectations are matched. Major malfunctioning may block the robot, with a perception of "death" that should be avoided and can be prevented only with robust robots. If the cause of malfunctioning is the player him/herself, the sense of responsibility may trigger negative moods and reactions. Again, a robust design of the robot together with a careful definition of the play activity, which may integrate possible malfunctioning among the events that "may happen", may reduce negative effects.

9.4 Privacy

Privacy issues are ruled in Europe by the General Data Protection Regulation (GDPR), which is becoming a general standpoint also for other countries. ISO/IEC 29134:2017 is one of the documents that establish some guidelines for conducting a privacy impact assessment. Regulations are clear about the record, use, and maintenance of data, as well as about the rights of the subjects: if data are recorded they have to be properly treated.

If data are elaborated by the robot with computational power available on board and are not recorded, nobody has access to them, so this situation is compatible with GDPR and would not require any special treatment.

If data are collected by the robot and recorded for analysis and elaboration, e.g., for clinical assessment, they are subject to the same rules as data collected by the caregivers to perform their sessions and should be treated according to the GDPR.

A critical situation may arise when data are sent to the cloud to be elaborated (e.g., to interpret natural language sentences, or to answer questions), since it is not always clear who is managing data in this case nor whether they are recording them. There have been episodes where speaking dolls were suspected to be the way to collect personal information through the interaction with young players. These dolls have been banned in some countries. This triggered in many toy manufacturers a quite strong attention to the use of Internet or the cloud for their products, possibly reducing the capabilities of toys in exchange for a proper data treatment. Other manufacturers decided to ask explicitly to the customers the permission to manage their data, as it is commonly done for home assistants and social networks, in exchange to the possibility of accessing a service, which, in this case, is a highly performing toy.

A large number of interesting playing activities can now be implemented without the need of cloud services external to the robot, so avoiding to bring data outside the robot and eliminating issues about privacy. This is often in contrast with the interests of robot producers, who may be interested in an internet connection to monitor the customer and collect data, but the enforcement of data management rules may at least make clear the type of relationship that is set between producers and customers.

Chapter 10
To Infinity and Beyond

Andrea Bonarini

Abstract In this chapter, whose title is inspired by the motto of Buzz Lightyear, the robot toy appearing in the "Toy Story" movies, we put in evidence the open issues, and the developments that are being enabled both by the advancement of technology and by the results of the many experiences that are being done. We envision how playful robots and not yet implemented robotic games could be realized in the very next future, and we also present wishful thinking about desirable robotic games that may suggest further developments.

10.1 Dream Robots

Technology advancements are starting to enable functions that could support great play experiences with robots. Many of these functions are not reliable enough to be used in play, yet, they may take too much time to produce their results, or may require computational power that cannot run on cheap robots and may require network connection to big servers. We would like to stress here that a believable and trustful play companion should timely produce high quality actions, and a necessary condition for this is that the robot should have enough, good quality information from its sensors in a proper time. However, we may expect that in few years posture and activity recognition, speech recognition, sight direction recognition, emotion recognition, and natural language dialogue management may be available on board. These features have interest for many applications, not only robotic, and the research community is working hard to develop them. Most of the expected functionalities refer to sensing capabilities, which are still not adequate for the purposes, while actuation capabilities can already reach a sufficient performance, at least in some configurations.

At the same time, hardware development is progressing and there are high expectations to have handheld large computational possibilities in the very next future that could be integrated in robots and, to a certain extent, into cheap devices. Given the fast development of relatively affordable and cheap hardware designed for machine learning, also the choice to include them in the robot architecture is more frequent. For instance, the last version of Oimi, the robot developed at AIRLab-POLIMI and

A. Bonarini and S. Besio, *Robot Play for All*, Research for Development,
https://doi.org/10.1007/978-3-031-05042-8_10

introduced in Sect. 6.3 includes a NVIDIA Nano board enabling both activity recognition, emotion recognition from face, and object recognition, so making it possible not only to detect critical situations, like the insurgence of tantrums, but also to implement play activities that do not require exact gestures, always problematic to be recognized.

A further issue that should be faced to have these devices is electrical power, since the computational power requires to be fed with electrical energy. Battery development is one of the main targets for the whole technological market, from phones, to IoT (Internet of Things) devices, to cars, to robots, and, again, a lot of resources are invested in this and will soon bring results.

The availability of these features may enable robots to play with sensing abilities as close as possible to those of human players and the development of new play activities involving robots will be made possible. However, the main motivations for the implementation of playing robots will have to be kept in mind: robots are not substitutes for human play companions, but tools to improve experience and knowledge.

One of the requirements still poorly satisfied is the adaptation of the play experience to the specific player. More sophisticated sensors and interpretation software may enable to capture from the interaction the information needed to model the player behaviour and adapt the robot's behaviour online, so to obtain playful experiences always automatically tuned to the abilities, and the mood of the player. For instance, detecting a lack of interaction either by a camera or by the accelerometer, or problems in manipulation, or problems in finalization of the play activity may trigger in the robot some recovery behaviour, either supporting the player (e.g., reducing its speed if it is running), still maintaining the proper role in the play (so adapting the challenge to the player's detected abilities), or suggesting what to do.

It will also be possible to develop play activities where the player is not required to wear sensors or special cloths, but the robot will be able to understand with its own sensors all that is needed to play. This will free the play experience from settings that, although possibly included in the "start ceremony" that may be held at the beginning of the play activity, may not be always accepted by the players.

Improvements in actuation may also make the development of new experiences possible. Humanoids may start to be able to run and jump, thus making it possible to have a human-shaped robot able to escape in a tag game, or to play real soccer, possibly passing the ball always in the right way.

We mentioned that robots may have many shapes, not necessarily humanoid. Fantastic shapes with special abilities may be interesting. Even simple shapes like a net, maybe sustaining balls like in *Knitted Wonder Spare 2* by Toshiko Horiuchi MacAdam, a permanent playground/artwork at Hakone Open Air Museum[1] (see Fig. 10.1[2]).

[1] https://www.archdaily.com/297941/meet-the-artist-behind-those-amazing-hand-knitted-play grounds.

[2] Picture by Roberta Carabalona. This work is licensed under a Creative Commons Attribution 4.0 International License (http://creativecommons.org/licenses/by/4.0/).

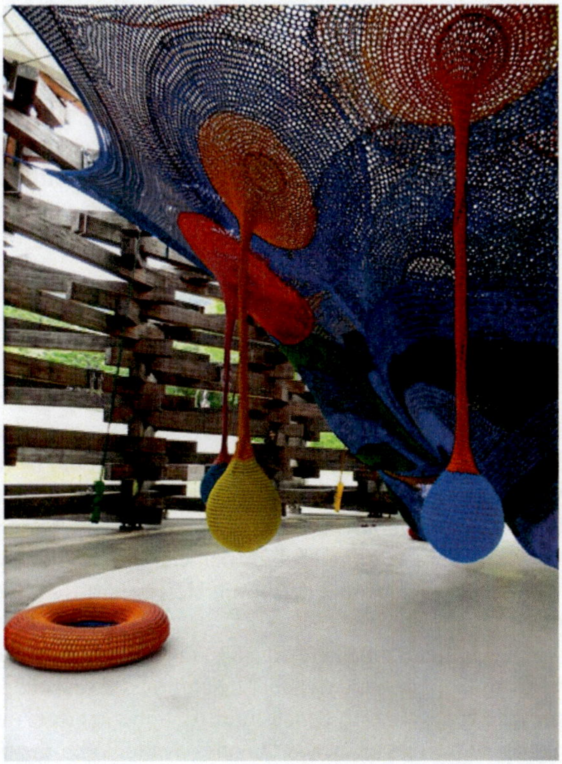

Fig. 10.1 Knitted Wonder Spare 2 at Hakone Open Air Museum, an inspiration to implement an inclusive active playground

Kids enjoy to interact with these coloured nets and big balls by physically exploring their relationship with them, entering their cavities and holding on the ball suspensions. Installations like this are presently passive, but may become active and reactive to the players on the playground, possibly enabling them to explore possibilities according to their abilities. The same may be done with ground fountains that are appearing in many cities, where nowadays kids enjoy the interaction with water that is split with a given pattern by many holes on the ground, but might be made reactive to the situation and the behaviour of the players, so becoming even more engaging.

Robot shape exploration can be done according to the principles discussed in Chap. 4 to further improve engagement and compliance to the user needs. Soft robots can have different shapes and textures to explore different ways of touching and obtaining reactions, at different levels of detail to implement the proper challenge for the specific player. It may be interesting, mostly for people with visual impairments, but not only, to have robots able to change their shape so to put in evidence characteristics that could be associated, for instance, to animals, and, when the animal is recognized, give a feedback with the animal cry.

Unusual shapes may also be devised. For instance, we are planning to implement a semi-cylindrical, 2 metres high shape made of white Lycra, behind which a robot can move a ball pushing on the surface. The player would interact with this entity through the tissue, possibly touching the ball, but also experiencing what happens when getting close to it or playing with the elasticity of the medium elsewhere. The robot will react, maintaining the neutral separation of the fabric surface, which may reassure people that may have issues to sustain an open face interaction. Projections or moving LED lights may integrate the experience.

10.2 Dream Play

Dream play is oriented to cover disabilities that presently we cannot cover with augmented playful objects. For instance, it would be interesting to have a ball that, when thrown to another player, actually reaches he/him whatever the quality of the launch. At the moment, this would in principle be possible if the ball rolls on the floor, since we have ball robots that can move automatically and could be provided with sensors for people detection. However, a free flying ball is a dream still to be realized.

Other potentially interesting dream play activities may be enabled by exoskeletons worn by people with physical disabilities. Exoskeleton technology is now able to provide only walking capabilities to some subjects, and it is still hard to have an exoskeleton for kids, since the ones available on the market (at a high price) try to match a population as large as possible, so they are designed for adults, with the somatic characteristics typical of the corresponding market areas (e.g., Japan, or North Europe). Exoskeletons that could enable kids to run would open a wide range of traditional games to these children.

On a similar track, transducers from visual signal to touch or auditory signals for people with vision impairments, and from sound to visual or touch signals for people with hearing impairments, would give access to these people to play activities that require the channel they cannot use. This is analogous to what is done with assistive technology devices for people with movement impairments. For instance, one of the limitations for blind people is that they are not fully aware of what is around, they may feel they are alone when others are moving away and they may not be confident in autonomously moving in the play space [269]. If they could be equipped with a bracelet sending auditory or vibratory signals to signal the presence of companions or specific toys, they may be supported in a richer play experience. This will need to have the bracelet interfaced with a set of IoT sensors so as to be able to detect the situations to be communicated to the player, or even with sensors similar to the ones developed at IBM already mentioned in Chap. 6. A setting like this has to be properly designed. For instance, if more people are wearing the bracelet, sound may be interesting for direct interaction, while it may be better to have vibration for "personal" information to reduce cross-talk in the room.

Chapter 11
Conclusion

Andrea Bonarini and Serenella Besio

Abstract This book would like to be a contribution to support the engineered development of robotic devices able to play with people, including people affected by disabilities, and the corresponding play activities. We have shown how it is possible to design a robot that can play a role in the development of new play experiences in the physical world and could be affordable for everybody. We have proposed a framework to analyse the different aspects involved in this activity and guide the development of such robots and play activities, and we have discussed how this can be applied to existing robots and to the ones that could be realized. In this chapter, we summarize what has been presented and propose guidelines for the development process.

11.1 Conclusion

Play is the natural activity in everybody's life, and an avalanche of literature has demonstrated its importance for overall development and growth. Through play children learn, of course, but they also make friends, take risks, experience emotions and feelings, learn to feel self-competent, practice through repetition, and invent through problem-solving. Play is irreplaceable in the individual's life: it is the door to irony and humour, to relational skills, and to know oneself deeply. All of this while having fun!

We have discussed how play for children with disability is not always easy, at least at the level and in the ways they may like. There are types of play or games that they know their peers do play, but that are not accessible to them. There are play situations that nobody offers them to enter in. They may not be able to initiate playing with peers. Often the children with a disability end up being satisfied by watching the play of others, but play does not really exist without acting as protagonists of one's own play activity. This book would like to be a contribution to support the engineered development of play activities involving robotic devices and including persons with disabilities. We have seen how robots, and the design of play activities based on robots, may be tools to offer new play possibilities to everybody, and, in particular, how they may support the reduction of the gaps that may hinder a satisfactory play

A. Bonarini and S. Besio, *Robot Play for All*, Research for Development,
https://doi.org/10.1007/978-3-031-05042-8_11

experience for persons with disabilities. We have shown how it is possible to design a robot that can play a role in the development of new play experiences in the physical world and could be affordable for everybody. We have proposed a framework to analyse and guide the development of such robots and play activities, and we have discussed how this can be applied to existing robots and to the ones that could be realized.

11.2 Guidelines for the Development of Play Activities

To finalize our presentation, we would like to propose a sort of guideline for the development of play experiences based on robots, so that they can respond to the need and the wish of the person with disabilities and at the same time represent an appropriate and satisfying play proposal as to the robot characteristics, the interaction modalities, the type of play and activity, the actors involved and their roles. These guidelines are mainly addressed to developers, but they may be useful also for educators, teachers, and professionals in the field of disability who intend to improve the play of the children they work with, considering robots as interesting tools.

The implementation process we propose implies the involvement of all the concerned actors, for the unavoidable reason that each of them can provide useful information for the process itself, and can bring interesting perspectives, important suggestions and warnings, but also specific competence to face the problem.

Most of the robots presented in this book have been developed by multidisciplinary teams, although often the final users have not been involved. Developing a robot, and the corresponding play activities, requires non-secondary inventiveness, and the creative process should integrate opinions and suggestions from all the involved actors.

The participation of the final player him/herself in this group should not be an option, rather a must: as the UNCRPD stresses when it indicates the full participation of persons with disabilities to what concerns them, the involvement of the players brings to this particular process the key-information, that is what they intend for "playing", how they would like to play, what they may like and dislike in playing.

The guidelines are organized into six steps, each of them containing subsequent phases, presented in the form of objectives to accomplish, but any Step is always strictly related with each other, and loops among phases are possible and often needed. For each Step some phases are described, as well as related methodological tools, including possible warnings. The reported tools and methodologies are relevant and well-known in the field of human research. Children with disabilities must have the opportunity to participate to the various phases by using the support systems they normally use if they are appropriate to overcome their impairment.

These guidelines are intended for planning the design of a robot device that can play with the children, in whatever way, but for the sake of play. Playing with the children also to obtain other goals is always possible. These guidelines can also support play-like activities, after few—but crucial—changes.

Preamble

Before developing a play tool, a designer should adopt a theoretical approach on play, and particularly on the types of play and their internal relationships. In Part I of this book all the main issues concerning play have been presented in detail: definitions, facets, interpretations, functions, characteristics, and types.

To give research on play and with play a scientific and methodologically appropriate approach, it is necessary to start from a solid basis, which can be shared with researchers at large, and can lead to well-founded studies, with repeatable and comparable outcomes.

Play should no more be considered as a passepartout word, that anyone understands and thus does not require further clarification. Such indeterminacy has often led to confusion in the involved sectors, both Humanities and Technology. Making background choices is a fundamental starting point for the development process.

STEP 1. The Player

What child? What type of disability? What age? The first Step consists in the identification of the target of the play experience and robot that we would like to develop. This usually happens because of requests coming from families, schools, rehabilitation professionals, etc. Sometimes, the request comes from an association of persons with disabilities and in this case more children might be involved in the process. This Step implies the following phases.

- To know the characteristics of the type of impairment that will be involved as well as previous related research experiences.
  - Knowledge is obtained through studying in-depth the related literature, particularly that strictly related to play and the type of impairment taken into consideration.
- To know the functional limitations of the specific child (or children) as well as the supports (technical, assistive, robotics, etc.) they are actually using; to know the popularity and social inclusion of the child (or children) within the group of peers (at school, in other contexts).
  - Interviews with parents, relatives, professionals
    - Warning: it is very important that during the interviews any positive information is valued and exploited: what the children are able to do, how they are able to do things, if they use assistive technologies, aids, supports, other forms of help.
    - Warning: it is better to make separate interviews (e.g., parents/professionals) because the collected information can be uneven with respect to different contexts of life (the children can experience less or more limitations in different contexts and within different relationships).

- To know the user(s), their play wishes and their play experiences.
  - Interviews, focus group (in the case of parents or group of teachers/educators; they should be requested what they know and they think about the play wishes and experiences of the child).
    - Warning: the interview with the child may be difficult due to communication or language impairment, or should be done with the mediation of communication devices or supports. Sometimes the presence of an assistant can prove useful.
    - Warning: the interviews and the focus groups with parents and/or professionals should be led with a firm attention to the goal of deepening play for the sake of play, and not play for other purposes. Professionals and parents are often strictly and solely interested in functional improvement and learning acquisition. This recommendation can be relaxed if it is decided to develop play-like experiences.
- To know the play abilities and modalities of the child and the preferred play tools and activities. This phase involves direct observation by the researcher; it can be done also by using video recording. Modalities should be chosen in accordance with the developmental plan of the robot device. The child should be requested to play as he/she prefers but can also be requested to face with new toys, tools, and play situations. The same for the observation in a group. Depending on the research objectives, the researcher might intervene, play with the child, and give suggestions or not.
  - Observation in the context, alone
  - Observation in the context, with one or more adults
  - Observation in the context, in group
  - Interview with parents and/or professionals.

STEP 2. What Objective for the Play Activity?

The accomplishment of Step 1 produces some ideas on the type of play and type of activities that should be implemented. It is not definitive, at this point. Discussion is open and useful within the group, but only in specific moments devoted to this scope and not during the observation phases. In what follows, alternative objectives are presented.

- To be able to carry out a desired type of play (or, a specific type of activity afferent to that type).
  - Targeted observation in the context (see Step 3).

  - Brainstorming within the working groups, to develop hypotheses on the following points: why this type of play (activity) cannot be done? What are potential obstacles? What type of intervention, tool, support could let them emerge or develop?

- To improve or to widen the player's competences and the abilities within a type of play, or get accustomed to shift from one type to another type, or within the same type of play gain a further more complex step.

  - Targeted observation in the context (see Step 3).
  - Brainstorming within the working groups, to develop hypotheses on the following points: what causes these difficulties in play? What type of intervention, tool, or support could let it emerge or develop?

- To improve the play activity when it happens in a group or in a dyad.

  - Targeted observation in the context (see Step 3).
  - Possible interviews or free conversation with the peers.

STEP 3. What Assessment Tool to Adopt for Evaluating the Play Activity?

This book presents a wealth of existing assessment tools in the field, but most of them are not addressed to evaluate play as such, rather the outcomes of play activities. In most cases they are tools that support the overall child assessment, where play is one of the observed areas due to its driving potential of development.

Some scales, questionnaires and other kinds of tools are also available, and in most cases, they have been developed on purpose since they are addressed to a specific population. On the contrary, despite they have not yet been used for the sole purposes of play, some particularly interesting tools exist that present a detail of various evolutionary stages within the single type of play, and they are very promising for the study of play for the sake of play.

Tools are also available to evaluate the attitude towards robots and technology as well as the effectiveness of the robot use by the child. e.g. with respect to the use of traditional toys and can be used both with the final users and the other members of the play activity. Other tools are available to evaluate and support the development of accessible and usable devices. It is important to select the evaluation procedures at this point of the development, since in many cases they put in evidence aspects that should be addressed in the design, so they can support the next steps, even before being applied for evaluation.

- To know the existing tools in relation to the considered situation, with the related literature.

  - Knowledge can be reached through the study of the literature, possibly exploiting what has been presented in this book and in those cited, and particularly through a direct analysis and comparison of the various existing tools, with the possible constraints they imply, e.g., in administration procedures or contexts of application.

- To envisage the opportunity to adapt the chosen assessment tool to the characteristics and needs of the child involved in the design plan (e.g., in case of sensory impairment).
  - Warning: an adaptation procedure is very welcome to know more precisely what types of play the child and his/her peers are able and used to play. Nevertheless, being the assessment a formal procedure, careful attention should be paid in avoiding that the procured adaptations introduce changes or variations to the items proposed. This risk is discussed in the methodological literature.
- To verify that the identified assessment tool is correctly addressed to measure the objectives that have been singled out.
  - Warning: some inaccuracies have also been found in the literature in this regard. Some studies have extrapolated parts related to play from tests that measure the development of the child as a whole, but this produces difficulties in measuring results. The concept of playfulness, adopted in the test with the same name, refers to an individual personality trait, while in some cases the concept of playfulness has been used differently: it is necessary to be precise and cautious in choosing the instrument.
- To consider the possibility and the opportunity to develop an ad hoc tool for the specific needs of the considered situation.

STEP 4. What Play Activity?

To implement this Step the participation of the whole group the entire group of researchers and professionals involved in the project is very useful, so that the information collected through the previous steps can be correlated in an effective and significant way. Furthermore, the construction of the idea for a play activity is an inventive process, favoured by discussion and confrontation. Ultimately, sharing the initial idea and participating to its implementation and monitoring process, creates a climate of collaboration that increases the feeling of belonging to the developmental plan.

As sustained in this book, a play activity emerges and develops within a ludic framework formed by child/ren, environment, tool/s, adult/s and their reciprocal relationships. The play activity is the glue that holds everything together; if it all works, then there is fun and, in case of a group play acitvity, there is a general feeling of inclusion.

- To indicate precisely the type of play to which the to-be-invented play activity belongs.
- To define the modalities for the implementation of the activity.

- To define what the child is expected to do, what he/she is proposed to do, with respect to the objectives and the modalities of the activities, to the objects and to the robot device, as well as to the environment.
- To define what the peers are expected to do, what they are proposed to do and how the relationships within the group will be regulated.

  Warning: To create an inclusive play activity, in the case that there is a gap—e.g., cognitive—between the child with a disability and the peers, the needed adaptations, supports, or tricks within the play should be prepared, so that the child can be equally protagonist with the others. If this aspect is not finely adjusted, the general fun will decrease and the child with disability risks to be isolated.

- To define what is the role of the adult within the activity.
  Many roles can be played by the adult within a play activity, and they are described in literature. Choosing the most adequate to the situation is sometimes related to what concretely happens during the activity itself. Nevertheless, a well-planned play activity should attribute the adult his/her role from the start; the developing situation may require changes.
- To define the characteristics of the environment where the activity will take place. The environment should be accessible and safe and should offer the opportunity to carry out the activity at its best and without obstacles. The perfect organization of the environment according to a good planning will give every child the opportunity to feel free to play as he/she prefers.

STEP 5. The Robot

What robot is suitable to support the devised activity? How can it support? How is the devised activity organized? In this step the robot is designed to be part of the devised activity, considering the possibilities offered by the technology and what has been defined about the player. Most of the steps listed here below have to be done in parallel in an integrated design process.

- To define the physical aspect of the robot. The physical aspect should be functional to the activity and compatible with the possible preferences of the player. All the related aspects should be considered: dimensions, colour, material, shape, etc.
- To design the interaction needs to implement the devised activity. This step is mostly aimed at defining the specifications of what is expected to obtain by the robot, which can be implemented once sensors and actuators are selected.
- To define the sensor capabilities of the robot that are needed to implement the devised activity.
  - Warning: if no sensors can provide the signals needed to reliably implement the devised activity, this should be revised.

- To define the actuator capabilities of the robot that are needed to implement the devised activity.
  - Warning: if it is not possible to achieve the desired performance the devised activity should be revised to match the available possibilities.
- To evaluate whether a robot is available on the market that could cover the requirements at a cost compatible with the setting. If this is available, it may be selected considering that the development of a robot would be much more resource demanding than its acquisition from the market.
  - Warning: when selecting a product it is needed to consider also how much this could be modified to adapt it to the play activity and to the specific player. Often products are sold as they are, except for some possibility to program some of them at a certain extent.
- To evaluate whether there are the resources to develop a robot satisfying the requirements.
  - Warning: the resources needed are money, capability, materials, time.
- To implement the robot in the play activity. Any robot, either developed or purchased should be integrated in the devised play activity.

STEP 6. Assessment

As we have seen, a thorough assessment of play activity is not an easy task, and it should be done according to the guidelines that have been presented, using the tools that have been selected in Step 3.

This means that, according to the overall objectives of the play activity, the assessment process might evaluate, among others, the effectiveness of the play activity in terms of: a) fun and playability; b) increased play ability of the child/ren; c) robot-child/ren interaction; d) robot functionality; d) quality of inclusion; e) appropriateness of the environment; f) quality and modalities of adults' participation, and so on. Each area of investigation can be analysed and studied in more detail, according to the child/ren's needs, the research objectives, the specific constraints and opportunities.

- Warning: The developed play activity must be tested in different sessions, probably with different players. In fact, many play activities may have success due to the novelty of interacting with a robot. The real success of play activity is obtained when the novelty effect is diluted and the real drivers to fun and engagements are emerging.

11.3 Farewell

In this book, we have provided a quite large amount of knowledge and information about the development of interactive robots that could participate in interesting play activities also with people with disability. We expect that this material will inspire the development of many interesting play activities and robots that will be used not only by persons with disabilities, but for the enjoyment of anyone. Playing with a robot, in the real, physical world gives us the possibility to interact with another kind of being, with its capabilities and limitations, so to explore new interaction possibilities that may enhance our abilities to face the issues arising in the real world. In the play context, this interaction is also bringing all the positive aspects that characterize play, including fun.

Enjoy!

References

1. Abu-Amara, F., Bensefia, A., Mohammad, H., Tamimi, H.: Robot and virtual reality-based intervention in autism: a comprehensive review. Int. J. Inf. Technol. 1–13 (2021)
2. Adams, K., Alvarez, L., Rios, A.: Robotic systems for augmentative manipulation to promote cognitive development, play, and education. In: Robotic Assistive Technologies, pp. 219–261. CRC Press, Boca Raton, US-FL (2017)
3. Ahmetovic, D., Sato, D., Oh, U., Ishihara, T., Kitani, K., Asakawa, C.: ReCog: Supporting Blind People in Reçognizing Personal Objects, pp. 1–12. Association for Computing Machinery, New York, US-NY (2020)
4. Ainscow, M., Conteh, J., Dyson, A., Gallannaugh, F.: Children in primary education: Demography, culture, diversity, inclusion. In: Alexander, R. J., Doddington, C., Gray, J., Hargreaves, L., Kershner, R. (eds.) The Cambridge Primary Review Research Surveys, pp. 215–236. Routledge, London, UK (2012)
5. Ajuwon, P.M., Meeks, M.K., Griffin-Shirley, N., Okungu, P.A.: Reflections of teachers of visually impaired students on their assistive technology competencies. J. Vis. Impairment & Blindness **110**(2), 128–134 (2016)
6. Aktürk Ablan, H.: Developing toy design criteria for visually impaired children: A new play set design. Master's thesis, Izmir Institute of Technology (2013). https://gcris.iyte.edu.tr/bitstream/11147/3604/1/10011472.pdf
7. Alayli, A.: Sequential development of theory of mind and relations with receptive language, self-regulation, aggressive behavior and social competence in hearing impaired Turkish children. Master's thesis, Sosyal Bilimler Enstitüsü (2015). https://acikbilim.yok.gov.tr/bitstream/handle/20.500.12812/168434/yokAcikBilim_10092501.pdf?sequence=-1&isAllowed=y
8. Alhaddad, A.Y., Cabibihan, J.J., Bonarini, A.: Recognition of aggressive interactions of children toward robotic toys. 2019 28th IEEE International Conference on Robot and Human Interactive Communication (RO-MAN), pp. 1–8. IEEE (2019)
9. Alhaddad, A.Y., Cabibihan, J.J., Bonarini, A.: Influence of reaction time in the emotional response of a companion robot to a child's aggressive interaction. Int. J. Soc. Robot. 1279–1291 (2020)
10. Alhaddad, A.Y., Cabibihan, J.J., Hayek, A., Bonarini, A.: Influence of the shape and mass of a small robot when thrown to a dummy human head. SN Appl. Sci. **1**(11), 1–9 (2019)
11. Allievi, A.G., Arichi, T., Gordon, A.L., Burdet, E.: Technology-aided assessment of sensorimotor function in early infancy. Front. Neurol. **5**, 197 (2014)

A. Bonarini and S. Besio, *Robot Play for All*, Research for Development,
https://doi.org/10.1007/978-3-031-05042-8

12. de Almeida Soares, D., von Hofsten, C., Tudella, E.: Development of exploratory behavior in late preterm infants. Infant Behav. Dev. **35**(4), 912–915 (2012)
13. Amabile, T.M., Collins, M., Conti, R., Phillips, E.: Creativity in context. Update to the Social Psychology of Creativity. Westview Press, Boulder, US-CO (1996)
14. American Association on Intellectual and Developmental Disabilities (AAIDD): Diagnostic and statistical manual of mental disorders: DSM-5. American Association on Intellectual and Developmental Disabilities, Arlington, VA (2012)
15. Anazi, S., Maddirevula, S., Salpietro, V., Asi, Y.T., Alsahli, S., Alhashem, A., Shamseldin, H.E., Al Zahrani, F., Patel, N., Ibrahim, N., et al.: Expanding the genetic heterogeneity of intellectual disability. Hum. Genet. **136**(11), 1419–1429 (2017)
16. Andersen, E.S., Dunlea, A., Kekelis, L.S.: Blind children's language: resolving some differences. J. Child Lang. **11**(3), 645–664 (1984)
17. Andreeva, A., Celo, P., Vian, N.: Play in children with hearing impairments. In: Besio, S., Bulgarelli, D., Stancheva-Popkostadinova, V. (eds.) Play Development in Children with Disabilities, pp. 94–101. De Gruyter Open Warsaw, PL (2017)
18. Angel-Fernandez, J.M., Bonarini, A.: Robots showing emotions - emotion representation with no bio-inspired body. Interact. Stud. **17**(3), 408–437 (2016)
19. Angelin, A.C., Sposito, A.M., Pfeifer, L.I.: Influence of functional mobility and manual function on play in preschool children with cerebral palsy. Hong Kong J. Occup. Ther. **31**(1), 46–53 (2018)
20. Arens, K., Cress, C.J., Marvin, C.A.: Gaze-shift patterns of young children with developmental disabilities who are at risk for being nonspeaking. Education and Training in Developmental Disabilities, **40**(2), 158–170 (2005)
21. Argyropoulou, Z., Papoudi, D.: The training of a child with autism in a greek preschool inclusive class through intensive interaction: a case study. Eur. J. Spec. Needs Educ. **27**(1), 99–114 (2012)
22. Arias, V.B., Gómez, L.E., Morán, M.L., Alcedo, M.Á., Monsalve, A., Fontanil, Y.: Does quality of life differ for children with autism spectrum disorder and intellectual disability compared to peers without autism? J. Autism Dev. Disord. **48**(1), 123–136 (2018)
23. Aries, P.: Centuries of Childhood. Jonathan Cape, London, UK (1962)
24. Arrasvuori, J., Korhonen, H., Montola, M.: Understanding playful user experience through digital games. In: International Conference on Designing Pleasurable Products and Interfaces (2010)
25. Ashman, A.F., Conway, R.N.: Cognitive Strategies for Special Education: Process-Based Instruction. Routledge, London, UK (2017)
26. Astramovich, R.L., Lyons, C., Hamilton, N.J.: Play therapy for children with intellectual disabilities. J. Child and Adolesc. Couns. **1**(1), 27–36 (2015)
27. Ayton, L.N., Allen, P.J., Abbott, C.J., Petoe, M.A.: Technologies for vision impairment: Bionic eyes and sensory substitution devices. In: Ravenscroft, J. (ed.) The Routledge Handbook of Visual Impairment, pp. 392–411. Routledge, London, UK (2019)
28. Azevedo, L.: Play and augmentative mobility: the INMAC (inclusive mobility for all children) vehicle. In: Presentation at the 15th AAATE Conference, Special Thematic Session "Play, Children with Disabilities, and Robotics. State of the Art and New Developments". AAATE (2019)
29. Bach-y-Rita, P., Collins, C.C., Saunders, F.A., White, B., Scadden, L.: Vision substitution by tactile image projection. Nature **221**(5184), 963–964 (1969)
30. Bach-y-Rita, P., Tyler, M.E., Kaczmarek, K.A.: Seeing with the brain. Int. J. Hum.-Comput. Interact. **15**(2), 285–295 (2003)
31. Baghdadli, A., Brisot-Dubois, J.: Entraînement Aux Habiletés Sociales Appliqué a L'autisme. Elsevier Masson, Paris, FR (2011)
32. Bagnato, S.J., Neisworth, J.T., Pretti-Frontczak, K.: LINKing Authentic Assessment and Early Childhood Intervention: Best Measures for Best Practice. Paul H Brookes Publishing, Baltimora, US-MD (2010)

33. Baird, G., Charman, T., Baron-Cohen, S., Cox, A., Swettenham, J., Wheelwright, S., Drew, A.: A screening instrument for autism at 18 months of age: a 6-year follow-up study. J. Am. Acad. Child Adolesc. Psychiatry **39**(6), 694–702 (2000)
34. Baker, R., Knight, P.: Total communication–current policy and practice. In: Gregory, S. (ed.) Issues in deaf education, pp. 215–224. Routledge, London, UK (1998)
35. Balogh, R.: Educational robotic platform based on arduino. In: Proceedings of the 1st International Conference on Robotics in Education, RiE2010. FEI STU, Slovakia, pp. 119–122 (2010)
36. Bana, S., Sajedi, F., Mirzaie, H., Rezasoltani, P.: The efficacy of cognitive behavioral play therapy on self esteem of children with intellectual disability. Iran. Rehabil. J. **15**(3), 235–242 (2017)
37. Bandler, R., Grinder, J.: The Structure of Magic, vol. 1. Science and Behavior Books Palo Alto, US-CA (1975)
38. Barakova, E.I., Lourens, T.: Expressing and interpreting emotional movements in social games with robots. Pers. Ubiquit. Comput. **14**(5), 457–467 (2010)
39. Barbeau, M.: Processus interactifs mnésiques et comportementaux après coma posttraumatique chez l'enfant. ANAE **2**, 20–22 (1990)
40. Barnett, L.A.: The playful child: measurement of a disposition to play. Play and Culture **4**(1), 51–74 (1991)
41. Barnett, L.A.: The inculcation of adult playfulness: from west to east. Int. J. Play **6**(3), 255–271 (2017)
42. Barnett, W.S., Jung, K., Yarosz, D.J., Thomas, J., Hornbeck, A., Stechuk, R., Burns, S.: Educational effects of the tools of the mind curriculum: a randomized trial. Early Childhood Res. Quart. **23**(3), 299–313 (2008)
43. Baron-Cohen, S.: From attention-goal psychology to belief-desire psychology: The development of a theory of mind and its dysfunction. In: Baron-Cohen, S., Tager-Flusberg, H., Cohen, D. (eds.) Understanding Other Minds: Perspectives from Autism, pp. 59–82. Oxford University Press, Oxford, UK (1993)
44. Barron, C., Beckett, A., Coussens, M., Desoete, A., Cannon Jones, N., Lynch, H., Prellwitz, M., Fenney Salkeld, D.: Barriers to Play and Recreation for Children and Young People with Disabilities: Exploring Environmental Factors. De Gruyter, Warsaw, PL (2017)
45. Bartneck, C., Croft, E., Kulic, D.: Measurement instruments for the anthropomorphism, animacy, likeability, perceived intelligence, and perceived safety of robots. Int. J. Soc. Robot. **1**(1), 71–81 (2009)
46. Bartneck, C., Kanda, T., Mubin, O., Al Mahmud, A.: Does the design of a robot influence its animacy and perceived intelligence? Int. J. Soc. Robot. **1**(2), 195–204 (2009)
47. Bartneck, C., Reichenbach, J., Breemen, v.A.: In your face, robot! the influence of a character's embodiment on how users perceive its emotional expressions. In: Proceedings of Design and Emotion, pp. 1–19 (2004)
48. Bateson, G.: The message "This is play.". Group processes **2**, 145–241 (1956)
49. Bateson, G.: A Theory of Play and Fantasy. MIT Press, Boston, US-MA (1972)
50. Batorowicz, B., Stadskleiv, K., von Tetzchner, S., Missiuna, C.: Children who use communication aids instructing peer and adult partners during play-based activity. Augment. Altern. Commun. **32**(2), 105–119 (2016)
51. Baumeister, R.F., Vohs, K.D.: Self-regulation and the executive function of the self. In: Leary, M.R., Tangney, J.P. (eds.) Handbook of Self and Identity 2nd Ed., pp. 180–197. Guilford Press, London, UK (2012)
52. Becker-Asano, C., Ishiguro, H.: Evaluating facial displays of emotion for the android robot geminoid F. In: 2011 IEEE Workshop on Affective Computational Intelligence (WACI), pp. 1–8. IEEE (2011)
53. Beeghly, M.: Emergence of symbolic play: Perspectives from typical and atypical development. In: Burack, J.A., Hodapp, R.M., Zigler, E. (eds.) Handbook of mental retardation and development, pp. 240–289. Cambridge University Press, Cambridge, UK (1998)

54. Beer, J.M., Prakash, A., Mitzner, T.L., Rogers, W.A.: Understanding robot acceptance. Tech. rep. Georgia Institute of Technology (2011)
55. Bekoff, M.: Social play behaviour. cooperation, fairness, trust, and the evolution of morality. Journal of Consciousness Studies **8**(2), 81–90 (2001)
56. Bekoff, M.: Wild justice and fair play: Cooperation, forgiveness, and morality in animals. Biol. Philos. **19**(4), 489–520 (2004)
57. Belsky, J., Most, R.K.: From exploration to play: a cross-sectional study of infant free play behavior. Dev. Psychol. **17**(5), 630 (1981)
58. Ben-Sasson, A., Hen, L., Fluss, R., Cermak, S.A., Engel-Yeger, B., Gal, E.: A meta-analysis of sensory modulation symptoms in individuals with autism spectrum disorders. J. Autism Dev. Disord. **39**(1), 1–11 (2009)
59. Benson, J.D., Nicka, M.N., Stern, P.: How does a child with sensory processing problems play? Internet Journal of Allied Health Sciences and Practice **4**(4), 1–4 (2006)
60. Bergen, D.: Play, technology toy affordances, and brain development-research needs and policy issues. In: Waite-Stupiansky, S., Cohen, L. (eds.) Play: A polyphony of research, theories and issues, vol. 12, pp. 163–73. Information Age, Lanham, US-MD (2012)
61. Bergen, D.: Infant sensorimotor play: Development of sociocultural competence and enactive cognition. In: P. Smith, J. Roopnarine (eds.) The Cambridge Handbook of Play, pp. 125–141. Cambridge University Press, Cambridge, UK (2019)
62. Bergeron, F., Berland, A., Demers, D., Gobeil, S.: Contemporary speech and oral language care for deaf and hard-of-hearing children using hearing devices. J. Clin. Med. **9**(2), 378 (2020)
63. Berghänel, A., Schülke, O., Ostner, J.: Locomotor play drives motor skill acquisition at the expense of growth: A life history trade-off. Science advances **1**(7) (2015)
64. Bernardini, M.G.: Disabilità, giustizia, diritto. Itinerari tra filosofia del diritto e Disability Studies, vol. 124. G. Giappichelli Editore, Torino, IT (2016)
65. Bertel, L.B., Rasmussen, D.M.: Peers at play: A case study on persuasive educational and entertainment robotics in autism education. In: Proceedings of the International Workshop on EuroPLOT Persuasive Technology for Learning, Education, and Teaching IWEPLET, pp. 161–168 (2013)
66. Besio, S.: Analysis of critical factors involved uin using interactive robots for education and therapy of children with disabilities: IROMEC, Interactive robotic social mediators as companions, IST-FP6-045356. UNIservice, Trento, IT (2008)
67. Besio, S.: The need for play for the sake of play. In: S. Besio, D. Bulgarelli, V. Stancheva-Popkostadinova (eds.) Play development in children with disabilities, pp. 9–52. De Gruyter Open, Warsaw, PL (2017)
68. Besio, S.: Play for the sake of play: in pursuit of a dream? In: S. Besio, T. Zappaterra (eds.) Children's play. Multifaceted aspects, p. 43-70. ETS, Firenze, IT (2018)
69. Besio, S.: Gioco e robotica. In: A. Bobbio, A. Bondioli (eds.) Gioco e infanzia. Teorie e scenari educativi, pp. 127–160. Carocci, Roma, IT (2019)
70. Besio, S.: Ricercare la disabilità. In: N. Bianquin (ed.) L'ICF a supporto di percorsi personalizzati lungo l'arco della vita, pp. 9–19. Pensa Multimedia, Lecce, IT (2020)
71. Besio, S.: Il gioco del bambino con disabilitá, trasformatore del gioco di tutti. In: Polenghi, S., Cereda, F., Zini, P. (eds.) La responsabilitá della pedagogia nelle trasformazioni dei rapporti sociali, pp. 229–237. Pensa Multimedia, Lecce, IT (2021)
72. Besio, S., Amelina, N.: Play in children with physical impairment. In: Besio, S., Bulgarelli, D., Stancheva-Popkostadinova, V. (eds.) Play development in children with disabilities. De Gruyter Open, Warsaw, PL (2017)
73. Besio, S., Bianquin, N.: Il paradigma inclusivo fra approcci teorici, pratiche e corpi agiti. Nuova Secondaria Ricerca **10**, 91–98 (2019)
74. Besio, S., Bonarini, A., Lynch, H., Molina, P., Veronese, F., Bulgarelli, D.: Mainstream robotic toys and children with physical impairment: what about playfulness? In: Proceedings of the 7th International Conference on Software Development and Technologies for Enhancing Accessibility and Fighting Info-exclusion, pp. 208–215 (2016)

75. Besio, S., Bulgarelli, D., Stancheva-Popkostadinova, V., et al.: Evaluation of children's play. Tools and methods. De Gruyter Open, Warsaw, PL (2018)
76. Bethel, C.L., Henkel, Z., Darrow, S., Baugus, K.: Therabot-an adaptive therapeutic support robot. In: 2018 World Symposium on Digital Intelligence for Systems and Machines (DISA), pp. 23–30. IEEE (2018)
77. Beyer, J., Gammeltoft, L.: Autism and play. Kingsley Publishers, London, UK (2000)
78. Bianquin, N.: How can I, as an adult, facilitate play? In: Encarnação, P., Ray-Kaeser, S., Bianquin, N. (eds.) Guidelines for supporting children with disabilities' play: Methodologies, tools, and contexts, pp. 50–58. De Gruyter Open, Warsaw, PL (2018)
79. Bianquin, N.: Le jeu de l'enfant: un droit encore a réaliser. In: Besio, S., Zappaterra, T. (eds.) Children's play. Multifaceted aspects, pp. 15–42. ETS, Firenze, IT (2018)
80. Bickenbach, J.E.: Assistive technology and the international classification of functioning, disability, and health. The Engineering Handbook of Smart Technology for Aging, Disability, and Independence p. 81 (2008)
81. Bickenbach, J.E., Chatterji, S., Badley, E.M., Üstün, T.B.: Models of disablement, universalism and the international classification of impairments, disabilities and handicaps. Social science & medicine **48**(9), 1173–1187 (1999)
82. Bickford, R.G., Daly, D., Keith, H.M.: Convulsive effects of light stimulation in children. A.M.A. Am. J. Dis. Child. **86**(2), 170–183 (1953)
83. Bigelow, A.E.: The development of reaching in blind children. Br. J. Dev. Psychol. **4**(4), 355–366 (1986)
84. Bigelow, A.E.: The development of joint attention in blind infants. Dev. Psychopathol. **15**(2), 259–275 (2003)
85. Billstedt, E., Gillberg, I.C., Gillberg, C.: Aspects of quality of life in adults diagnosed with autism in childhood: A population-based study. Autism **15**(1), 7–20 (2011)
86. Black-Hawkins, K., Florian, L.: Classroom teachers' craft knowledge of their inclusive practice. Teachers and Teaching **18**(5), 567–584 (2012)
87. Blair, C.: School readiness: Integrating cognition and emotion in a neurobiological conceptualization of children's functioning at school entry. Am. Psychol. **57**(2), 111 (2002)
88. Blair, C., Raver, C.C.: Closing the achievement gap through modification of neurocognitive and neuroendocrine function: Results from a cluster randomized controlled trial of an innovative approach to the education of children in kindergarten. PLoS ONE **9**(11), e112393 (2014)
89. Blanc, R., Adrien, J.L., Roux, S., Barthélémy, C.: Dysregulation of pretend play and communication development in children with autism. Autism **9**(3), 229–245 (2005)
90. Blanche, E.I.: Play in children with cerebral palsy: Doing with-not doing to. In: Parham, L.D., Fazio, L.S. (eds.) Play in occupational therapy for children, pp. 375–393. Mosby Elsevier, St. Louis, US-MO (2008)
91. Blum, E.J., Fields, B.C., Scharfman, H., Silber, D.: Development of symbolic play in deaf children aged 1 to 3. In: Slade, A., Palmer Wolf, D. (eds.) Children at play: Clinical and Developmental Approaches to Meaning and Representation, pp. 238–259, New York, US-NY (1994)
92. Blumstein, D.T., Chung, L.K., Smith, J.E.: Early play may predict later dominance relationships in yellow-bellied marmots (marmota flaviventris). Proceedings of the Royal Society B: Biological Sciences **280**(1759), 20130485 (2013)
93. Bobzien, J., Richels, C., Raver, S.A., Hester, P., Browning, E., Morin, L.: An observational study of social communication skills in eight preschoolers with and without hearing loss during cooperative play. Early Childhood Educ. J. **41**(5), 339–346 (2013)
94. Bodrova, E., Leong, D.J.: Tools of the mind: Vygotskian approach to early childhood education. Merrill Prentice Hall, Columbus, US-OH (2006)
95. Bodrova, E., Leong, D.J.: Standing "a head taller than himself": Vygotskian and post-vygotskian views on children's play. In: Johnson, J.E., Eberle, S.G., Henricks, T.S. (eds.) The Handbook of the Study of Play, vol. 7, pp. 203–214. Rowman & Littlefield Publishing Group, Lanham, US-MD (2015)

96. Bodrova, E., Leong, D.J., Germeroth, C., Day-Hess, C.: Leading children in their & "leading activity": A vygotskian approach to play. In: Smith, P., Roopnarine, J. (eds.) The Cambridge Handbook of Play, pp. 436–456. Cambridge University Press, Cambridge, UK (2019)
97. Bonani, M., Oliveira, R., Correia, F., Rodrigues, A., Guerreiro, T., Paiva, A.: What my eyes can't see, a robot can show me: Exploring the collaboration between blind people and robots. In: Proceedings of the 20th International ACM SIGACCESS Conference on Computers and Accessibility, pp. 15–27 (2018)
98. Bonarini, A., Boriero, S., de Oliveira, E.L.S.: Robot player adaptation to human opponents in physical, competitive robogames. In: 2020 29th IEEE International Conference on Robot and Human Interactive Communication (RO-MAN), pp. 851–856. IEEE (2020)
99. Bonarini, A., Ceriani, S., Fontana, G., Matteucci, M.: On the development of a multi-modal autonomous wheelchair. In: Handbook of Research on ICTs for Human-Centered Healthcare and Social Care Services, pp. 727–748. IGI Global (2013)
100. Bonarini, A., Garzotto, F., Gelsomini, M., Romero, M., Clasadonte, F., Yilmaz, A.N.Ç.: A huggable, mobile robot for developmental disorder interventions in a multi-modal interaction space. In: 25th IEEE International Symposium on Robot and Human Interactive Communication (RO-MAN 2016), pp. 823–830. IEEE, Piscataway, NJ (2016). Winner of the Kazuo Tamie award 2016
101. Bonarini, A., Lavatelli, D., Matteucci, M.: A composite system for real-time robust whistle recognition. In: Robot Soccer World Cup, pp. 130–141. Springer, Berlin, D (2005)
102. Bondioli, A.: Gioco e educazione. FrancoAngeli, Milano, IT (1996)
103. Booth, T., Ainscow, M.: From them to us: An international study of inclusion in education. Routledge, London, UK (1998)
104. Bornstein, M.H., Selmi, A.M., Haynes, O., Painter, K.M., Marx, E.S.: Representational abilities and the hearing status of child/mother dyads. Child Dev. **70**(4), 833–852 (1999)
105. Bottos, M., Ferrari, A.: Le soluzioni chirurgiche: significato e limiti in PCI: dalla "guarigione" all'autonomia. Diagnosi e proposte riabilitative. Piccin, Padova, IT (2003)
106. Bower, T.: The perceptual world of the child. Harvard University Press, Cambridge, US-MA (1977)
107. Boyette, A.H.: Play in foraging societies. In: Smith, P., Roopnarine, J. (eds.) The Cambridge Handbook of Play, pp. 302–321. Cambridge University Press, Cambridge, UK (2019)
108. Bozena, M.: Exploratory play and cognitive activity. Garant, Antwerp, BE (2007)
109. Brambring, M.: Lo sviluppo nei bambini non vedenti. Osservazione e intervento precoce, vol. 41. FrancoAngeli, Milano, IT (2004)
110. Brambring, M.: Assessing developmental differences in blind versus sighted children. Conference report - ICEVI International Council of Education for People with Visual Impairment: Education - aiming for excellence, pp. 18–23. Chemnitz, D (2005)
111. Bravo, F.A., Gonzalez, E., Di Blas, N., Bonarini, A.: Robots at school: supporting humanities teaching through robots-based storytelling. In: EdMedia+ Innovate Learning. pp 162–175. Association for the Advancement of Computing in Education (AACE) (2019)
112. Breazeal, C.L.: Designing sociable robots. MIT Press, Cambridge, US-MA (2002)
113. van Breemen, A., Yan, X., Meerbeek, B.: ICAT: an animated user-interface robot with personality. In: Proceedings of the fourth international joint conference on Autonomous agents and multiagent systems, pp. 143–144 (2005)
114. Brivio, A., Rogacheva, K., Lucchelli, M., Bonarini, A.: A soft, mobile, autonomous robot to develop skills through play in autistic children. Paladyn, Journal of Behavioral Robotics **12**(1), 187–198 (2021)
115. Brodin, J.: Diversity of aspects on play in children with profound multiple disabilities. Early Child Dev. Care **175**(7–8), 635–646 (2005)
116. Bronfenbrenner, U.: The ecology of human development: natural and planned experiments. Harvard University Press, Cambridge, US-MA (1979)
117. Bronson, M.R., Bundy, A.C.: A correlational study of a test of playfulness and a test of environmental supportiveness for play. The Occupational Therapy Journal of Research **21**(4), 241–259 (2001)

118. Brown, A.L., Campione, J.C.: Psychological theory and the study of learning disabilities. Am. Psychol. **41**(10), 1059 (1986)
119. Brown, C.S., Emmett, S.D., Robler, S.K., Tucci, D.L.: Global hearing loss prevention. Otolaryngol. Clin. North Am. **51**(3), 575–592 (2018)
120. Brown, D.J., Proulx, M.J., Chen, L., Lin, C.: Increased signal complexity improves the breadth of generalization in auditory perceptual learning. Journal of Neural Transplantation & Plasticity, **2013** (2013)
121. Brown, D.J., Proulx, M.J.: Audio-vision substitution for blind individuals: Addressing human information processing capacity limitations. IEEE Journal of Selected Topics in Signal Processing **10**(5), 924–931 (2016)
122. Brown, P., Rickards, F., Jeanes, R.: The symbolic play of hearing impaired and normally hearing four year olds. The Australian Teacher of the Deaf **32**, 1–13 (1992)
123. Brown, P.M., Bortoli, A.: Play and children with sensory impairments. In: Smith, P., Roopnarine, J. (eds.) The Cambridge Handbook of Play, pp. 580–596. Cambridge University Press, Cambridge, UK (2019)
124. Brown, P.M., Prescott, S.J., Rickards, F.W., Paterson, M.M.: Communicating about pretend play: A comparison of the utterances of 4-year-old normally hearing and deaf or hard-of-hearing children in an integrated kindergarten. The Volta Review **99**(1), 5–17 (1997)
125. Brown, P.M., Remine, M.D.: Building pretend play skills in toddlers with and without hearing loss: Maternal scaffolding styles. Deafness & Education International **6**(3), 129–153 (2004)
126. Brown, P.M., Rickards, F.W., Bortoli, A.: Structures underpinning pretend play and word production in young hearing children and children with hearing loss. J. Deaf Stud. Deaf Educ. **6**(1), 15–31 (2001)
127. Brown, S.L.: Play: How it shapes the brain, opens the imagination, and invigorates the soul. Penguin, London, UK (2009)
128. Bruce, A., Knight, J., Nourbakhsh, I.R.: Robot improv: Using drama to create believable agents. In: In AAAI Workshop Technical Report WS-99-15 of the 8th Mobile Robot Competition and Exhibition. AAAI Press, Menlo, pp. 27–33 (2000)
129. Bruner, J.: Actual minds, possible worlds. Harvard University Press, Cambridge, US-MA (1986)
130. Bruner, J.S.: Processes of cognitive growth: Infancy. Clark University Press, Worcester, US-MA (1968)
131. Bucci, P., Zhang, L., Cang, X.L., MacLean, K.E.: Is it happy? Behavioural and narrative frame complexity impact perceptions of a simple furry robot's emotions. Proceedings of the 2018 CHI Conference on Human Factors in Computing Systems, pp. 1–11. ACM Press (2018)
132. Buchs, C., Butera, F.: Cooperative learning and social skills development. In: Gillies, R.M. (ed.) Collaborative learning: Developments in research and practice, pp. 201–217. Nova Science, Hauppauge, US-NY (2015)
133. Budoff, M.: The validity of learning potential assessment. Guilford Press, New York, US-NY (1987)
134. Bulgarelli, D., Bianquin, N.: Conceptual review of play. In: Besio, S., Bulgarelli, D., Stancheva-Popkostadinova, V. (eds.) Play evelopment in children with disabilities, pp. 58–70. De Gruyter Open, Warsaw, PL (2017)
135. Bulgarelli, D., Bianquin, N.: Playfulness. criticità di un costrutto e della sua misurazione nel caso della disabilità. Atti del Convegno Nazionale del Gruppo di lavoro SIPED - Teoria e Metodi della Ricerca Empirica in Educazione Dipartimento di Scienze per la Qualitá della Vita, p. 329-339. Dipartimento di Scienze per la Qualità della Vita, Alma Mater Studiorum Università di Bologna (2017)
136. Bulgarelli, D., Stancheva-Popkostadinova, V.: Play in children with intellectual disabilities. In: Besio, S., Bulgarelli, D. Stancheva-Popkostadinova, V. (eds.) Play development in children with disabilities, pp. 88–93. De Gruyter Open, Warsaw, PL (2017)
137. Bundy, A.: Test of Playfulness, version 3. Colorado State University, Ft Collins, US-CO (1997)

138. Bundy, A.: Can I play too? In: Kids can be Kids, p. 28–43. Davis Company, Philadelphia, US-FA (2012)
139. Bundy, A.C., Nelson, L., Metzger, M., Bingaman, K.: Validity and reliability of a test of playfulness. The Occupational Therapy Journal of Research **21**(4), 276–292 (2001)
140. Burghardt, G.: A brief glimpse at the long evolutionary history of play. Animal behavior and cognition **1**(2), 90–98 (2014)
141. Burghardt, G.M.: The genesis of animal play: Testing the limits. MIT Press, Cambridge, US-MA (2005)
142. Burghardt, G.M., Albright, J.D., Davis, K.M.: Motivation, development and object play: comparative perspectives with lessons from dogs. Behaviour **153**(6–7), 767–793 (2016)
143. Burghardt, G.M., Pellis, S.M.: New directions in studying the evolution of play. In: Smith, P., Roopnarine, J. (eds.) The Cambridge Handbook of Play, pp. 11–29. Cambridge University Press, Cambridge, UK (2019)
144. Butler, C.: Effects of powered mobility on self-initiated behaviors of very young children with locomotor disability. Developmental Medicine & Child Neurology **28**(3), 325–332 (1986)
145. Byers, J.A., Walker, C.: Refining the motor training hypothesis for the evolution of play. Am. Nat. **146**(1), 25–40 (1995)
146. Byers, J.A. Play in ungulates. In: Smith, P.K. (ed.) Play in Animals and Humans, pp. 44–65. Basil Blackwell, Oxford, UK (1984)
147. Caballo, C., Verdugo, M.Á.: Social skills assessment of children and adolescents with visual impairment: Identifying relevant skills to improve quality of social relationships. Psychological reports **100**(3_suppl), 1101–1106 (2007)
148. Cabibihan, J.J., Javed, H., Ang, M., Jr., Aljunied, S.M.: Why robots? a survey on the roles and benefits of social robots in the therapy of children with autism. Int. J. Soc. Robot. **5**(4), 593–618 (2013)
149. Caillois, R.: Les jeux et les hommes Le masque et le vertige. Gallimard, Paris, FR (1967)
150. Cairney, J.: Developmental coordination disorder and its consequences. University of Toronto Press, Toronto, CA (2015)
151. Calder, L., Hill, V., Pellicano, E.: 'Sometimes i want to play by myself': Understanding what friendship means to children with autism in mainstream primary schools. Autism **17**(3), 296–316 (2013)
152. Cameron, D., Leslie, M., Teplicky, R., Pollock, N., Stewart, D., Toal, C., Gaik, S.: The clinical utility of the test of playfulness. Can. J. Occup. Ther. **68**(2), 104–111 (2001)
153. Cameron, E.Z., Linklater, W.L., Stafford, K.J., Minot, E.O.: Maternal investment results in better foal condition through increased play behaviour in horses. Anim. Behav. **76**(5), 1511–1518 (2008)
154. Cameron, C.B., Patten, M.M. A Typology of Play in Medical Settings. In: Smith, P.K., Roopnarine, J.L. (eds.) The Cambridge Handbook of Play, pp. 615–629. Cambridge University Press, Cambridge, UK (2019)
155. Campione, J.C.: Assisted assessment: A taxonomy of approaches and an outline of strengths and weaknesses. J. Learn. Disabil. **22**(3), 151–165 (1989)
156. Campos, J.J., Anderson, D.I., Barbu-Roth, M.A., Hubbard, E.M., Hertenstein, M.J., Witherington, D.: Travel broadens the mind. Infancy **1**(2), 149–219 (2000)
157. Camurri, A., Lagerlöf, I., Volpe, G.: Recognizing emotion from dance movement: comparison of spectator recognition and automated techniques. Int. J. Hum Comput Stud. **59**(1–2), 213–225 (2003)
158. Cannao, M.: Ipovisione. i problemi dell'età evolutiva. La Nostra Famiglia Editore, Bosisio Parini, I (1989)
159. Capio, C.M., Mak, T., Tse, M., Masters, R.: Fundamental movement skills and balance of children with down syndrome. J. Intellect. Disabil. Res. **62**(3), 225–236 (2018)
160. Card, R., Dodd, B.: The phonological awareness abilities of children with cerebral palsy who do not speak. Augment. Altern. Commun. **22**(3), 149–159 (2006)
161. Cardoso, L.F.F., Santos, V.C.A., Francês, R.S.K., Prudêncio, R.B.C., Alves, R.C.O.: Decoding machine learning benchmarks. In: Cerri, R., Prati, R.C. (eds.) Intelligent Systems, pp. 412–425. Springer International Publishing, Berlin, DE (2020)

162. Carr, M.: Technological affordance, social practice and learning narratives in an early childhood setting. Int. J. Technol. Des. Educ. **10**(1), 61–80 (2000)
163. Casby, M.W.: Symbolic play of children with language impairment: A critical review. J. Speech Lang. Hear. Res. **40**(3), 468–479 (1997)
164. Cattaneo, Z., Fantino, M., Tinti, C., Pascual-Leone, A., Silvanto, J., Vecchi, T.: Spatial biases in peripersonal space in sighted and blind individuals revealed by a haptic line bisection paradigm. J. Exp. Psychol. Hum. Percept. Perform. **37**(4), 1110 (2011)
165. Cejas, I., Barker, D.H., Quittner, A.L., Niparko, J.K.: Development of joint engagement in young deaf and hearing children: Effects of chronological age and language skills. J. Speech Lang. Hear. Res. **57**(5), 1831–1841 (2014)
166. Celeste, M.: Play behaviors and social interactions of a child who is blind: In theory and practice. Journal of visual impairment & Blindness **100**(2), 75–90 (2006)
167. Ceppi, G., Zini, M.: Children. Spaces. Metaproject for an Environment for Young Children. Reggio Children Publisher, Reggio Emilia, I (1998)
168. Ceres, R., Pons, J.L., Calderon, L., Jimenez, A.R., Azevedo, L.: A robotic vehicle for disabled children. IEEE Eng. Med. Biol. Mag. **24**(6), 55–63 (2005)
169. Chan, P.C., Chen, C.T., Feng, H., Lee, Y.C., Chen, K.L.: Theory of mind deficit is associated with pretend play performance, but not playfulness, in children with autism spectrum disorder. Hong Kong J. Occup. Ther. **28**, 43–52 (2016)
170. Chang, P.Y.: Understanding taiwanese children's play via constructing and reconstructing: A prospective vision. In: Roopnarine, J., Patte, M., Johnson, J. (eds.) International perspective on children's play, pp. 119–133. Open University Press, New York, US-NY (2015)
171. Charman, T.: Why is joint attention a pivotal skill in autism? Philosophical Transactions of the Royal Society of London. Series B: Biological Sciences **358**(1430), 315–324 (2003)
172. Charman, T., Swettenham, J., Baron-Cohen, S., Cox, A., Baird, G., Drew, A.: Infants with autism: an investigation of empathy, pretend play, joint attention, and imitation. Dev. Psychol. **33**(5), 781 (1997)
173. Chebat, D.R., Rainville, C., Kupers, R., Ptito, M.: Tactile-'visual'acuity of the tongue in early blind individuals. NeuroReport **18**(18), 1901–1904 (2007)
174. Chebat, D.R., Schneider, F.C., Kupers, R., Ptito, M.: Navigation with a sensory substitution device in congenitally blind individuals. NeuroReport **22**(7), 342–347 (2011)
175. Chen, D.: Parent-infant communication: Early intervention for very young children with visual impairment or hearing loss. Infants & Young Children **9**(2), 1–12 (1996)
176. Cho, E., Josol, C.K.: Dynamic assessment in schools: What, why, and how. Information Age Publishing, Inc., Charlotte, US-NC (2021)
177. Chudacoff, H.P.: Children at play: An American history. New York University Press, New York, US-NY (2007)
178. Ciani, F., Dall'Olio, S., Stanyon, R., Palagi, E.: Social tolerance and adult play in macaque societies: a comparison with different human cultures. Anim. Behav. **84**(6), 1313–1322 (2012)
179. Cicchetti, D., Ganiban, J.: The organization and coherence of developmental processes in infants and children with down syndrome. In: Hodapp, R.M., Burack, J.A., Zigler, E. (eds.) Issues in the developmental approach to mental retardation, pp. 169–225. Cambridge University Press, Cambridge, UK (1990)
180. Cioni, G., Paolicelli, P.B., Sordi, C., Vinter, A.: Sensorimotor development in cerebral-palsied infants assessed with the uzgiris-hunt scales. Developmental Medicine & Child Neurology **35**(12), 1055–1066 (1993)
181. Claparède, E.: L'éducation fonctionnelle. Delachaux et Niestlé, Neuchâtel, CH (1931)
182. Clarke, M., Kirton, A.: Patterns of interaction between children with physical disabilities using augmentative and alternative communication systems and their peers. Child Language Teaching and Therapy **19**(2), 135–151 (2003)
183. Clarke, M., Newton, C., Petrides, K., Griffiths, T., Lysley, A., Price, K.: An examination of relations between participation, communication and age in children with complex communication needs. Augment. Altern. Commun. **28**(1), 44–51 (2012)

184. Clarke, M., Wilkinson, R.: The collaborative construction of non-serious episodes of interaction by non-speaking children with cerebral palsy and their peers. Clinical linguistics & phonetics **23**(8), 583–597 (2009)
185. Coeckelbergh, M., Pop, C., Simut, R., Peca, A., Pintea, S., David, D., Vanderborght, B.: A survey of expectations about the role of robots in robot-assisted therapy for children with asd: ethical acceptability, trust, sociability, appearance, and attachment. Sci. Eng. Ethics **22**(1), 47–65 (2016)
186. Cohen, E., Chazan, S. E., Lerner, M., Maimon, E. Post-traumatic play in young children exposed to terrorism: An empirical study. Infant Mental Health Journal, **31**(2), 1–23 (2010)
187. Cohen, E. Political Violence (War and Terrorism) and Children's Play. In: Smith, P.K., Roopnarine, J.L. (eds.) The Cambridge Handbook of Play, pp. 649–663. Cambridge University Press, Cambridge, London, UK (2019)
188. Cook, A., Polgar, J.M. Assistive Technology. Principles and Pratices. Elsevier, Philadeplpia, US-PA (2015)
189. Cooper, J.O., Heron, T.E., Heward, W.L., et al.: Applied behavior analysis. Pearson/Merrill-Prentice Hall, Upper Saddle River, US-NJ (2007)
190. Cordoni, G.: Social play in captive wolves (canis lupus): not only an immature affair. Behaviour **146**(10), 1363–1385 (2009)
191. Corneliussen, B.: Blind children's participation in the natural flow of play. In: Hillesøy, S., Killi, E., Kristoffersen, A.E. (eds.) Togetherness in Play and Learning, pp. 142–153. Statped, Oslo, NO (2020)
192. Costa, M., Périno, O., Ray-Kaeser, S.: Tuet–toys and games usability evaluation tool. manual, questionnaire and development process (2018). http://www.tuet.eu
193. Couzens, D., Cuskelly, M.: Cognitive strengths and weaknesses for informing educational practice. In: Faragher, R., Clarke, B. (eds.) Educating learners with Down syndrome, pp. 54–73. Routledge, London, UK (2013)
194. Cress, C.: Expanding children's early augmented behaviors to support symbolic development. In: Reichle, J., Beukelman, D.R., Light, J.C. (eds.) Exemplary practices for beginning communicators: Implications for AAC, vol. 2. Paul H. Brookes Baltimore, US-MD (2002)
195. Cress, C.: Play and children with sensory impairments. In: Smith, P., Roopnarine, J. (eds.) The Cambridge Handbook of Play, pp. 597–614. Cambridge University Press, Cambridge, UK (2019)
196. Cress, C., Shapley, K., Linke, M., Havelka, S., Dietrich, C., Elliott, J., Clark, J.: Characteristics of intentional communication in young children with physical impairments. In: International Conference of the Society for Augmentative and Alternative Communication (2000)
197. Crocker, A.D., Orr, R.R.: Social behaviors of children with visual impairments enrolled in preschool programs. Except. Child. **62**(5), 451–462 (1996)
198. Crossman, M.K., Kazdin, A.E., Kitt, E.R.: The influence of a socially assistive robot on mood, anxiety, and arousal in children. Prof. Psychol. Res. Pract. **49**(1), 48 (2018)
199. Csikszentmihalyi, M., Abuhamdeh, S., Nakamura, J.: Flow. In: Csikszentmihalyi, M., Reed L. (eds.) Flow and the foundations of positive psychology, pp. 227–238. Springer, Berlin, DE (2014)
200. Csikszentmihályi, M.: Finding flow: The psychology of engagement with everyday life. Basic Books, New York, US-NY (1997)
201. Curry, J., Exner, C.: Comparison of tactile preferences in children with and without cerebral palsy. Am. J. Occup. Ther. **42**(6), 371–377 (1988)
202. Dale, N.: Early signs of developmental setback and autism in infants with severe visual impairment. In: Pring, L. (ed.) Autism and blindness: Research and reflections, pp. 74–98. Whurr Publishers, London, UK (2005)
203. Dallas, E., Stevenson, J., McGurk, H.: Cerebral-palsied children's interactions with siblings-II. interactional structure. Journal of Child Psychology and Psychiatry **34**(5), 621–647 (1993)
204. Damiano, D.L., Longo, E., deCampos, A.C., Forssberg, H., Rauch, A.: Systematic review of clinical guidelines related to care of individuals with cerebral palsy as part of the world health organization efforts to develop a global package of interventions for rehabilitation. Arch. Phys. Med. Rehabil. **102**(9), 1764–1774 (2021)

205. Danis, A., Kutluk, M.G.: The evolution of cerebral palsy publications and global productivity: a bibliometric analysis between 1980 and 2019. Acta Neurol. Belg. **121**(6), 1807–1814 (2021)
206. Dapporto, L., Palagi, E.: Il gioco delle vespe. Le scienze **457**, 94–100 (2006)
207. Dapretto, M., Davies, M.S., Pfeifer, J.H., Scott, A.A., Sigman, M., Bookheimer, S.Y., Iacoboni, M.: Understanding emotions in others: mirror neuron dysfunction in children with autism spectrum disorders. Nat. Neurosci. **9**(1), 28–30 (2006)
208. Darbyshire, J.O.: Play patterns in young children with impaired hearing. Volta Review **79**(1), 19–26 (1977)
209. Dautenhahn, K., Ogden, B., Quick, T.: From embodied to socially embedded agents-implications for interaction-aware robots. Cogn. Syst. Res. **3**(3), 397–428 (2002)
210. Dautenhahn, K., Werry, I.: Towards interactive robots in autism therapy: Background, motivation and challenges. Pragmatics & Cognition **12**(1), 1–35 (2004)
211. Davis, R., Proulx, R., van Schrojenstein Lantman-de Valk, H.: Health issues for people with intellectual disabilities: the evidence base. In: L. Taggart, W. Cousins (eds.) Health promotion for people with intellectual and developmental disabilities, pp. 7–14. McGraw-Hill Education, London, UK (2014)
212. De Falco, S., Esposito, G., Venuti, P., Bornstein, M.: Fathers' play with their down syndrome children. J. Intellect. Disabil. Res. **52**(6), 490–502 (2008)
213. DeKoven, B.: The well-played game: A player's philosophy. Cambridge, US-MA (2013)
214. Deleau, M.: Communication and the development of symbolic play: The need for a pragmatic perspective. In: Nadel, J., Camaioni, L. (eds.) New perspectives in early communicative development, pp. 97–115. Routledge, London, UK (2017)
215. DeLuzio, J., Girolametto, L.: Peer interactions of preschool children with and without hearing loss. Journal of Speech, Language, and Hearing Research **54**(4), 1197–1210 (2011)
216. Deutsch, K.W.: Creativity in a scientific civilization. Bank Street College of Education, Publications, New York, US-NY (1981)
217. Diamond, A.: The early development of executive functions. In: Bjialystock, C., Craik, F.I.M. (eds.) Lifespan cognition: Mechanisms of change, pp. 70–95. Oxford University Press, London, UK (2006)
218. Diamond, A., Barnett, W.S., Thomas, J., Munro, S.: Preschool program improves cognitive control. Science **318**(5855), 1387 (2007)
219. DiBianca Fasoli, A.: To play or not to play: diverse motives for Latino and Euro-American parent-child play in a children's museum. Infant Child Dev. **23**(6), 605–621 (2014)
220. Dignum, V.: Ethics in artificial intelligence: introduction to the special issue. Ethics Inf. Technol. **20**(1), 1–3 (2018)
221. Dimcovic, N.: Why is the change in the task difficult for blind children? Eur. J. Psychol. Educ. **7**(3), 231–244 (1992)
222. DiSalvo, C.F., Gemperle, F., Forlizzi, J., Kiesler, S.: All robots are not created equal: The design and perception of humanoid robot heads. Proceedings of the 4th Conference on Designing Interactive Systems: Processes, Practices, Methods, and Techniques, DIS '02, p. 321-326. Association for Computing Machinery, New York, NY, USA (2002)
223. D'Souza, H., Karmiloff-Smith, A.: Neurodevelopmental disorders. Cognit. Sci. **8**(1–2), e1398 (2017)
224. Dučić, B., Gligorović, M., Kaljača, S.: Relation between working memory and self-regulation capacities and the level of social skills acquisition in people with moderate intellectual disability. J. Appl. Res. Intellect. Disabil. **31**(2), 296–307 (2018)
225. Duquette, A., Michaud, F., Mercier, H.: Exploring the use of a mobile robot as an imitation agent with children with low-functioning autism. Auton. Robot. **24**(2), 147–157 (2008)
226. Dutton, G.N., Bauer, C.M.: Cerebral (cortical) visual impairment in children: a perspective. In: Ravenscroft, J. (ed.) The Routledge Handbook of Visual Impairment, pp. 53–69. Routledge, London, UK (2019)
227. Dutton, G.N., Jacobson, L.K.: Cerebral visual impairment in children. Seminars in Neonatology, **6**(6), 477–485 (2001)

228. Eberle, S.G.: The elements of play: toward a philosophy and a definition of play. Am. J. Play **6**(2), 214–233 (2014)
229. Edwards, C., Gandini, L., Forman, G.: The Hundred Languages of Children: The Reggio Emilia Experience in Transformation. ABC-CLIO, Santa Barbara, US-CA (2011)
230. Edwards, C.P.: Three approaches from Europe: Waldorf, Montessori, and Reggio Emilia. Early Child. Res. Pract. **4**(1) (2002)
231. Elkonin, D.B.: Chapter 2: On the historical origin of role play. J. Russ. East Eur. Psychol. **43**(1), 49–89 (2005)
232. Emerson, E., Baines, S.: The estimated prevalence of autism among adults with learning disabilities in England. Technical report, Improving Health and Lives: Learning Disabilities Observatory (2010). https://improvinghealthandlives.org.uk/
233. Encarnação, P., Cook, A. Robotic Assistive Technology. Principles and Practice. CRC Press, Boca Raton, US-FL (2017)
234. Encarnação, P., Ray-Kaeser, S., Bianquin, N.: Guidelines for Supporting Children with Disabilities' Play: Methodologies, Tools, and Contexts. De Gruyter, Warsaw, PL (2018)
235. Erikson, E.H.: Childhood and Society. WW Norton & Company, New York, US-NY (1963)
236. Escobar, J.P., Castro, C., Garolera, M., Sepúlveda, A., Cruz, M.S., Rosas, R.: Testing of a drawing toy for children with blindness: The kuwu experience. Int. J. Early Child. Spec. Educ. **13**(1) (2021)
237. Esposito, B.G., Koorland, M.A.: Play behavior of hearing impaired children: Integrated and segregated settings. Except. Child. **55**(5), 412–419 (1989)
238. Evans, T., Whittingham, K., Sanders, M., Colditz, P., Boyd, R.N.: Are parenting interventions effective in improving the relationship between mothers and their preterm infants? Infant Behav. Dev. **37**(2), 131–154 (2014)
239. Evenhuis, H., Theunissen, M., Denkers, I., Verschuure, H., Kemme, H.: Prevalence of visual and hearing impairment in a Dutch institutionalized population with intellectual disability. J. Intellect. Disabil. Res. **45**(5), 457–464 (2001)
240. Fagen, R., Fagen, J.: Play behaviour and multi-year juvenile survival in free-ranging brown bears, ursus arctos. Evol. Ecol. Res. **11**(7), 1053–1067 (2009)
241. Fairclough, N.: Language and Globalization. Routledge, London, UK (2009)
242. Fantuzzo, J., Sutton-Smith, B., Coolahan, K.C., Manz, P.H., Canning, S., Debnam, D.: Assessment of preschool play interaction behaviors in young low-income children: Penn interactive peer play scale. Early Child. Res. Quart. **10**(1), 105–120 (1995)
243. Fantuzzo, J.W., Hampton, V.R.: Penn Interactive Peer Play Scale: A Parent and Teacher Rating System for Young Children. Wiley, Hoboken, US-NJ (2000)
244. Faragher, R., Robertson, P., Bird, G.: International Guidelines for the Education of Learners with Down Syndrome. Down Syndrome International, Teddington, UK (2020)
245. Fazzi, E.M., Lanners, J., Martini, A., Pagliano, E., Telesca, C., Lanzi, G.: Il bambino cieco: sviluppo neuromotorio e cognitivo nei primi 3 anni di vita. PI-ME, Pavia, IT (1994)
246. Feil-Seifer, D., Skinner, K., Matarić, M.J.: Benchmarks for evaluating socially assistive robotics. Interact. Stud. **8**(3), 423–439 (2007)
247. Feng, H.: Organization of theory of mind (tom) test, the development of tom in children with autism, and the effect of tom training on social skills in children with high-functioning autism in central Taiwan. National Science Council Project Reports: NSC89-2413-H-018-026 (2001)
248. Ferland, F.: The Ludic Model - Play, Children with Physical Disabilities and Occupational Therapy. Canadian Association of Occupational Therapists, Ottawa, Canada (2005)
249. Ferrari, M., Ferrari, G.: Building robots with LEGO Mindstorms NXT. Syngress, Waltham, US-MA (2011)
250. Fewell, R.: Play assessment scale (5th rev.). Technical report, University of Washington, Seattle, WA (1986)
251. Fielder, J.C., Proulx, M.J.: Psychological representation of visual impairment: Perception and how visually impaired people "see" the world. In: Ravenscroft, J. (ed.) The Routledge Handbook of Visual Impairment, pp. 18–35. Routledge, London, UK (2019)

252. Fikes, R.E., Nilsson, N.J.: Strips: A new approach to the application of theorem proving to problem solving. Artif. Intell. **2**(3–4), 189–208 (1971)
253. Fink, E.: Oase des Glücks Gedanken Zu Einer Ontologie des Spiels. Verlag Karl Alber, Freiburg, D (1957)
254. Fitzpatrick, E.M., Hamel, C., Stevens, A., Pratt, M., Moher, D., Doucet, S.P., Neuss, D., Bernstein, A., Na, E.: Sign language and spoken language for children with hearing loss: a systematic review. Pediatrics **137**(1) (2016)
255. Fjørtoft, I.: Landscape as playscape: the effects of natural environments on children's play and motor development. Child. Youth Environ. **14**(2), 21–44 (2004)
256. Fleer, M.: Play and learning in everyday family contexts. In: Smith, P., Roopnarine, J. (eds.) The Cambridge Handbook of Play, pp. 419–435. Cambridge University Press, Cambridge, UK (2019)
257. Florian, L., Black-Hawkins, K.: Exploring inclusive pedagogy. Br. Edu. Res. J. **37**(5), 813–828 (2011)
258. Folmer, E.: Exploring the use of an aerial robot to guide blind runners. ACM SIGACCESS Access. Comput. **112**, 3–7 (2015)
259. Fombonne, E.: The epidemiology of autism: a review. Psychol. Med. **29**(4), 769–786 (1999)
260. Fombonne, E.: Past and future perspectives on autism epidemiology. In: Moldin, S.O., Rubenstein, J.L.R. (eds.) Understanding Autism: From Basic Neuroscience to Treatment. CRC Press - Routledge - Taylor & Francis Group (2006)
261. Fong, T., Nourbakhsh, I., Dautenhahn, K.: A survey of socially interactive robots. Robot. Auton. Syst. **42**(3), 143–166 (2003)
262. Fornari, F.: La vita affettiva originaria del bambino, vol. 9. Feltrinelli, Milano, IT (1969)
263. Fortes, R.P.M., de Lima Salgado, A., de Souza Santos, F., Agostini do Amaral, L., Nogueira da Silva, E.A.: Game accessibility evaluation methods: A literature survey. In: Antona Margheritaand Stephanidis, C. (ed.) Universal Access in Human–Computer Interaction. Design and Development Approaches and Methods, pp. 182–192. Springer International Publishing, Berlin, DE (2017)
264. Fosch-Villaronga, E.: Robots, Healthcare, and the Law: Regulating Automation in Personal Care. Routledge, London, UK (2019)
265. Fosch-Villaronga, E., Albo-Canals, J.: "I'll take care of you", said the robot. Paladyn, J. Behav. Robot. **10**(1), 77–93 (2019)
266. Fraiberg, S.: Insights from the Blind. Basic Books, New York, US-NY (1977)
267. Fraiberg, S., Adelson, E.: Self-representation in language and play: Observations of blind children. Psychoanal. Q. **42**(4), 539–562 (1973)
268. Fraser, N.: Ten things we've learned from Blockly. In: 2015 IEEE Blocks and Beyond Workshop, pp. 49–50. IEEE Computer press (2015)
269. Freeman, E., Brewster, S.: Using sound to help visually impaired children play independently. In: Proceedings of the 2016 CHI Conference Extended Abstracts on Human Factors in Computing Systems, pp. 1670–1676 (2016)
270. Freud, S.: Jenseits des lustprinzips. Internationaler Psychoanalytischer Verlag, **2** (1920)
271. Freud, S.: On creativity and the unconscious. Harper and Row, New York, US-NY (1958)
272. Frid, E., Bresin, R., Alexanderson, S.: Perception of mechanical sounds inherent to expressive gestures of a NAO robot-implications for movement sonification of humanoids. Sound and Music Computing (2018)
273. Frith, U.: Autism: Explaining the Enigma. Blackwell Publishing, Hoboken, US-NJ (2003)
274. Fröbel, F.: Die Menschenerziehung, die Erziehungs-, Unterrichts-und Lehrkunst: angestrebt in der allgemeinen deutschen Erziehungsanstalt zu Keilhau, vol. 1. Verlag der Allgemeinen Dt, Erziehungsanst (1826)
275. Frost, J.L., Wortham, S.C., Reifel, R.S.: Play and Child Development. Pearson/Merrill Prentice Hall, Upper Saddle River, US-NJ (2008)
276. Gadamer, H.G.: Truth and method. J. Aesthet. Art Criticism **36**(4) (1975)
277. Galati, D.: Vedere con la mente: conoscenza, affettività, adattamento nei non vedenti. FrancoAngeli, Milano, IT (1992)

278. Garvey, C.: Some properties of social play. In: Bruner, S., Jolly, A., S. K. (eds.) Play. Its role in Development and Evolution, pp. 570–584. Basic Books, New York, US-NY (1976)
279. Garvey, C.: Play, vol. 27. Harvard University Press, Cambridge, US-MA (1990)
280. Gaskins, S.: Yucatec mayan children's play. In: Roopnarine, J., Patte, M., Johnson, J., Kuschner, D. (eds.) International perspectives on children's play, pp. 11–22. McGraw Hill, New York, US-NY (2014)
281. Gaskins, S., Haight, W., Lancy, D.F.: The cultural construction of play. In: Goncu, A., Gaskins, S. (eds.) Play and development: Evolutionary, sociocultural, and functional perspectives. Psychology Press, London, UK (2007)
282. Getzels, J.W., Jackson, P.W.: Creativity and Intelligence: Explorations with Gifted Students. Wiley, Hoboken, US-NJ (1962)
283. Giangreco, M.F.: Expanding opportunities for students with intellectual disability. Differences **74**(7) (2017)
284. Giannopulu, I., Pradel, G.: Multimodal interactions in free game play of children with autism and a mobile toy robot. NeuroRehabilitation **27**(4), 305–311 (2010)
285. Gibson, E.J.: Principles of Perceptual Learning and Development. Appleton-Century-Crofts, Norwalk, US-CT (1969)
286. Gibson, J.J.: The Ecological Approach to Visual Perception Houghton Mifflin. Boston, US-MA (1979)
287. Giezen, M.: Speech and sign perception in deaf children with cochlear implants. Sign language & linguistics, **14**(2), 277–283 (2011)
288. Gilbert, C., Foster, A.: Childhood blindness in the context of vision 2020: the right to sight. Bull. World Health Organ. **79**, 227–232 (2001)
289. Glidden, L.M., Warner, D.A.: Semantic processing and recall improvement of EMR adolescents. Am. J, Mental Defic **88**(1), 96–105 (1983)
290. Goffman, E.: Frame Analysis: An Essay on the Organization of Experience. Harvard University Press, Cambridge, US-MA (1974)
291. Gomendio, M.: The development of different types of play in gazelles: implications for the nature and functions of play. Anim. Behav. **36**(3), 825–836 (1988)
292. Göncü, A., Jain, J., Tuermer, U.: Children's play as cultural interpretation. In: Goncu, A., Gaskins, S. (eds.) Play and development: Evolutionary, sociocultural, and functional perspectives. pp. 160–183. Psychology Press, London, UK (2007)
293. Gopnik, A., Kuhl, K., Meltzoff, A.: The Scientist in the Crib: What Early Learning Tells Us About the Mind. HarperCollins Publishers, New York, US-NY (2001)
294. Gori, M., Cappagli, G., Tonelli, A., Baud-Bovy, G., Finocchietti, S.: Devices for visually impaired people: high technological devices with low user acceptance and no adaptability for children. Neurosci. Biobehav. Rev. **69**, 79–88 (2016)
295. Gosso, Y., Resende, B.D., Carvalho, A.M.: Play in south american indigenous children. In: Smith, P., Roopnarine, J. (eds.) The Cambridge Handbook of Play, pp. 322–342. Cambridge University Press, Cambridge, UK (2019)
296. Gouaillier, D., Hugel, V., Blazevic, P., Kilner, C., Monceaux, J., Lafourcade, P., Marnier, B., Serre, J., Maisonnier, B.: The NAO humanoid: a combination of performance and affordability. CoRR abs/0807.3223 (2008)
297. Gowen, J.W., Johnson-Martin, N., Goldman, B.D., Hussey, B.: Object play and exploration in children with and without disabilities: a longitudinal study. Am. J. Ment. Retard. **97**(1), 21–38 (1992)
298. Graham, D., Paget, S.P., Wimalasundera, N.: Current thinking in the health care management of children with cerebral palsy. Med. J. Aust. **210**(3), 129–135 (2019)
299. Gray, P.: The play theory of hunter-gatherer egalitarianism. In: Narvaez, D., Valentino, K., Fuentes, A., McKenna, J.J., Gray, P. (eds) Ancestral Landscapes in Human Evolution: Culture, Childrearing and Social Wellbeing, pp. 190–213, Oxford University Press, Oxford, UK (2014)
300. Gray, P.: Evolutionary functions of play: Practice, resilience, innovation, and cooperation. In: Smith, P., Roopnarine, J. (eds.) The Cambridge Handbook of Play, pp. 83–102. Cambridge University Press, Cambridge, UK (2019)

301. Greenwald, A.G., McGhee, D.E., Schwartz, J.L.: Measuring individual differences in implicit cognition: the implicit association test. J. Pers. Soc. Psychol. **74**(6), 1464 (1998)
302. Gregory, S., Mogford, K.: The development of symbolic play in young deaf children. In: The Acquisition of Symbolic Skills, pp. 221–231. Springer, Berlin, DE (1983)
303. Groos, K.: The Play of Animals. D. Appleton and Company, Boston, US-MA (1898)
304. Grosjean, F.: Parler plusieurs langues: le monde des bilingues. Albin Michel, Paris. F (2015)
305. Gudareva, O.: Psikhologicheskie osobennosti suzhetno-rolevoy igry sovremennykh doshkol'nikov [Psychological features of make-believe play in today's preschoolers]. Unpublished doctoral dissertation. Moscow City University for Psychology and Education, Moscow (2005)
306. Gulati, S., Sondhi, V.: Cerebral palsy: an overview. Indian J. Pediat. **85**(11), 1006–1016 (2018)
307. Guralnick, M.J.: Family and child influences on the peer-related social competence of young children with developmental delays. Ment. Retard. Dev. Disabil. Res. Rev. **5**(1), 21–29 (1999)
308. Guralnick, M.J.: Peer relationships and the mental health of young children with intellectual delays. J. Policy Pract. Intell. Disabil. **3**(1), 49–56 (2006)
309. Guralnick, M.J., Groom, J.M.: Correlates of peer-related social competence of developmentally delayed preschool children. Am. J, Mental Defic, **90**(2), 140–150 (1985)
310. Guralnick, M.J., Groom, J.M.: The peer relations of mildly delayed and nonhandicapped preschool children in mainstreamed playgroups. Child Development, **58**(6), 1556–1572
311. Haigh, A., Brown, D.J., Meijer, P., Proulx, M.J.: How well do you see what you hear? The acuity of visual-to-auditory sensory substitution. Front. Psychol. **4**, 330 (2013)
312. Hakkarainen, P., Brėdikytė, M.: The adult as a mediator of development in children's play. In: Smith, P., Roopnarine, J. (eds.) The Cambridge Handbook of Play, pp. 457–474. Cambridge University Press, Cambridge, UK (2019)
313. Haley, S.M., Coster, W., Ludlow, L.H., Haltiwanger, J.T., Andrellos, P.J.: Pediatric evaluation of disability inventory (PEDI). Development, Standardization and Administration Manual. Boston, MA: Trustees of Boston University (1992)
314. Halevi, G., Djalovski, A., Vengrober, A., Feldman, R. Risk and resilience trajectories in war-exposed children across the first decade of life. Journal of Child Psychology and Psychiatry, **57**(10), 1183–1193 (2016)
315. Hansell, M., Ruxton, G.D.: Setting tool use within the context of animal construction behaviour. Trends Ecol. Evolut. **23**(2), 73–78 (2008)
316. Hanzlik, J.R.: Nonverbal interaction patterns of mothers and their infants with cerebral palsy. Education and Training in Mental Retardation, **25**(4), 333–343 (1990)
317. Happé, F.: Autism: cognitive deficit or cognitive style? Trends Cognit. Sci. **3**(6), 216–222 (1999)
318. Haring, K.S., Watanabe, K., Velonaki, M., Tossell, C.C., Finomore, V.: Ffab-the form function attribution bias in human-robot interaction. IEEE Trans. Cognit. Dev. Syst. **10**(4), 843–851 (2018)
319. Harkness, L., Bundy, A.C.: The test of playfulness and children with physical disabilities. Occup. Therapy J. Res. **21**(2), 73–89 (2001)
320. Harper, L.V., McCluskey, K.S.: Caregiver and peer responses to children with language and motor disabilities in inclusive preschool programs. Early Child. Res. Quart. **17**(2), 148–166 (2002)
321. Harris, P.L.: The Work of the Imagination. Basil Blackwell, Oxford, UK (2000)
322. Harrison, P.: Oakland T: Adaptive Behavior Assessment System ed 2. Psychological Corporation, San Antonio, TX (2003)
323. Hart, J.L., Tannock, M.T.: Playful aggression in early childhood settings. Child. Aust. **38**(3), 106–114 (2013)
324. Hart, J.L., Tannock, M.T.: Rough play: Past, present and potential. In: Smith, P., Roopnarine, J. (eds.) The Cambridge Handbook of Play, pp. 200–221. Cambridge University Press, Cambridge, UK (2019)
325. Hartup, W.W.: Social relationships and their developmental significance. Am. Psychol. **44**(2), 120 (1989)

326. Hatwell, Y.: Elaborazione dei dati spaziali e sviluppo cognitivo nei non vedenti. In: Galati, D. (ed.) Vedere con la mente, pp. 87–112. Franco Angeli, Milano, IT (1992)
327. Hauser-Cram, P., Howell, A.: The development of young children with disabilities and their families. In: Lerner, R.M., Jacobs, F., Wertlieb, D. (eds.) Handbook of Applied Developmental Science, vol. 1, pp. 259–279. Sage, Thousand Oaks, US-CA (2003)
328. Hay, D.F., Payne, A., Chadwick, A.: Peer relations in childhood. J. Child Psychol. Psych. **45**(1), 84–108 (2004)
329. Hedegaard, M., Fleer, M.: Play, Learning, and Children's Development: Everyday Life in Families and Transition to School. Cambridge University Press, Cambridge, UK (2013)
330. Heelan, A.: Universal design for learning (UDL): Implications for education. (2015). http://arrow.dit.ie/cgi/viewcontent.cgi?article=1000&context=exdesthe4
331. Hellendoorn, J., van der Kooij, R., Sutton-Smith, B.: Play and Intervention. SUNY Press, Albany, US-NY (1994)
332. Henricks, T.S.: Play Reconsidered: Sociological Perspectives on Human Expression. University of Illinois Press (2006)
333. Henricks, T.S.: Play and the rhetorics of time: Progress, regression, and the meanings of the present. In: Kuschner, D. (ed.) From Children to Red Hatters: Diverse Images and Issues of Play, pp. 14–38. United Press of America, Lanham, USA (2009)
334. Henricks, T.S.: Play as a pathway of behavior. Am. J. Play **4**(2), 225–253 (2011)
335. Henricks, T.S.: Play as self-realization: toward a general theory of play. Am. J. Play **6**(2), 190–213 (2014)
336. Henricks, T.S.: Play and the Human Condition. University of Illinois Press, Champaign, US-IL (2015)
337. Henricks, T.S.: Classic theories of play. In: Smith, P., Roopnarine, J. (eds.) The Cambridge Handbook of Play, pp. 361–382. Cambridge University Press, Cambridge, UK (2019)
338. Henricks, T.S.: Play and the Human Condition. University of Illinois Press, Champaign, US-IL (2019)
339. Hernandez, H.A., Ye, Z., Graham, T.N., Fehlings, D., Switzer, L.: Designing action-based exergames for children with cerebral palsy. Proceedings of the SIGCHI Conference on Human Factors in Computing Systems, pp. 1261–1270 (2013)
340. van den Heuvel, R.J., Lexis, M.A., Gelderblom, G.J., Jansens, R.M., de Witte, L.P.: Robots and ICT to support play in children with severe physical disabilities: a systematic review. Disabil. Rehabil. Assist. Technol. **11**(2), 103–116 (2016)
341. Hewett, D.: The Intensive Interaction Handbook. Sage, Thousand Oaks, US-CA (2018)
342. Hewett, D., Nind, M.: Interaction in Action: Reflections on the Use of Intensive Interaction. David Fulton Publishers, London, UK (1998)
343. Hewett, V.M.: Examining the Reggio Emilia approach to early childhood education. Early Child. Educ. J. **29**(2), 95–100 (2001)
344. Higginbotham, D.J., Baker, B.M., et al.: Social participation and cognitive play differences in hearing-impaired and normal hearing preschoolers. Master's thesis, University of Louisville, USA (1979). http://a.xueshu.baidu.com/usercenter/paper/show?paperid=1j4h0vw00s2q02a0k75b0as0fm265760
345. Hill, P.M., McCune-Nicolich, L.: Pretend play and patterns of cognition in down's syndrome children. Child Development, **52**(2), 611–617 (1981)
346. Hobson, J.A., Hobson, R.P., Malik, S., Bargiota, K., Caló, S.: The relation between social engagement and pretend play in autism. Br. J. Dev. Psychol. **31**(1), 114–127 (2013)
347. Hobson, R.P., et al.: Autism and the Development of Mind. Taylor & Francis, Abingdon-on-Thames, UK (1993)
348. Hockings, C.: Inclusive Learning and Teaching in Higher Education: A Synthesis of Research. Higher Education Academy (2010). https://www.plymouth.ac.uk/uploads/production/document/path/2/2735/Inclusive_teaching_and_learning_in_HEsynthesis_.pdf
349. Hofmann, W., Schmeichel, B.J., Baddeley, A.D.: Executive functions and self-regulation. Trends Cognit. Sci. **16**(3), 174–180 (2012)

350. Hogan, K.: Nonverbal Thinking, Communication, Imitation, and Play Skills from a Developmental Perspective. ERIC Document no. ED412690 (1997). https://eric.ed.gov/?id=ED412690
351. Howes, C.: Peer play scale as an index of complexity of peer interaction. Dev. Psychol. **16**(4), 371 (1980)
352. Hughes, B., Paterson, K.: The social model of disability and the disappearing body: towards a sociology of impairment. Disabil. Soc. **12**(3), 325–340 (1997)
353. Hughes, F.P.: Children, Play, and Development. SAGE Publications, Thousand Oaks, US-CA (2021)
354. Hughes, L.A.: A conceptual framework for the study of children's gaming. Play Cult. **4**(3), 284–301 (1991)
355. Hughes, M., Dote-Kwan, J., Dolendo, J.: A close look at the cognitive play of preschoolers with visual impairments in the home. Except. Child. **64**(4), 451–462 (1998)
356. Huizinga, J.: Homo Ludens: A study of the play element in culture. Routledge, London, UK (1949)
357. Hulme, I., Lunzer, E.: Play, language and reasoning in subnormal children. J. Child Psychol. Psych. **7**(2), 107–123 (1966)
358. Imms, C., Reilly, S., Carlin, J., Dodd, K.: Diversity of participation in children with cerebral palsy. Dev. Med. Child Neurol. **50**(5), 363–369 (2008)
359. Imray, P., Hadfield, M.: Equals sld (semi-formal) curriculum schemes of work: My play and leisure. http://equals.co.uk/wp-content/uploads/2016/12/Semi-Formal-SLD-Curriculum-SoW-My-Play-and-Leisure-Preview.pdf(2017). Accessed on January 22, 2022
360. Imray, P., Hinchcliffe, V.: Curricula for Teaching Children and Young People with Severe or Profound and Multiple Learning Difficulties: Practical Strategies for Educational professionals. Routledge, London, UK (2013)
361. Ingersoll, B., Gergans, S.: The effect of a parent-implemented imitation intervention on spontaneous imitation skills in young children with autism. Res. Dev. Disabil. **28**(2), 163–175 (2007)
362. Institute of Electronics and Electrical Engineers: IEEE standard ontologies for robotics and automation. IEEE Std. **1872–2015**, 1–60 (2015)
363. ISO - International Organization of Standards 8373:2012 – Robots and robotic devices - Vocabulary. (2012)
364. ISO - International Organization of Standardization: Ergonomics of human-system interaction - Part 11: Usability: definitions and concepts (2018)
365. ISO - International Organization of Standardization - IEC: Guide 71 - Guide for addressing accessibility in standards (2014)
366. James, S., Ma, Z., Arrojo, D.R., Davison, A.J.: Rlbench: the robot learning benchmark and learning environment. IEEE Robot. Autom. Lett. **5**(2), 3019–3026 (2020)
367. Jansens, R., Bonarini, A.: Guidelines for parents, professionals, designers, makers and researchers on toys and technologies for play for children with disabilities: How to take usability and accessibility aspects into consideration? In: Bulgarelli, D. (ed.) Perspectives and Research on Play for Children with Disabilities, pp. 106–145. De Gruyter, Warsaw, PL (2020)
368. Jansens, R., Bonarini, A.: Usability and accessibility of toys and technologies for play for children with disabilities: Scoping review of guidelines and tools. In: Bulgarelli, D. (ed.) Perspectives and Research on Play for Children with Disabilities, pp. 83–105. De Gruyter, Warsaw, PL (2020)
369. Jee, E.S., Jeong, Y.J., Kim, C.H., Kobayashi, H.: Sound design for emotion and intention expression of socially interactive robots. Intel. Serv. Robot. **3**(3), 199–206 (2010)
370. Jeong, S., Breazeal, C., Logan, D., Weinstock, P.: Huggable: impact of embodiment on promoting verbal and physical engagement for young pediatric inpatients. 2017 26th IEEE International Symposium on Robot and Human Interactive Communication (RO-MAN), pp. 121–126. IEEE (2017)

371. Johansson, B., Tjøstheim, T.A., Balkenius, C.: Epi: an open humanoid platform for developmental robotics. Int. J. Adv. Rob. Syst. **17**(2), 1729881420911498 (2020)
372. Johnson, J.E., Christie, J.F., Wardle, F.: Play, Development, and Early Education. Pearson/Allyn and Bacon (2005)
373. Johnson, J.E., Dong, P.I.: Methods of studying play. In: Smith, P., Roopnarine, J. (eds.) The Cambridge Handbook of Play, pp. 399–415. Cambridge University Press, Cambridge, UK (2019)
374. Johnston, O., Thomas, F.: The Illusion of Life: Disney Animation. Disney Editions, New York, US-NY (1981)
375. Jones, H.A., Horn, E.M., Warren, S.F.: The effects of motor skill acquisition on the development of intentional communication. J. Early Interv. **22**(1), 25–37 (1999)
376. Jordan, R.: Autism with Severe Learning Difficulties. Souvenir Press Ltd, London, UK (2013)
377. Juffer, F.E., Bakermans-Kranenburg, M.J., Van Ijzendoorn, M.H.: Promoting Positive Parenting: An Attachment-Based Intervention. Taylor & Francis Group/Lawrence Erlbaum Associates, Milton Park, UK (2008)
378. Jung, E., Han, S.: Play in societies influenced by confucian values. In: Smith, P., Roopnarine, J. (eds.) The Cambridge Handbook of Play, pp. 343–358. Cambridge University Press, Cambridge, UK (2019)
379. Kabacińska, K., Prescott, T.J., Robillard, J.M.: Socially assistive robots as mental health interventions for children: a scoping review. Int. J. Soc. Robot. **13**(5), 919–935 (2021)
380. Kahn, P.H., Friedman, B., Perez-Granados, D.R., Freier, N.G.: Robotic pets in the lives of preschool children. Interact. Stud. **7**(3), 405–436 (2006)
381. Kahn, P.H., Jr., Ishiguro, H., Friedman, B., Kanda, T., Freier, N.G., Severson, R.L., Miller, J.: What is a human?: Toward psychological benchmarks in the field of human-robot interaction. Interact. Stud. **8**(3), 363–390 (2007)
382. Kana, R.K., Wadsworth, H.M., Travers, B.G.: A systems level analysis of the mirror neuron hypothesis and imitation impairments in autism spectrum disorders. Neurosci. Biobehav. Rev. **35**(3), 894–902 (2011)
383. Karasik, L.B., Tamis-LeMonda, C.S., Adolph, K.E.: Transition from crawling to walking and infants' actions with objects and people. Child Dev. **82**(4), 1199–1209 (2011)
384. Karpov, Y.V.: Three-to six-year-olds: Sociodramatic play as the leading activity during the period of early childhood. In: Karpov, J.V., Karpov, Y.V. (eds.) The Neo-Vygotskian Approach to Child Development, pp. 139–170. Cambridge University Press, Cambridge, UK (2005)
385. Kasari, C., Chang, Y.C., Patterson, S.: Pretending to play or playing to pretend: The case of autism. Am. J. Play **6**(1), 124 (2013)
386. Kasari, C., Gulsrud, A., Paparella, T., Hellemann, G., Berry, K.: Randomized comparative efficacy study of parent-mediated interventions for toddlers with autism. J. Consult. Clin. Psychol. **83**(3), 554 (2015)
387. Kasari, C., Huynh, L., Gulsrud, A.: Play interventions for children with autism. In: Russ, S.W., Niec, L.N. (eds.) Play in Clinical Practice: Evidence Based Approaches, pp. 201–217. Guilford Press, London, UK (2011)
388. Kazou, K.: Analysing the definition of disability in the un convention on the rights of persons with disabilities: is it really based on a'social model'approach? Int. J. Mental Health Capacit. Law **23**, 25–48 (2017)
389. Keeffe, J.: Global data on vision loss: implications for services. In: Ravenscroft, J. (ed.) The Routledge Handbook of Visual Impairment, pp. 11–17. Routledge, London, UK (2019)
390. Kellogg, E.C.: Young children who are deaf or hard of hearing and have autism spectrum disorder: Three case studies, Graduate Thesis Dissertation (2013). https://scholar.colorado.edu/concern/graduate_thesis_or_dissertations/41687h66b
391. Kelly-Vance, L., Ryalls, B.O.: A systematic, reliable approach to play assessment in preschoolers. Sch. Psychol. Int. **26**(4), 398–412 (2005)
392. Kelly-Vance, L., Ryalls, B.O.: Best Practices in Play Assessment and Intervention. In: Thomas A., Grimes J. (eds). Best Practices in School Psychology. Vol 2. pp. 549–559. National Association of School Psychologists, Bethesda, MD (2008)

393. Kennedy-Behr, A., Rodger, S., Mickan, S.: A comparison of the play skills of preschool children with and without developmental coordination disorder. OTJR: Occup. Particip. Health **33**(4), 198–208 (2013)
394. Khadka, J., Ryan, B., Margrain, T.H., Woodhouse, J.M., Davies, N.: Listening to voices of children with a visual impairment: A focus group study. Br. J. Vis. Impair. **30**(3), 182–196 (2012)
395. Klawonn, M.A., Klamar, K., Turk, M.A.: Trends in publications about cerebral palsy 1990 to 2020. J. Pediat. Rehabil. Med. **13**(2), 107–117 (2020)
396. Klin, A., Jones, W., Schultz, R., Volkmar, F.: The enactive mind, or from actions to cognition: lessons from autism. Philos. Trans. Roy. Soc. Lond. Ser. B: Biol. Sci. **358**(1430), 345–360 (2004)
397. Knox, S.: Development and current use of the knox preschool play scale. In: Parham, L.D., Fazio, L. (eds.) Play Occupational Therapy for Children, pp. 35–51, Elsevier, Amsterdam, NL (1997)
398. Knox, S.: Avaliação lúdica de pré-escolares: a escala Knox. In: Parham, L.D., Fazio, L. (eds.) A recreação na terapia ocupacional pediátrica., pp. 2–22. Santos, São Paulo, BR (2002)
399. Koch, S.C.: Basic principles of movement analysis: Steps toward validation of the kmp. In: Bender, S., Koch, S. (eds.) Movement Analysis. The Legacy of Laban, Bartenieff, Lamb and Kestenberg. Logos, Berlin, DE (2007)
400. Koller, D., Pouesard, M.L., Rummens, J.A.: Defining social inclusion for children with disabilities: a critical literature review. Child. Soc. **32**(1), 1–13 (2018)
401. Kozima, H., Michalowski, M.P., Nakagawa, C.: Keepon. a playful robot for research, therapy, and entertainment. Int. J. Soc. Robot. **1**(1), 3–18 (2009)
402. Kozima, H., Nakagawa, C.: Interactive robots as facilitators of childrens social development. INTECH Open Access Publisher (2006)
403. Koziol, L.F., Budding, D.E., Chidekel, D.: From movement to thought: executive function, embodied cognition, and the cerebellum. The Cerebellum **11**(2), 505–525 (2012)
404. Krakow, J.B., Kopp, C.B.: The effects of developmental delay on sustained attention in young children. Child Development, **54**(5):1143–1155 (1983)
405. Kral, A., O'Donoghue, G.M.: Profound deafness in childhood. N. Engl. J. Med. **363**(15), 1438–1450 (2010)
406. Kupers, R., Ptito, M.: Insights from darkness: what the study of blindness has taught us about brain structure and function. Prog. Brain Res. **192**, 17–31 (2011)
407. Kuschner, D.: Play is natural to childhood but school is not: the problem of integrating play into the curriculum. Int. J. Play **1**(3), 242–249 (2012)
408. Laban, R.: Modern Educational Dance. MacDonald and Evans (First published 1948). London, UK (1963)
409. Lammer, L., Huber, A., Weiss, A., Vincze, M.: Mutual care: How older adults react when they should help their care robot. AISB2014 Proceedings of the 3rd International Symposium on New Frontiers in Human–Robot Interaction, pp. 1–4. Routledge, London, UK (2014)
410. Lancioni, G.E.: Employment of normal third and fourth graders for training retarded children to solve problems dealing with quantity. Education and Training of the Mentally Retarded, **17**(2), 93–102 (1982)
411. Landry, S.H., Chapieski, M.L.: Joint attention and infant toy exploration: effects of down syndrome and prematurity. In: Child Development, **60**(1), 103–118 (1989)
412. Lane, A.E., Young, R.L., Baker, A.E., Angley, M.T.: Sensory processing subtypes in autism: association with adaptive behavior. J. Autism Dev. Disord. **40**(1), 112–122 (2010)
413. Lapeyre, M.: Poppy: open-source, 3d printed and fully-modular robotic platform for science, art and education. Ph.D. thesis, Université de Bordeaux (2014)
414. Lasseter, J.: Principles of traditional animation applied to 3d computer animation. Proceedings of the 14th Annual Conference on Computer Graphics and Interactive Techniques, pp. 35–44 (1987)
415. Law, M., King, G., King, S., Kertoy, M., Hurley, P., Rosenbaum, P., Young, N., Hanna, S.: Patterns of participation in recreational and leisure activities among children with complex physical disabilities. Dev. Med. Child Neurol. **48**(5), 337–342 (2006)

416. Leech, B.E.R., Cress, C.J.: Indirect facilitation of speech in a late talking child by prompted production of picture symbols or signs. Augment. Altern. Commun. **27**(1), 40–52 (2011)
417. Lender, W.L., Goodman, J.F., Linn, M.I.: Repetitive activity in the play of children with mental retardation. J. Early Interv. **21**(4), 308–322 (1998)
418. Leslie, A.M.: Pretense and representation: the origins of "theory of mind." Psychol. Rev. **94**(4), 412 (1987)
419. Lesperance, A., Blain, S., Chau, T.: An integrated approach to detecting communicative intent amid hyperkinetic movements in children. Augment. Altern. Commun. **27**(3), 150–162 (2011)
420. Levi, G., Penge, R., Romani, R.: Disturbi dello sviluppo: verso il DSM 5 e verso l'ICD 11. Psichiatria dell'infanzia e dell'adolescenza **79**(1), 3–13 (2012)
421. Levine, L.M., Antia, S.D.: The effect of partner hearing status on social and cognitive play. J. Early Interv. **21**(1), 21–35 (1997)
422. Lewis, V., Boucher, J.: The Test of Pretend Play: ToPP. Psychological Corporation (1997)
423. Lewis, V., Norgate, S., Collis, G., Reynolds, R.: The consequences of visual impairment for children's symbolic and functional play. Br. J. Dev. Psychol. **18**(3), 449–464 (2000)
424. Libby, S., Powell, S., Messer, D., Jordan, R.: Imitation of pretend play acts by children with autism and down syndrome. J. Autism Dev. Disord. **27**(4), 365–383 (1997)
425. Lieberman, J.N.: Playfulness: Its Relationship to Imagination and Creativity. Academic, New York, US-NY (1977)
426. Lieberman, L.J.: Visual impairments. In: Winnick, J.P. (ed.) Adapted Physical Education and Sport, pp. 205–220. Human Kinetics Publisher, Champaign, US-IL (2005)
427. Lifter, K.: Linking assessment to intervention for children with developmental disabilities or at-risk for developmental delay: The developmental play assessment (dpa) instrument. Play Diagn. Assess. **2**, 228–261 (2000)
428. Lifter, K., Mason, E.J., Cannarella, A.M., Cameron, A.D.: Developmental Play Assessment for Practitioners (DPA-P) Guidebook and Training Website. Routledge, London, UK (2022)
429. Lifter, K., Sulzer-Azaroff, B., Anderson, S.R., Cowdery, G.E.: Teaching play activities to preschool children with disabilities: the importance of developmental considerations. J. Early Interv. **17**(2), 139–159 (1993)
430. Lillard, A., Pinkham, A.M., Smith, E.: Pretend play and cognitive development. In: Goswami, U. (ed.) The Wiley-Blackwell Handbook of Childhood Cognitive Development, pp. 285–311. Wiley-Blackwell, Hoboken, US-NJ (2011)
431. Lillard, A.S.: Mother-child fantasy play. In: Pellegrini, A.S. (ed.) The Oxford Handbook of the Development of Play, pp. 284–295. Oxford University Press, Oxford, UK (2019)
432. Lillard, A.S., Lerner, M.D., Hopkins, E.J., Dore, R.A., Smith, E.D., Palmquist, C.M.: The impact of pretend play on children's development: a review of the evidence. Psychol. Bull. **139**(1), 1 (2013)
433. Lin, S.K., Tsai, C.H., Li, H.J., Huang, C.Y., Chen, K.L.: Theory of mind predominantly associated with the quality, not quantity, of pretend play in children with autism spectrum disorder. Eur. Child Adolesc. Psych. **26**(10), 1187–1196 (2017)
434. Linder, T.: Transdisciplinary Play-Based Assessment. Wiley, Hoboken, US-NJ (2000)
435. Linder, T., Linas, K.: A functional, holistic approach to developmental assessment through play: the transdisciplinary play-based assessment. Zero to Three (J) **30**(1), 28–33 (2009)
436. Linder, T.W.: Transdisciplinary Play-Based Assessment: A Functional Approach to Working with Young Children. Paul H Brookes Publishing, Baltimore, US-MD (1993)
437. Linn, M.I., Goodman, J.F., Lender, W.L.: Played out? passive behavior by children with down syndrome during unstructured play. J. Early Interv. **23**(4), 264–278 (2000)
438. Logan, D.E., Breazeal, C., Goodwin, M.S., Jeong, S., O'Connell, B., Smith-Freedman, D., Heathers, J., Weinstock, P.: Social robots for hospitalized children. Pediatrics **144**(1) (2019)
439. Løokken, G.: Tracing the social style of toddler peers. Scand. J. Educ. Res. **44**(2), 163–176 (2000)
440. Lord, C., Rutter, M., DiLavore, P., Risi, S., Gotham, K., Bishop, S.: Autism Diagnostic Observation Schedule. Western Psychological Services, Los Angeles, US-CA (2009)

441. Lorenz, K.: Psychology and phylogeny. In: Bruner, J.S., Jolly, A., Sylva, K. (eds.) Play: Its Role in Development and Evolution, pp. 132–152. Basic Books, New York, US-NY (1976)
442. Louv, R.: The Nature Principle: Reconnecting with Life in a Virtual Age. Algonquin Books, Chapel Hill, US-NC (2012)
443. Lovaas, O.I.: Behavioral treatment and normal educational and intellectual functioning in young autistic children. J. Consult. Clin. Psychol. **55**(1), 3 (1987)
444. Luckett, T., Bundy, A., Roberts, J.: Do behavioural approaches teach children with autism to play or are they pretending? Autism **11**(4), 365–388 (2007)
445. Ludi, S., Ellis, L., Jordan, S.: An accessible robotics programming environment for visually impaired users. Proceedings of the 16th international ACM SIGACCESS conference on Computers & Accessibility, pp. 237–238 (2014)
446. Lund, H.: Playware e robotica modulare per il gioco. Italian J. Educ. Technol. **17**(2), 15–15 (2009)
447. Lund, H.H.: Disrupting the industry with play. J. Robot. Netw. Artif. Life **3**(1), 13–16 (2016)
448. Lupetti, M.L., Norese, M.F., Wu, X., Mi, H.: A video-based assessment of likeability and usability in a play application of robots for children. Meas. Bus. Excell. **23**(2), 110–120 (2019)
449. Luttropp, A., Granlund, M.: Interaction-it depends-a comparative study of interaction in preschools between children with intellectual disability and children with typical development. Scand. J. Disabil. Res. **12**(3), 151–164 (2010)
450. Lynch, H.: Which playspaces are appropriate for our children? In: Encarnação, P., Ray-Kaeser, S., Bianquin, N. (eds.) Guidelines for Supporting Children with Disabilities Play: Methodologies, Tools and Contexts, pp. 98–108. De Gruyter, Warsaw, PL (2018)
451. Lyon, M.: Symbolic play and language development in young deaf children. Deafness Educ. **21**(2), 10–20 (1997)
452. Lyytinen, P.: Developmental trends in children's pretend play. Child: Care, Health Dev. **17**(1), 9–25 (1991)
453. Macpherson, K., Charlop, M.H., Miltenberger, C.A.: Using portable video modeling technology to increase the compliment behaviors of children with autism during athletic group play. J. Autism Dev. Disord. **45**(12), 3836–3845 (2015)
454. Macy, M., Bagnato, S.J.: Keeping it "REAL" with authentic assessment. NHSA Dialog **13**(1), 1–20 (2010)
455. Maguire, E., Mulryan, N., Sheerin, F., McCallion, P., McCarron, M.: Autism spectrum disorder in older adults with intellectual disability: a scoping review. Irish J. Psychol. Med., **6**, 1–14 (2021)
456. Malaby, T.M.: Anthropology and play: the contours of playful experience. New Lit. Hist. **40**(1), 205–218 (2009)
457. Malaguzzi, L.: Fragments.Commentaries for a code to reading the exhibition. Scuole e Nidi d'infanzia - Istituzione of the Municipality of Reggio Emilia and Reggio Children, Reggio Emilia, I (2020)
458. Malone, D.M., Landers, M.A.: Mothers' perceptions of the toy play of preschoolers with intellectual disabilities. Int. J. Disabil. Dev. Educ. **48**(1), 91–102 (2001)
459. Malone, D.M., Stoneman, Z.: Cognitive play of mentally retarded preschoolers: Observations in the home and school. Am. J. Ment. Retard. **94**(5), 475–487 (1990)
460. Malone, M.: Patterns of home-and classroom-based toy play of preschoolers with and without intellectual disabilities. Int. J. Disabil. Dev. Educ. **56**(4), 333–347 (2009)
461. Martelo, A.B., Villaronga, E.F.: Child-robot interaction studies: from lessons learned to guidelines. Proceedings of the third Workshop on Child-Robot Interaction, CRI 2017: Research, Methodology and Best Practices at HRI 2017. HRI - Human Robot Interaction, Vienna, Austria (2017)
462. Martín, F.A., Castro-González, Á., Salichs, M.Á., et al.: Sound synthesis for communicating nonverbal expressive cues. IEEE Access **5**, 1941–1957 (2017)
463. Martinoia, D., Calandriello, D., Bonarini, A.: Physically interactive robogames: Definition and design guidelines. Robot. Auton. Syst. **61**(8), 739–748 (2013)

464. Martinoni, M., Scascighini, G.: Pedagogia specializzata e informatica. Esperienze e realizzazioni in Ticino, Edizioni del Segretariato svizzero di pedagogia curativa e speciale, Lucerna, CH (1997)
465. Mastyukova, E.M.: Speech Impairments of Children with Cerebral Palsy. Prosvesheniye, Moscow, RU (1985)
466. Mathur, S.: The ecology of play among young children of Mexican origin and seasonal farmworkers. In: Roopnarine, L., Patte, J.M., Johnson, K.D. (eds.) International Perspective on Children's Play, pp. 49–61. Open University Press/McGraw Hill, London, UK (2015)
467. Matson, J.L., Shoemaker, M.: Intellectual disability and its relationship to autism spectrum disorders. Res. Dev. Disabil. **30**(6), 1107–1114 (2009)
468. Matsumaru, T.: Friendly amusing mobile function for human-robot interaction. 19th International Symposium in Robot and Human Interactive Communication, pp. 88–93. IEEE (2010)
469. Mazzeo, M.: Il bambino cieco: introduzione allo sviluppo cognitivo. Anicia, Roma, IT (1988)
470. McCune, L.: A normative study of representational play in the transition to language. Dev. Psychol. **31**(2), 198 (1995)
471. McGillicuddy-De Lisi, A.V.: Sibling interactions and children's communicative competency. J. Appl. Dev. Psychol. **14**(3), 365–383 (1993)
472. McNeill, E., Sheehan, P., Marder, L.: Hearing issues. In: Newton, R.W., Puri, S., Marder, L. (eds.) Down Syndrome: Current Perspectives, pp. 70–76. Mac Keith Press, London, UK (2015)
473. McPartland, J.C., Reichow, B., Volkmar, F.R.: Sensitivity and specificity of proposed dsm-5 diagnostic criteria for autism spectrum disorder. J. Am. Acad. Child Adolesc. Psych. **51**(4), 368–383 (2012)
474. Medeiros, K.F., Cress, C.J.: Differences in maternal responsive and directive behavior during free play with and without aided aac. Augment. Altern. Commun. **32**(2), 151–161 (2016)
475. Merabet, L.B., Pascual-Leone, A.: Neural reorganization following sensory loss: the opportunity of change. Nat. Rev. Neurosci. **11**(1), 44–52 (2010)
476. Messier, J., Ferland, F., Majnemer, A.: Play behavior of school age children with intellectual disability: their capacities, interests and attitude. J. Dev. Phys. Disabil. **20**(2), 193–207 (2008)
477. Metatla, O., Bryan-Kinns, N., Stockman, T., Martin, F.: Designing with and for people living with visual impairments: audio-tactile mock-ups, audio diaries and participatory prototyping. CoDesign **11**(1), 35–48 (2015)
478. Metra, M.: Approches théoriques du jeu. IUFM, Lyon, FR. http://www2.ac-lyon.fr/etab/ien/ain/bourg2/IMG/pdf/Approches_theoriques_du_jeu.pdf (2006). Accessed: 2022-01-21
479. Michaud, F., Caron, S.: Roball, the rolling robot. Auton. Robot. **12**(2), 211–222 (2002)
480. Michaud, F., Laplante, J.F., Larouche, H., Duquette, A., Caron, S., Létourneau, D., Masson, P.: Autonomous spherical mobile robot for child-development studies. IEEE Trans. Syst. Man Cybernet.-Part A: Syst. Hum. **35**(4), 471–480 (2005)
481. Mikula, M.: Games, Toys, and Pastimes. Greenwood Press, Westport, US-CT (2007)
482. Miller, P.H.: Piaget's theory: Past, present, and future. In: Goswami, U. (ed.) The Wiley-Blackwell Handbook of Childhood Cognitive Development, pp. 649–672. Wiley-Blackwell, Hoboken, US-NJ (2011)
483. Miller, S.: Ends, means, and galumphing: some leitmotifs of play 1. Am. Anthropol. **75**(1), 87–98 (1973)
484. Miot, S., Akbaraly, T., Michelon, C., Couderc, S., Crepiat, S., Loubersac, J., Picot, M.C., Pernon, É., Gonnier, V., Jeandel, C., et al.: Comorbidity burden in adults with autism spectrum disorders and intellectual disabilities-a report from the efaar (frailty assessment in ageing adults with autism spectrum and intellectual disabilities) study. Front. Psych. **10**, 617 (2019)
485. Mirzaie Ranjbarr, R., Norouzi, G., Abedi, A., Ashori, M.: The effectiveness of intervention based on play therapy on the social skills and problems behaviors in children with intellectual and developmental disabilities (meta-analysis). Middle East. J. Disabil. Stud. **8**, 29–29 (2018)
486. Monceaux, J., Becker, J., Boudier, C., Mazel, A.: First steps in emotional expression of the humanoid robot nao. Proceedings of the 2009 International Conference on Multimodal Interfaces, pp. 235–236 (2009)

487. Morelli, T., Foley, J., Columna, L., Lieberman, L., Folmer, E.: Vi-tennis: a vibrotactile/audio exergame for players who are visually impaired. Proceedings of the Fifth International Conference on the Foundations of Digital Games, pp. 147–154 (2010)
488. Morgenstern, F.: Psychological handicaps in the play of handicapped children. Dev. Med. Child Neurol. **10**(1), 115–120 (1968)
489. Mori, M., MacDorman, K.F., Kageki, N.: The uncanny valley [from the field]. IEEE Robot. Autom. Mag. **19**(2), 98–100 (2012)
490. Motti, F., Cicchetti, D., Sroufe, L.A.: From infant affect expression to symbolic play: the coherence of development in down syndrome children. Child Dev. **54**(5), 1168–1175 (1983)
491. Moyson, T., Roeyers, H.: 'The overall quality of my life as a sibling is all right, but of course, it could always be better'. Quality of life of siblings of children with intellectual disability: The siblings' perspectives. Journal of Intellectual Disability Research **56**(1), 87–101 (2012)
492. Mundy, P., Neal, R.: Neural plasticity, joint attention and autistic developmental pathology. Int. Rev. Res. Mental Retard. **23**(139), 68 (2001)
493. Mundy, P., Sigman, M., Ungerer, J., Sherman, T.: Defining the social deficits of autism: the contribution of non-verbal communication measures. J. Child Psychol. Psych. **27**(5), 657–669 (1986)
494. Mundy, P., Sigman, M., Ungerer, J., Sherman, T.: Nonverbal communication and play correlates of language development in autistic children. J. Autism Dev. Disord. **17**(3), 349–364 (1987)
495. Muñoz, J.E., Dautenhahn, K.: Robo ludens: a game design taxonomy for multiplayer games using socially interactive robots. ACM Trans. Hum. Robot Interact. (THRI) **10**(4), 1–28 (2021)
496. Murdock, L.C., Ganz, J., Crittendon, J.: Use of an ipad play story to increase play dialogue of preschoolers with autism spectrum disorders. J. Autism Dev. Disord. **43**(9), 2174–2189 (2013)
497. Muys, V., Rodger, S., Bundy, A.C.: Assessment of playfulness in children with autistic disorder: A comparison of the children's playfulness scale and the test of playfulness. OTJR: Occup. Particip. Health **26**(4), 159–170 (2006)
498. Nadel, J.: Imitation and imitation recognition: Functional use in preverbal infants and nonverbal children with autism. In: Meltzoff, A.N., Prinz, W. (eds.) The Imitative Mind: Development, Evolution, and Brain Bases, pp. 42–62, Cambridge University Press, Cambridge, UK (2002)
499. Nader-Grosbois, N., Vieillevoye, S.: Variability of self-regulatory strategies in children with intellectual disability and typically developing children in pretend play situations. J. Intellect. Disabil. Res. **56**(2), 140–156 (2012)
500. Nakadoi, Y.: Usefulness of animal type robot assisted therapy for autism spectrum disorder in the child and adolescent psychiatric ward. JSAI International Symposium on Artificial Intelligence, pp. 478–482. Springer, Berlin, DE (2015)
501. Nevala, N., Pehkonen, I., Koskela, I., Ruusuvuori, J., Anttila, H.: Workplace accommodation among persons with disabilities: a systematic review of its effectiveness and barriers or facilitators. J. Occup. Rehabil. **25**(2), 432–448 (2015)
502. Newell, A.: Unified Theories of Cognition. Harvard University Press, Cambridge, US-MA (1990)
503. Nicolopoulou, A., Roopnarine, J., Smith, P.: Pretend and social pretend play: complexities, continuities, and controversies of a research field. In: Smith, P., Roopnarine, J. (eds.) The Cambridge Handbook of Play, pp. 183–199. Cambridge University Press, Cambridge, UK (2019)
504. Nikopoulos, C.K., Keenan, M.: Effects of video modeling on social initiations by children with autism. J. Appl. Behav. Anal. **37**(1), 93–96 (2004)
505. Nind, M.: Intensive interaction and autism: a useful approach? Br. J. Spec. Educ. **26**(2), 96–102 (1999)
506. Nomura, T., Suzuki, T., Kanda, T., Kato, K.: Measurement of anxiety toward robots. ROMAN 2006-The 15th IEEE International Symposium on Robot and Human Interactive Communication, pp. 372–377. IEEE Computer Press (2006)

507. Nomura, T., Suzuki, T., Kanda, T., Kato, K.: Measurement of negative attitudes toward robots. Interact. Stud. **7**(3), 437–454 (2006)
508. Oberman, L.M., Ramachandran, V.S.: The simulating social mind: the role of the mirror neuron system and simulation in the social and communicative deficits of autism spectrum disorders. Psychol. Bull. **133**(2), 310 (2007)
509. Okimoto, A.M., Bundy, A., Hanzlik, J.: Playfulness in children with and without disability: measurement and intervention. Am. J. Occup. Ther. **54**(1), 73–82 (2000)
510. de Oliveira, E., Donadoni, L., Boriero, S., Bonarini, A.: Deceptive actions to improve the attribution of rationality to playing robotic agents. Int. J. Soc. Robot. **13**(2), 391–405 (2021)
511. Oliveira, R., Arriaga, P., Correia, F., Paiva, A.: Looking beyond collaboration: socioemotional positive, negative and task-oriented behaviors in human-robot group interactions. Int. J. Soc. Robot. **12**(2), 505–518 (2020)
512. Oliverio, A.: The acting mind. the role of motricity in mental representation processes. In: Dompè, E., Tabasso, M.L., Trabalzini, P. (eds.) Proceedings of the Montessori Centenary Conference, 1907–2007, pp. 27–34. Opera Nazionale Montessori, Roma, IT (2007)
513. Olswang, L.B., Pinder, G.L.: Preverbal functional communication and the role of object play in children with cerebral palsy. Infant-Toddler Interv.: Transdiscipl. J. **5**(3), 277–99 (1995)
514. Ortibus, E., Fazzi, E., Dale, N.: Cerebral visual impairment and clinical assessment: the European perspective. Seminars in Pediatric Neurology, **31**, 15–24 (2019)
515. Owens, R.E., Jr.: Language Development: An Introduction. Pearson, Boston, US-MA (2016)
516. Ozaydin, L.: Teaching play skills to visually impaired preschool children: its effect on social interaction. Educ. Sci.: Theory Pract. **15**(4), 1021–1038 (2015)
517. Ozonoff, S., Goodlin-Jones, B.L., Solomon, M.: Evidence-based assessment of autism spectrum disorders in children and adolescents. J. Clin. Child Adolesc. Psychol. **34**(3), 523–540 (2005)
518. Pandey, A.K., Gelin, R.: A mass-produced sociable humanoid robot: Pepper, the first machine of its kind. IEEE Robot. Autom. Mag. **25**(3), 40–48 (2018)
519. Papoudi, D.: Interpersonal play and communication between young autistic children and their mothers. Ph.D. thesis, University of Edinburgh (1993). https://era.ed.ac.uk/handle/1842/20088?show=full
520. Papoudi, D.: The inclusion of children with Asperger disorder in the mainstream school. Hellenic Rev. Spec. Educ. **1**, 195–207 (2008)
521. Papoudi, D.: The Intersubjective Motives of Play: The Case of Autism. Elefterna, Special Issue: Intersubjective Paths to Interpersonal Relationships and Learning, **VII**(202), 204–239 (2015)
522. Papoudi, D., Kossyvaki, L.: Play and children with autism. insights from research and implications for practice. In: Smith, P., Roopnarine, J. (eds.) The Cambridge Handbook of Play, pp. 563–574. Cambridge University Press, Cambridge, UK (2019)
523. Parasuraman, A., Colby, C.L.: An updated and streamlined technology readiness index: Tri 2.0. J. Ser. Res. **18**(1), 59–74 (2015)
524. Paris, S.G., Oka, E.R.: Self-regulated learning among exceptional children. Except. Child. **53**(2), 103–108 (1986)
525. Parkes, J., White-Koning, M., Dickinson, H.O., Thyen, U., Arnaud, C., Beckung, E., Fauconnier, J., Marcelli, M., McManus, V., Michelsen, S.I., et al.: Psychological problems in children with cerebral palsy: a cross-sectional European study. J. Child Psychol. Psych. **49**(4), 405–413 (2008)
526. Parmenter, T.: Comparisons of the effects of teaching direct and indirect strategies on acquisition of reading skills by mildly developmentally disabled adolescents. Perspect. Prog. Mental Retardation **1**, 293–301 (1984)
527. Parsons, S.: Function of play in low vision children (part 1): a review of the research and literature. J. Vis. Impairment Blindness **80**(3), 627–630 (1986)
528. Parten, M.B.: Social participation among pre-school children. Psychol. Sci. Public Interest **27**(3), 243 (1932)

529. Pasternak, E., Fenichel, R., Marshall, A.N.: Tips for creating a block language with blockly. In: 2017 IEEE Blocks and Beyond Workshop (B B), pp. 21–24. IEEE Computer press (2017)
530. Patel, D.R., Cabral, M.D., Ho, A., Merrick, J.: A clinical primer on intellectual disability. Transl. Pediat. **9**(Suppl 1), S23 (2020)
531. Paterson, C.R., Arco, L.: Using video modeling for generalizing toy play in children with autism. Behav. Modif. **31**(5), 660–681 (2007)
532. Pedersen, J., Schelde, T.: Behavioral aspects of infantile autism: an ethological description. Eur. Child Adolesc. Psych. **6**(2), 96–106 (1997)
533. Peeters, M., Verhoeven, L., de Moor, J., Van Balkom, H.: Importance of speech production for phonological awareness and word decoding: The case of children with cerebral palsy. Res. Dev. Disabil. **30**(4), 712–726 (2009)
534. Pellegrini, A.D.: Object use in childhood: development and possible functions. In: Smith, P., Roopnarine, J. (eds.) The Cambridge Handbook of Play, pp. 165–182. Cambridge University Press, Cambridge, UK (2019)
535. Pellegrini, A.D., Hou, Y.: The development of preschool children's (homo sapiens) uses of objects and their role in peer group centrality. J. Comp. Psychol. **125**(2), 239 (2011)
536. Pellis, S.M., Pellis, V.C.: Rough-and-Tumble Play: Training and Using the Social Brain. Oxford University Press, Oxford, UK (2011)
537. Pellis, S.M., Pellis, V.C.: Play and cognition: the final frontier. In: Olmstead, M.C. (ed.) Animal Cognition: Principles, Evolution, and Development, pp. 201–230. Nova Science Publishers, New York, US-NY (2016)
538. Pellis, S.M., Pellis, V.C., Himmler, B.T.: How play makes for a more adaptable brain: a comparative and neural perspective. Am. J. Play **7**(1), 73–98 (2014)
539. Pereira, A., Martinho, C., Leite, I., Paiva, A.: ICAT, the chess player: the influence of embodiment in the enjoyment of a game. Proceedings of the 7th International Joint Conference on Autonomous Agents and Multiagent Systems, vol. 3, pp. 1253–1256 (2008)
540. Peres, L.W., Leite, A.C.A.B., de Andrade Alvarenga, W., Al, M.M., Ghazaoui, T.M.R., Nascimento, L.C.: Play therapy strategies in motor rehabilitation of children with cerebral palsy: an integrative review. Rev. Eletr. Enf. **20**, 20–25 (2018)
541. Périno, O.: Des espaces pour jouer. Erès, Lyon, FR (2016)
542. Périno, O., Besio, S.: Mainstream toys for play. In: Besio, S., Bulgarelli, D., Stancheva-Popkostadinova, V. (eds.) Play Development in Children with Disabilities, pp. 181–200. De Gruyter Open, Warsaw, PL (2017)
543. Peterson, C.C., Siegal, M.: Insights into theory of mind from deafness and autism. Mind Lang. **15**(1), 123–145 (2000)
544. Pfeifer, L.I., Pacciulio, A.M., Santos, C.A.d., Santos, J.L.d., Stagnitti, K.E.: Pretend play of children with cerebral palsy. Phys. Occupat. Therapy Pediat. **31**(4), 390–402 (2011)
545. Pfeifer, L.P., Cruz, D.M.C.: Play assessments and their evidences to practice of occupational therapist into special education. In: Almeida, M.A., Gonçalves, E.G., Hayashi, M. (eds.) Topic in Special Education: Multiple View (Temas em educação Especial: mùltiplos olhares), pp. 403–412. Junqueira & Marin, Brasılia, BR (2008)
546. Pfeifer, R., Bongard, J.: How the Body Shapes the Way We Think: A New View of Intelligence. MIT Press, Cambridge, US-MA (2006)
547. Piaget, J.: The Child's Conception of the World. Routledge and Kegan Paul, London, UK (1928)
548. Piaget, J.: Play, Dreams and Imitation in Childhood. Heinemann, Portsmouth, UK (1945)
549. Piaget, J.: Symbolic play. In: Bruner, J.S., Jolly, A., Sylva, K. (eds.) Play: Its Role in Development and Evolution. Penguin, London, UK (1976)
550. Pickersgill, M.: Bilingualism, current policy and practice. Issues Deaf Educ. **1**, 88–97 (1998)
551. Pierucci, J.M., Barber, A.B., Gilpin, A.T., Crisler, M.E., Klinger, L.G.: Play assessments and developmental skills in young children with autism spectrum disorders. Focus Autism Other Dev. Disabil. **30**(1), 35–43 (2015)
552. Pijnacker, J., Vervloed, M.P., Steenbergen, B.: Pragmatic abilities in children with congenital visual impairment: An exploration of non-literal language and advanced theory of mind understanding. J. Autism Dev. Disord. **42**(11), 2440–2449 (2012)

553. Pioggia, G., Igliozzi, R., Sica, M.L., Ferro, M., Muratori, F., Ahluwalia, A., De Rossi, D.: Exploring emotional and imitational android-based interactions in autistic spectrum disorders. J. Cyber, Therapy Rehabil. **1**(1), 49–61 (2008)
554. Pizzo, L., Bruce, S.M.: Language and play in students with multiple disabilities and visual impairments or deaf-blindness. J. Vis. Impairment Blindness **104**(5), 287–297 (2010)
555. Pollock, L.: Children at play in western Europe, 1500–1800. In: Smith, P., Roopnarine, J. (eds.) The Cambridge Handbook of Play, pp. 281–300. Cambridge University Press, Cambridge, UK (2019)
556. Pollock, N., Stewart, D., Law, M., Sahagian-Whalen, S., Harvey, S., Toal, C.: The meaning of play for young people with physical disabilities. Can. J. Occup. Ther. **64**(1), 25–31 (1997)
557. Poulin-Dubois, D., Lepage, A., Ferland, D.: Infants' concept of animacy. Cognit. Dev. **11**(1), 19–36 (1996)
558. Powers, M.: The smallest remainder: Benjamin and freud on play. MLN **133**(3), 720–742 (2018)
559. Pratt, S.R.: Nonverbal play interaction between hearing mothers and young deaf children. Ear Hear. **12**(5), 328–326 (1991)
560. Preisler, G.: The development of communication and language in deaf and severely hard of hearing children: implications for the future. Int. J. Pediatr. Otorhinolaryngol. **49**, S39–S43 (1999)
561. Preisler, G.M.: A descriptive study of blind children in nurseries with sighted children. Child: Care, Health Dev. **19**(5), 295–315 (1993)
562. Prellwitz, M., Skär, L.: How children with restricted mobility perceive the accessibility and usability of their home environment. Occup. Ther. Int. **13**(4), 193–206 (2006)
563. Prezbindowski, A.K., Adamson, L.B., Lederberg, A.R.: Joint attention in deaf and hearing 22 month-old children and their hearing mothers. J. Appl. Dev. Psychol. **19**(3), 377–387 (1998)
564. Prizant, B.M., Wetherby, A.M.: Enhancing language and communication in autism: from theory to practice. In: Dawson, G. (ed.) Autism: Nature, Diagnosis, and Treatment, pp. 282–309. Guilford Press, New York, US-NY (1989)
565. Profice, C., Santos, G., Anjos, N.: Children and nature in Tukum village: indigenous education and biophilia. J. Child Adolesc. Behav. **4**(6), 1–6 (2016)
566. Proulx, M.J., Brown, D.J., Pasqualotto, A., Meijer, P.: Multisensory perceptual learning and sensory substitution. Neurosci. Biobehav. Rev. **41**, 16–25 (2014)
567. Proulx, M.J., Gwinnutt, J., Dell'Erba, S., Levy-Tzedek, S., de Sousa, A.A., Brown, D.J.: Other ways of seeing: from behavior to neural mechanisms in the online "visual" control of action with sensory substitution. Restor. Neurol. Neurosci. **34**(1), 29–44 (2016)
568. Provenzo, E.F. Friedrich Froebel's Gifts. Connecting the Spiritual and Aesthetic to the Real World of Play and Learning. American Journal of Play, Summer, 85–99 (2009)
569. Quigley, S., Paul, P.: Language and Deafness. Croom Helm, London, UK (1984)
570. Quittner, A.L., Cejas, I., Wang, N.Y., Niparko, J.K., Barker, D.H.: Symbolic play and novel noun learning in deaf and hearing children: longitudinal effects of access to sound on early precursors of language. PLoS ONE **11**(5), e0155964 (2016)
571. Quittner, A.L., Leibach, P., Marciel, K.: The impact of cochlear implants on young deaf children: new methods to assess cognitive and behavioral development. Arch. Otolaryngol.-Head & Neck Surg. **130**(5), 547–554 (2004)
572. Ramírez-Duque, A.A., Aycardi, L.F., Villa, A., Munera, M., Bastos, T., Belpaeme, T., Frizera-Neto, A., Cifuentes, C.A.: Collaborative and inclusive process with the autism community: a case study in Colombia about social robot design. Int. J. Soc. Robot. **13**(2), 153–167 (2021)
573. Ray-Kaeser, S., Châtelain, S., Kindler, V., Schneider, E.: The evaluation of play from occupational therapy and psychology perspectives. In: Besio, S., Bulgarelli, D., Stancheva-Popkostadinova, V. (eds.) Evaluation of Childrens' Play: Tools and Methods, pp. 19–57. De Gruyter, Warsaw, PL (2018)
574. Ray-Kaeser, S., Perino, O., Costa, M., Schneider, E., Kindler, V., Bonarini, A.: Which toys and games are appropriate for our children? In: Encarnação, P., Ray-Kaeser, S., Bianquin, N. (eds.) Guidelines for Supporting Children with Disabilities Play: Methodologies, Tools and Contexts, pp. 98–108. De Gruyter, Warsaw, PL (2018)

575. Read, R., Belpaeme, T.: People interpret robotic non-linguistic utterances categorically. Int. J. Soc. Robot. **8**(1), 31–50 (2016)
576. Recchia, S.: Establishing intersubjective experience: developmental challenges for young children with congenital blindness and autism and their caregivers. In Lewis, V. , Collis, G.M. (eds.), Blindness and psychological development in young children, pp. 116–136. BPS Books, Leicester, UK (1997)
577. Reid, D.: The influence of virtual reality on playfulness in children with cerebral palsy: a pilot study. Occup. Ther. Int. **11**(3), 131–144 (2004)
578. Reid, D., Campbell, K., et al.: The use of virtual reality with children with cerebral palsy: a pilot randomized trial. Ther. Recreation J. **40**(4), 255 (2006)
579. Reid, S.M., Meehan, E.M., Arnup, S.J., Reddihough, D.S.: Intellectual disability in cerebral palsy: a population-based retrospective study. Dev. Med. Child Neurol. **60**(7), 687–694 (2018)
580. Rembis, M.: Challenging the impairment/disability divide. In: Watson, N., Vehmas, S. (eds.) Routledge Handbook of Disability Studies, pp. 377–390. Routledge, London, UK (2019)
581. Remine, M., Brown, P.: Playing with peers: play partner preferences and acceptability into play for preschoolers with and without normal hearing. Aust. J. Educ. Deaf **2**(1), 30–5 (1996)
582. Resnick, M., Maloney, J., Monroy-Hernández, A., Rusk, N., Eastmond, E., Brennan, K., Millner, A., Rosenbaum, E., Silver, J., Silverman, B., et al.: Scratch: programming for all. Commun. ACM **52**(11), 60–67 (2009)
583. Ribeiro, T., Paiva, A.: The illusion of robotic life: principles and practices of animation for robots. Proceedings of the Seventh Annual ACM/IEEE International Conference on Human-Robot Interaction, pp. 383–390 (2012)
584. Rickard, C., Strother, M., Fox, B.A., Raymond, C.W.: Scaffolding embodied access for categorization in interactions between a blind child and her mother. Languages **4**(1), 2 (2019)
585. Rizzolatti, G., Fadiga, L., Gallese, V., Fogassi, L.: Premotor cortex and the recognition of motor actions. Cognit. Brain Res. **3**(2), 131–141 (1996)
586. Roach, M.A., Barratt, M.S., Miller, J.F., Leavitt, L.A.: The structure of mother-child play: young children with down syndrome and typically developing children. Dev. Psychol. **34**(1), 77 (1998)
587. Roberts, S., Brown, P., Rickards, F.: Social pretend play entry behaviors of preschoolers with and without impaired hearing. J. Early Interv. **20**(1), 52–64 (1996)
588. Robins, B., Dautenhahn, K., Te Boekhorst, R., Billard, A.: Robotic assistants in therapy and education of children with autism: can a small humanoid robot help encourage social interaction skills? Univ. Access Inf. Soc. **4**(2), 105–120 (2005)
589. Rogers, S.J.: Play interventions for young children with autism spectrum disorders. In: Reddy, L.A., Files-Hall, T.M., Schaefer, C.E. (eds.) Empirically Based Play Interventions for Children, pp. 215–238. American Psychological Association, Washington, US-DC (2005)
590. Rogers, S.J., Hepburn, S., Wehner, E.: Parent reports of sensory symptoms in toddlers with autism and those with other developmental disorders. J. Autism Dev. Disord. **33**(6), 631–642 (2003)
591. Rogers, S.J., Puchalski, C.B.: Development of symbolic play in visually impaired young children. Top. Early Child. Spec. Educ. **3**(4), 57–63 (1984)
592. Rogow, S.M.: Rhythms and rhymes: Developing communication in very young blind and multihandicapped children. Child: Care, Health Dev. **8**(5), 249–260 (1982)
593. Roopnarine, J., Patte, M., Johnson, J., Kuschner, D.: International Perspectives on Children's Play. McGraw-Hill Education, New York, US-NY (2014)
594. Roopnarine, J.L.: Play as culturally situated: diverse perspectives on its meaning and significance. In: Roopnarine, J., Patte, M., Johnson, J., Kuschner, D. (eds.) International Perspectives on Children's Play, pp. 1–7. Open University Press, New York, US-NY (2015)
595. Roskos, K.: Play and literacy: knowns and unknowns in a changing world. In: Smith, P., Roopnarine, J. (eds.) The Cambridge Handbook of Play, pp. 528–545. Cambridge University Press, Cambridge, UK (2019)
596. Rubin, K.H., Fein, G.G., Vanderberg, B.: Play. In: Mussen, P., Hetherington, E.M. (eds.) Handbook of Child Psychology, vol. 4, p. 693–774. Wiley, Hoboken, US-NJ (1983)

597. Russ, S.W.: Play in Child Development and Psychotherapy: Toward Empirically Supported Practice. Routledge, London, UK (2003)
598. Russell, J.A.: A circumplex model of affect. J. Pers. Soc. Psychol. **39**(6), 11–61 (1980)
599. Russell, J.E.: Autism as an Executive Disorder. Oxford University Press, Oxford, UK (1997)
600. Ryalls, B.O., Harbourne, R., Kelly-Vance, L., Wickstrom, J., Stergiou, N., Kyvelidou, A.: A perceptual motor intervention improves play behavior in children with moderate to severe cerebral palsy. Front. Psychol. **7**, 643 (2016)
601. Šabanović, S., Bennett, C.C., Chang, W.L., Huber, L.: PARO robot affects diverse interaction modalities in group sensory therapy for older adults with dementia. 2013 IEEE 13th International Conference on Rehabilitation Robotics (ICORR), pp. 1–6. IEEE (2013)
602. Sacchi, F.: Applicazioni mobili per le persone con disabilitá visiva: una review delle proposte disponibili sullo store google play. Nuova Secondaria Ricerca **37**(4), 146–157 (2019)
603. Sackett, D.L.: Evidence-based medicine. Semin. Perinatol. **21**(1), 3–5 (1997)
604. Saerbeck, M., Bartneck, C.: Perception of affect elicited by robot motion. In: 2010 5th ACM/IEEE International Conference on Human-Robot Interaction (HRI), pp. 53–60. IEEE (2010)
605. Sahlins, M.: Colors and Cultures. De Gruyter, Berlin, DE (1976)
606. Sanders, T.: Implicit attitudes toward robots. Proceedings of the Human Factors and Ergonomics Society Annual Meeting, vol. 60, pp. 1746–1749 (2016)
607. Sandseter, E.B.H., Kennair, L.E.O.: Children's risky play from an evolutionary perspective: the anti-phobic effects of thrilling experiences. Evolut. Psychol. **9**(2) (2011)
608. Scassellati, B., Admoni, H., Mataric, M.: Robots for use in autism research. Ann. Rev. Biomed. Eng. **14**, 275–294 (2012)
609. Schaaf, R.C., Mailloux, Z.: Clinician's Guide for Implementing Ayres Sensory Integration: Promoting Participation for Children with Autism. AOTA Press, The American Occupational Therapy Association, Incorporated Bethesda (2015)
610. Schaaf, R.C., Toth-Cohen, S., Johnson, S.L., Outten, G., Benevides, T.W.: The everyday routines of families of children with autism: Examining the impact of sensory processing difficulties on the family. Autism **15**(3), 373–389 (2011)
611. Schalock, R.L., Borthwick-Duffy, S.A., Bradley, V.J., Buntinx, W.H., Coulter, D.L., Craig, E.M., Gomez, S.C., Lachapelle, Y., Luckasson, R., Reeve, A., et al.: Intellectual Disability: Definition, Classification, and Systems of Supports. American Association on Intellectual & Developmental Disabilities (2010)
612. Schalock, R.L., Luckasson, R., Tassé, M.J., Verdugo, M.A.: A holistic theoretical approach to intellectual disability: going beyond the four current perspectives. Intellect. Dev. Disabil. **56**(2), 79–89 (2018)
613. Schalock, R.L., Verdugo, M.A.: A conceptual and measurement framework to guide policy development and systems change. J. Policy Pract. Intellect. Disabil. **9**(1), 63–72 (2012)
614. Scheller, M., Petrini, K., Proulx, M.J.: Perception and interactive technology. In: Serences, J.T. (ed.) Stevens' Handbook of Experimental Psychology and Cognitive Neuroscience **2**, 1–50, Wiley and sons, Hoboken, US-NJ (2018)
615. Schick, B., De Villiers, P., De Villiers, J., Hoffmeister, R.: Language and theory of mind: a study of deaf children. Child Dev. **78**(2), 376–396 (2007)
616. Schirmer, B.R.: Relationship between imaginative play and language development in hearing-impaired children. Am. Ann. Deaf **134**(3), 219–222 (1989)
617. Schlottmann, A.: Perception versus knowledge of cause and effect in children: when seeing is believing. Curr. Dir. Psychol. Sci. **10**(4), 111–115 (2001)
618. Schopler, E., Van Bourgondien, M.E., Wellman, G.J., Love, S.R.: Childhood Autism Rating Scale (CARS2-ST, 2nd edn). Western Psychological Services, Los Angeles, US-CA (2010)
619. Schuengel, C., de Schipper, J.C., Sterkenburg, P.S., Kef, S.: Attachment, intellectual disabilities and mental health: research, assessment and intervention. J. Appl. Res. Intellect. Disabil. **26**(1), 34–46 (2013)
620. Schulze, C., Methúsalemsdóttir, H.F., Lynch, H., Jones, N.C., Winklhofer, U., Barron, C.: Empowering and enabling play in differing settings. In: Bulgarelli, D. (ed.) Perspectives and Research on Play for Children with Disabilities. De Gruyter-Sciendo, Warsaw, PL (2020)

621. Schum, R.: Psychological assessment of children with additional disabilities [study]. The Volta Rev. **104**(4), 237–255 (2004)
622. Schwartzman, H.: The sociocultural context of play. In: Sutton-Smith, B. (ed.) Play and Learning: Result of the Johnson Johnson Baby Products Company Round Table Conference III. pp. 239–255. Gardner Press, New York, US-NY (1979)
623. Scoglio, A.A., Reilly, E.D., Gorman, J.A., Drebing, C.E.: Use of social robots in mental health and well-being research: systematic review. J. Med. Internet Res. **21**(7:e13322), 1–8 (2019)
624. Scott, F.: Troublesome binaries. play and learning on screen and off. In: Smith, P., Roopnarine, J. (eds.) The Cambridge Handbook of Play, pp. 240–257. Cambridge University Press, Cambridge, UK (2019)
625. Seach, D.: Interactive Play for Children with Autism. Routledge, London, UK (2012)
626. Shakespeare, T.: Disability Rights and Wrongs Revisited. Routledge, London, UK (2013)
627. Sharpe, L.L.: Fun, fur, and future fitness: the evolution of play in mammals. In: Smith, P., Roopnarine, J. (eds.) The Cambridge Handbook of Play, pp. 49–66. Cambridge University Press, Cambridge, UK (2019)
628. Sharpe, L.L., Cherry, M.I.: Social play does not reduce aggression in wild meerkats. Anim. Behav. **66**(5), 989–997 (2003)
629. Sherratt, D.: The importance of play. Good Autism Pract. **1**(2), 23–31 (1999)
630. Sherratt, D.: Developing pretend play in children with autism: a case study. Autism **6**(2), 169–179 (2002)
631. Sherratt, D., Peter, M.: Developing Play and Drama in Children with Autistic Spectrum Disorders. David Fulton Publishers, London, UK (2012)
632. Shibata, T., Irie, R.: Artificial emotional creature for human-robot interaction-a new direction for intelligent systems. Proceedings of IEEE/ASME International Conference on Advanced Intelligent Mechatronics, pp. 47–52. IEEE (1997)
633. Shif, Z.: Development of children in schools for the mentally retarded. A Handbook of Contemporary Soviet Psychology, pp. 326–353. Basic Books, New York, US-NY (1969)
634. Shikako-Thomas, K., Majnemer, A., Law, M., Lach, L.: Determinants of participation in leisure activities in children and youth with cerebral palsy: systematic review. Phys. Occupat. Therapy Pediatr. **28**(2), 155–169 (2008)
635. Short, E.J., Schindler, R.C., Obeid, R., Noeder, M.M., Hlavaty, L.E., Gross, S.I., Lewis, B., Russ, S., Manos, M.M.: Examining the role of language in play among children with and without developmental disabilities. Lang. Speech Hear. Serv. Sch. **51**(3), 795–806 (2020)
636. Sidhu, J., Barlas, N., Lifter, K.: On the meanings of functional play: a review and clarification of definitions. Topics in Early Childhood Special Education, pp. 1–13 December (2020). https://journals.sagepub.com/doi/abs/10.1177/0271121420951859?journalCode=teca
637. Sigafoos, J., O'Reilly, M.F., Lancioni, G.E., Lang, R., Didden, R.: Self-injurious behavior. In: Sturmey, P., Didden, R. (eds.). Evidence-Based Practice and Intellectual Disabilities, pp. 133–162, Wiley & Sons, Hoboken, US-NJ (2014)
638. Sigel, I.E.: Research to practice redefined. In: Renninger, A., Sigel, I. (eds.) Handbook of Child Psychology, vol. 4, pp. 1017–1023. Wiley, Hoboken, US-NJ (2006)
639. Simeonsson, R.J., Leonardi, M., Lollar, D., Bjorck-Akesson, E., Hollenweger, J., Martinuzzi, A.: Applying the international classification of functioning, disability and health (ICF) to measure childhood disability. Disabil. Rehabil. **25**(11–12), 602–610 (2003)
640. Simplican, S.C., Leader, G., Kosciulek, J., Leahy, M.: Defining social inclusion of people with intellectual and developmental disabilities: an ecological model of social networks and community participation. Res. Dev. Disabil. **38**, 18–29 (2015)
641. Singer, D.G., Singer, J.L., D'Agnostino, H., DeLong, R.: Children's pastimes and play in sixteen nations: is free-play declining? Am. J. Play **1**(3), 283–312 (2009)
642. Singer, J.L., et al.: The Child's World of Make-Believe: Experimental Studies of Imaginative Play. Academic (1973)
643. Singh, A., Young, J.E.: A dog tail for communicating robotic states. International Conference on Human-Robot Interaction, pp. 417–418 (2013)

644. Siviy, S.M.: A brain motivated to play: insights into the neurobiology of playfulness. Behaviour **153**(6–7), 819–844 (2016)
645. Skär, L.: Disabled children's perceptions of technical aids, assistance and peers in play situations. Scand. J. Caring Sci. **16**(1), 27–33 (2002)
646. Skellenger, A., Hill, E.: The preschool learner. In: Wiener, W.R., Welsh, R.L., Blasch, B.B. (eds.) Foundations of Orientation and Mobility, pp. 407–438. American Foundation for the Blind Press, New York, US-NY (2005)
647. Skellenger, A.C., Hill, M., Hill, E.: The Social Functioning of Children with Visual Impairments. In: Odom, S.L., McConnell, S.R., McEvoy. M.A. (eds.) Social Competence of Young Children with Disabilities, pp. 165–188. Paul H. Brookes Publishing, Baltimora, US-MD (1992)
648. Slade, A., Wolf, D., Wolf, D.P.: Children at Play: Clinical and Developmental approaches to Meaning and Representation. Oxford University Press, Oxford, UK (1999)
649. Sleeuwenhoek, H.C., Boter, R.D., Vermeer, A.: Perceptual-motor performance and the social development of visually impaired children. J. Vis. Impairment Blindness **89**(4), 359–367 (1995)
650. Smilansky, S.: The Effects of Sociodramatic Play on Disadvantaged Preschool Children. Wiley, Hoboken, US-NJ (1968)
651. Smirnova, E., Kotliar, I., Sokolova, M., Sheina, E.: The children's playground in the context of cultural-historical psychology. Cult.-Hist. Psychol. **12**(3), 269–279 (2016)
652. Smith, P., Roopnarine, J.: The Cambridge Handbook of Play. Cambridge University Press, Cambridge, UK (2019)
653. Smith, P.K.: Children and Play: Understanding Children's Worlds, vol. 12. Wiley, Hoboken, US-NJ (2010)
654. Smyth, M.M., Anderson, H.I.: Coping with clumsiness in the school playground: social and physical play in children with coordination impairments. Br. J. Dev. Psychol. **18**(3), 389–413 (2000)
655. Solish, A., Perry, A., Minnes, P.: Participation of children with and without disabilities in social, recreational and leisure activities. J. Appl. Res. Intellect. Disabil. **23**(3), 226–236 (2010)
656. Spencer, H.: A System of Synthetic Philosophy: The Principles of Psychology. 2, vol. 2. D. Appleton & Company, Boston, US-MA (1873)
657. Spencer, P., Deyo, D.: Cognitive and Social Aspects of Deaf Children's play. In: Marschark, M., Clark, M.D. (eds.), Psychological perspectives on deafness, pp. 65–91. Lawrence Erlbaum, Hillsdale, US-NJ (1993)
658. Spencer, P., Waxman, R.: Joint attention and maternal attention strategies: 9, 12, and 18 months. In: Maternal responsiveness and child competency in deaf and hearing children, Final Report. Grant H023C10077, OSERS, US Department of Education (1995)
659. Spencer, P.E.: The association between language and symbolic play at two years: evidence from deaf toddlers. Child Dev. **67**(3), 867–876 (1996)
660. Spencer, P.E., Deyo, D., Grindstaff, N.: Symbolic Play Behavior of Deaf and Hearing Toddlers. In: Moores, D.F., Meadow-Orleans, K.P. (eds.), Educational and Developmental Aspects of Hearing Impairment, pp. 390–406. Gallaudet University Press, Washington, US-DC (1990)
661. Spencer, P.E., Marschark, M.: Evidence-Based Practice in educating Deaf and Hard-of-Hearing Students. Oxford University Press, Oxford, UK (2010)
662. Spencer, P.E., Meadow-Orlans, K.P.: Play, language, and maternal responsiveness: a longitudinal study of deaf and hearing infants. Child Dev. **67**(6), 3176–3191 (1996)
663. Spencer-Cavaliere, N., Watkinson, E.J.: Inclusion understood from the perspectives of children with disability. Adapt. Phys. Activ. Q. **27**(4), 275–293 (2010)
664. Spinka, M., Newberry, R.C., Bekoff, M.: Mammalian play: training for the unexpected. Q. Rev. Biol. **76**(2), 141–168 (2001)
665. Sprinkle, J., Hammond, J.: Family, health, and developmental background of children with developmental coordination disorder. Educ. Dev. Psychol. **14**(1), 55–62 (1997)

666. Stagnitti, K.: The Child Initiated Pretend Play Assessment (ChIPPA)[kit]. Co-ordinates Publications (2007)
667. Stanton, C.M., Kahn, P.H., Severson, R.L., Ruckert, J.H., Gill, B.T.: Robotic animals might aid in the social development of children with autism. 2008 3rd ACM/IEEE International Conference on Human-Robot Interaction (HRI), pp. 271–278. IEEE (2008)
668. Steinfeld, E., Maisel, J.: Universal Design: Creating Inclusive Environments. Wiley, Hoboken, US-NJ (2012)
669. Sternberg, R.J., Grigorenko, E.L.: Testing dinamico. Armando Editore, Roma, IT (2004)
670. Sternberg, R.J., Spear, L.C.: A triarchic theory of mental retardation. International Review of Research in Mental Retardation, **13**, 301–326 (1985)
671. Sterr, A., Green, L., Elbert, T.: Blind braille readers mislocate tactile stimuli. Biol. Psychol. **63**(2), 117–127 (2003)
672. Stone, W.L., Coonrod, E.E., Ousley, O.Y.: Brief report: screening tool for autism in two-year-olds (STAT): development and preliminary data. J. Autism Dev. Disord. **30**(6), 607 (2000)
673. Stone, W.L., Coonrod, E.E., Turner, L.M., Pozdol, S.L.: Psychometric properties of the STAT for early autism screening. J. Autism Dev. Disord. **34**(6), 691–701 (2004)
674. Stoneman, Z., Brody, G.H., Davis, C.H., Crapps, J.M.: Role relations between children who are mentally retarded and their older siblings: observations in three in-home contexts. Res. Dev. Disabil. **10**(1), 61–76 (1989)
675. Stropahl, M., Chen, L.C., Debener, S.: Cortical reorganization in postlingually deaf cochlear implant users: intra-modal and cross-modal considerations. Hear. Res. **343**, 128–137 (2017)
676. Struiksma, M.E., Noordzij, M.L., Postma, A.: What is the link between language and spatial images? Behavioral and neural findings in blind and sighted individuals. Acta Physiol. (Oxf) **132**(2), 145–156 (2009)
677. Sturmey, P., Didden, R.: Evidence-Based Practice and Intellectual Disabilities. Wiley, Hoboken, US-NJ (2014)
678. Suguitan, M., Hoffman, G.: Blossom: a handcrafted open-source robot. ACM Trans. Hum.-Robot Interact. **8**, 1–27 (2019)
679. Sundqvist, A., Lyxell, B., Jönsson, R., Heimann, M.: Understanding minds: early cochlear implantation and the development of theory of mind in children with profound hearing impairment. Int. J. Pediatr. Otorhinolaryngol. **78**(3), 538–544 (2014)
680. Sutterby, J.A.: "I wish we could do whatever we want!": children subverting scaffolding in the preschool classroom. J. Early Childhood Teacher Educ. **25**(4), 349–357 (2005)
681. Sutterby, J.A.: What kids don't get to do anymore and why. Child. Educ. **85**(5), 289–292 (2009)
682. Sutterby, J.A.: Lay spaces, indoors and out. In: Smith, P., Roopnarine, J. (eds.) The Cambridge Handbook of Play, pp. 667–685. Cambridge University Press, Cambridge, UK (2019)
683. Sutton-Smith, B.: Piaget on play: a critique. Psychol. Rev. **73**(1), 104–110 (1966)
684. Sutton-Smith, B.: Die Dialektik des Spiels [The dialectics of play]. Verlag Karl Hoffmann, Schorndorf, DE (1978)
685. Sutton-Smith, B.: Toys as Culture. Gardner Press, New York, US-NY (1986)
686. Sutton-Smith, B.: The Ambiguity of Play. Harvard University Press, Cambridge, US-MA (1997)
687. Sutton-Smith, B.: Play theory: a personal journey and new thoughts. Am. J. Play **1**(1), 80–123 (2008)
688. Tadić, V., Pring, L., Dale, N.: Attentional processes in young children with congenital visual impairment. Br. J. Dev. Psychol. **27**(2), 311–330 (2009)
689. Tager-Flusberg, H.: The challenge of studying language development in children with autism. In: Menn, L., Nan Bernstein Ratner, N. (eds.) Methods for Studying Language Production, pp. 317–336. Psychology Press, London, UK (1999)
690. Taggart, L., Cousins, W.: Health Promotion for People with Intellectual and Developmental Disabilities. McGraw-Hill Education, New York, US-NY (2014)
691. Takayama, L., Dooley, D., Ju, W.: Expressing thought: Improving robot readability with animation principles. Proceedings of the International Conference on Human-Robot Interaction, pp. 69–76. ACM Press, Lausanne, CH (2011)

692. Tannock, R., Girolametto, L., Siegel, L.: Language intervention with children who have developmental delays: effects of an interactive approach. Am. J. Mental Retardation: AJMR **97**(2), 145–160 (1992)
693. Tanta, K.J., Knox, S.H.: Play. In: Case-Smith, J., Obrien, J. (eds.) Occupational Therapy for Children and Adolescents, 7th edn., pp. 483–495. Mosby, St. Louis, US-MO (2015)
694. Taylor, B.A., Levin, L., Jasper, S.: Increasing play-related statements in children with autism toward their siblings: effects of video modeling. J. Dev. Phys. Disabil. **11**(3), 253–264 (1999)
695. Taylor, R., Iacono, T.: AAC and scripting activities to facilitate communication and play. Adv. Speech Lang. Pathol. **5**(2), 79–93 (2003)
696. Ten Eycke, K.D., Müller, U.: Brief report: new evidence for a social-specific imagination deficit in children with autism spectrum disorder. J. Autism Dev. Disord. **45**(1), 213–220 (2015)
697. Thelen, E.: Dynamic systems theory and the complexity of change. Psychoanal. Dialogues **15**(2), 255–283 (2005)
698. Theodorou, F., Nind, M.: Inclusion in play: a case study of a child with autism in an inclusive nursery. J. Res. Spec. Educ. Needs **10**(2), 99–106 (2010)
699. Thiyagalingam, J., Shankar, M., Fox, G., Hey, T.: Scientific machine learning benchmarks (2021). arXiv:2110.12773
700. Thomas, G.: A review of thinking and research about inclusive education policy, with suggestions for a new kind of inclusive thinking. Br. Edu. Res. J. **39**(3), 473–490 (2013)
701. Thommen, E., Cartier-Nelles, B., Guidoux, A., Wiesendanger, S.: Les particularités cognitives dans le trouble du spectre de l'autisme. Swiss Archives of Neurol. Psychiatry **165**, 290–297 (2014)
702. Thommen, É., Suárez, M., Guidetti, M., Guidoux, A., Rogé, B., Reilly, J.S.: Comprendre les émotions chez les enfants atteints d'autisme: regards croisés selon les tâches. Enfance **3**, 319–337 (2010)
703. Tieman, B.L., Palisano, R.J., Gracely, E.J., Rosenbaum, P.L., Chiarello, L.A., O'Neil, M.E.: Changes in mobility of children with cerebral palsy over time and across environmental settings. Phys. Occupat. Therapy Pediatr. **24**(1-2), 109–128 (2004)
704. Tingle, M.M., Tingle, M.: The Motor Impaired Child. Routledge, London, UK (2003)
705. Tioli, E.: Dallo spazio aptico alla rappresentazione immaginativo-motoria. Tratto da Biblioteca Italiana per i Ciechi "Regina Margherita". (2006). www.bibciechi.it/pubblicazioni/tiflologia/200601/Tioli.rtfVai
706. Tomasello, M., Call, J.: Primate Cognition. Oxford University Press, Oxford, UK (1997)
707. Torrance, E.P.: Factors affecting creative thinking in children: an interim research report. Merrill-Palmer Quart. Behav. Dev. **7**(3), 171–180 (1961)
708. Treffert, D.A.: The savant syndrome: an extraordinary condition. a synopsis: past, present, future. Philos. Trans. R. Soc. B: Biol. Sci. **364**(1522), 1351–1357 (2009)
709. Trevarthen, C.: Children with Autism: Diagnosis and Interventions to Meet Their Needs. Jessica Kingsley Publishers, London, UK (1998)
710. Trezza, V., Achterberg, E., Vanderschuren, L.J.: The neurochemistry of social play behaviour in rats. In: Smith, P., Roopnarine, J. (eds.) The Cambridge Handbook of Play, pp. 30–48. Cambridge University Press, Cambridge, UK (2019)
711. Tröster, H., Brambring, M.: Early motor development in blind infants. J. Appl. Dev. Psychol. **14**(1), 83–106 (1993)
712. Tröster, H., Brambring, M.: The play behavior and play materials of blind and sighted infants and preschoolers. J. Vis, Impairment Blindness, **88**(5), 421–432 (1994)
713. Trovato, G., Paredes, R., Balvin, J., Cuellar, F., Thomsen, N.B., Bech, S., Tan, Z.H.: The sound or silence: investigating the influence of robot noise on proxemics. 2018 27th IEEE International Symposium on Robot and Human Interactive Communication (RO-MAN), pp. 713–718. IEEE (2018)
714. Truong, A., Zaharia, T.: Laban movement analysis and hidden Markov models for dynamic 3d gesture recognition. EURASIP J. Image Video Process. **2017**(1), 1–16 (2017)

715. Tulloch, R.: The construction of play: rules, restrictions, and the repressive hypothesis. Games Cult. **9**(5), 335–350 (2014)
716. Turkle, S., Breazeal, C., Dasté, O., Scassellati, B.: Encounters with kismet and cog: children respond to relational artifacts. Digital Media: Transf. Hum. Commun. **120** (2006)
717. Turner, I.F., Small, J.D.: Similarities and differences in behaviour between mentally handicapped and normal preschool children during play. Child: Care, Health Dev. **11**(6), 391–401 (1985)
718. Turvey, M.T.: Nature of motor control: not strictly "motor", not quite "control". Adv Exp Med Biol., **629**:3–6 (2009)
719. Tzuriel, D.: Dynamic assessment of young children: educational and intervention perspectives. Educ. Psychol. Rev. **12**(4), 385–435 (2000)
720. Tzvetkova-Arsova, M., Zappaterra, T.: Play in children with visual impairments. In: Besio, S., Bulgarelli, D., Stancheva-Popkostadinova, V. (eds.) Play Development in Children with Disabilities, pp. 102–110. De Gruyter Open, PL (2017)
721. ÜÇGÜL, M.: History and educational potential of LEGO Mindstorms NXT. Mersin Üniversitesi Eğitim Fakültesi Dergisi **9**(2), 127–137 (2013)
722. Ugaste, A.: The Child's Play World at Home and the Mother's Role in the Play, vol. 259. Doctoral dissertation University of Jyväskylä (2005). https://jyx.jyu.fi/handle/123456789/13360?show=full
723. Uren, N., Stagnitti, K.: Pretend play, social competence and involvement in children aged 5–7 years: the concurrent validity of the child-initiated pretend play assessment. Aust. Occup. Ther. J. **56**(1), 33–40 (2009)
724. Van Breemen, A.: Bringing robots to life: Applying principles of animation to robots. Proceedings of Shaping Human-Robot Interaction Workshop held at International Conference on Computer-Human Interaction, pp. 143–144. Citeseer (2004)
725. Van Hasselt, V.B., Hersey, M., Kazdin, A.E., Simon, J., Mastanuono, A.: Training blind adolescents in social skills. J Vis Impairment Blindness **77**(5), 199–203 (1983)
726. Vermeulen, P.: The practice of promoting happiness in autism. In: Jones, G., Hurley, E. (eds.) Promoting Happiness and Wellbeing in Autism, pp. 23–34, British Institute of Learning Difficulties. Birmingham, UK (2014)
727. Veronese, F., Bulgarelli, D., Besio, S., Bianquin, N., Bonarini, A.: Off-the-shelf, robotic toys and physically impaired children: an analysis and suggested improvements. Proceedings of the 7th International Conference on Software Development and Technologies for Enhancing Accessibility and Fighting Info-Exclusion, pp. 232–239 (2016)
728. Verschure, P.F., Althaus, P.: A real-world rational agent: unifying old and new AI. Cognit. Sci. **27**(4), 561–590 (2003)
729. Veruggio, G., Operto, F., Bekey, G.: Roboethics: Social and ethical implications. In: Springer Handbook of Robotics, pp. 2135–2160. Springer, Berlin, DE (2016)
730. Vimercati, S., Galli, M., Stella, G., Caiazzo, G., Ancillao, A., Albertini, G.: Clumsiness in fine motor tasks: evidence from the quantitative drawing evaluation of children with d own syndrome. J. Intellect. Disabil. Res. **59**(3), 248–256 (2015)
731. Visalberghi, A.: Esperienza e valutazione. Taylor, Torino, IT (1958)
732. Volkmar, F.R., Klin, A.: Issues in the Classification of Autism and Related Conditions. Wiley, Hoboken, US-NJ (2005)
733. Volterra, V.: Gestures, signs, & words at two years: when does communication become language? Sign Lang. Stud. **33**, 351–362 (1981)
734. Volterra, V., Caselli, M.C.: From gestures and vocalizations to signs and words. Sign Lang. Res. **83** (1985)
735. Volterra, V., Erting, C.J.: From Gesture to Language in Hearing and Deaf Children. Gallaudet University Press, Washington, US-DC (1994)
736. Vu, J.A., Han, M., Buell, M.J.: The effects of in-service training on teachers' beliefs and practices in children's play. Eur. Early Child. Educ. Res. J. **23**(4), 444–460 (2015)
737. Vygotskij, L.S.: Thinking and speech. In: Rieber, R.W., Carton, A.S. (eds.) The Collected Works of L.S. Vygotsky: Problems of General Psychology, vol. 1, pp. 39–285. Plenum Press, New York, US-NY (1987)

738. Vygotskij, L.S., Rieber, R.W., Minick, N.: The History of the Development of Higher Mental Functions. Plenum Press, New York, US-NY (1997)
739. Wada, K., Shibata, T.: Living with seal robots-its sociopsychological and physiological influences on the elderly at a care house. IEEE Trans. Rob. **23**(5), 972–980 (2007)
740. Wall, K.: Modern approaches to orientation and mobility: habilitation and rehabilitation. In: Ravenscroft, J. (ed.) The Routledge Handbook of Visual Impairment, pp. 333–359. Routledge, London, UK (2019)
741. Wan, C.Y., Wood, A.G., Reutens, D.C., Wilson, S.J.: Early but not late-blindness leads to enhanced auditory perception. Neuropsychologia **48**(1), 344–348 (2010)
742. Watling, R.L., Deitz, J., White, O.: Comparison of sensory profile scores of young children with and without autism spectrum disorders. Am. J. Occup. Ther. **55**(4), 416–423 (2001)
743. Wauters, L.N., Knoors, H.: Social integration of deaf children in inclusive settings. J. Deaf Stud. Deaf Educ. **13**(1), 21–36 (2008)
744. Webster, A., Roe, J.: Children with Visual Impairments: Social Interaction. Language and Learning. Routledge, London, UK (1998)
745. Weisberg, D.S., Gopnik, A.: Pretense, counterfactuals, and bayesian causal models: Why what is not real really matters. Cognit. Sci. **37**(7), 1368–1381 (2013)
746. Weiss, A., Bartneck, C.: Meta analysis of the usage of the godspeed questionnaire series. 2015 24th IEEE International Symposium on Robot and Human Interactive Communication (RO-MAN), pp. 381–388 (2015)
747. Weiss, P.L., Bialik, P., Kizony, R.: Virtual reality provides leisure time opportunities for young adults with physical and intellectual disabilities. CyberPsychol. Behav. **6**(3), 335–342 (2003)
748. Wetherby, A.M.: Understanding and measuring social communication in children with autism spectrum disorders. In: Charman, T., Stone, W. (eds.) Social and Communication Development in Autism Spectrum Disorders: Early Identification, Diagnosis, and Intervention, pp. 3–34, Guilford Press, New York, US-NY (2006)
749. Wetherby, A.M., Prizant, B.M.: Communication and Symbolic Behavior Scales: Developmental Profile. Paul H Brookes Publishing Co., Baltimora, US-MD (2002)
750. Whitebread, D.: The importance of play. toy industries of europe (TIE) (2012). http://www.csap.cam.ac.uk/media/uploads/files/1/david-whitebread-importance-of-play-report.pdf. Accessed: 2022-02-06
751. Whitmore, A.S., Romski, M.A., Sevcik, R.A.: Early augmented language intervention for children with developmental delays: Potential secondary motor outcomes. Augment. Altern. Commun. **30**(3), 200–212 (2014)
752. Whittingham, K., Fahey, M., Rawicki, B., Boyd, R.: The relationship between motor abilities and early social development in a preschool cohort of children with cerebral palsy. Res. Dev. Disabil. **31**(6), 1346–1351 (2010)
753. Wieder, S., Greenspan, S.I.: Climbing the symbolic ladder in the dir model through floor time/interactive play. Autism **7**(4), 425–435 (2003)
754. Wills, D.M.: Early speech development in blind children. Psychoanal. Study Child **34**(1), 85–117 (1979)
755. Winnicott, D.: Playing and Reality. Tavistock Publications, London, UK (1971)
756. Winther-Lindqvist, D.: Playing games with rules in early child care and beyond. In: Smith, P., Roopnarine, J. (eds.) The Cambridge Handbook of Play, pp. 222–239. Cambridge University Press, Cambridge, UK (2019)
757. Wishart, J.: Learning the hard way: avoidance strategies in young children with down syndrome. Down Syndr. Res. Pract. **1**(2), 47–55 (1993)
758. Wistort, R., Breazeal, C.: Tofu: a socially expressive robot character for child interaction. Proceedings of the 8th International Conference on Interaction Design and Children, pp. 292–293 (2009)
759. Wolfberg, P., Bottema-Beutel, K., DeWitt, M.: Including children with autism in social and imaginary play with typical peers: integrated play groups model. Am. J. Play **5**(1), 55–80 (2012)

760. Wolfberg, P.J.: Peer play and the autism spectrum: The art of guiding children's socialization and imagination. AAPC Publishing, Shawnee, US-KS (2003)
761. Wolfberg, P.J., Schuler, A.L.: Integrated play groups: a model for promoting the social and cognitive dimensions of play in children with autism. J. Autism Dev. Disord. **23**(3), 467–489 (1993)
762. Wolfberg, P.J., Schuler, A.L.: Promoting Social Reciprocity and Symbolic Representation in Children with Autism Spectrum Disorders: Designing Quality Peer Play Interventions. The Guilford Press, New York, US-NY (2006)
763. Wood, D., Bruner, J.S., Ross, G.: The role of tutoring in problem solving. J. Child Psychol. Psychiatry **17**(2), 89–100 (1976)
764. Wood, H., Glaser, B., Eliez, S.: L'autisme-les nouveaux programmes thérapeutiques. Swiss Archives of Neurology and Psychiatry **164**(1), 13–19 (2013)
765. World Health Organization: International Classification of Functioning, Disability, and Health: Children and Youth Version: ICF-CY. World Health Organization (2007)
766. World Health Organization: Better health, better lives: children and young people with intellectual disabilities and their families (2010)
767. World Health Organization: Deafness and hearing loss (2025)
768. World Health Organization: Deafness and hearing loss factsheet. http://www.who.int/mediacentre/factsheets/fs300/en(2025)
769. Wright, B.: Development in deaf and blind children. Psychiatry **7**(7), 286–289 (2008)
770. Wright, I., Lewis, V., Collis, G.M.: Imitation and representational development in young children with down syndrome. Br. J. Dev. Psychol. **24**(2), 429–450 (2006)
771. Yaser, A.A., Cabibihan, J.J., Bonarini, A.: Influence of reaction time in the emotional response of a companion robot to a child's aggressive interaction. Int. J. Soc. Robot. **12**(6), 1279–1291 (2020)
772. Yazıcı, M., Livanelioğlu, A., Gücüyener, K., Tekin, L., Sümer, E., Yakut, Y.: Effects of robotic rehabilitation on walking and balance in pediatric patients with hemiparetic cerebral palsy. Gait & Posture **70**, 397–402 (2019)
773. Yoder, P.J., Warren, S.F.: Maternal responsivity predicts the prelinguistic communication intervention that facilitates generalized intentional communication. J. Speech Lang. Hear. Res. **41**(5), 1207–1219 (1998)
774. Yoshinaga-Itano, C.: Language assessment of infants and toddlers with significant hearing loss. Seminars in Hearing, **15**(2), 128–140 (1994)
775. Yoshinaga-Itano, C., Sedey, A.L., Coulter, D.K., Mehl, A.L.: Language of early-and later-identified children with hearing loss. Pediatrics **102**(5), 1161–1171 (1998)
776. Yoshinaga-Itano, C., Snyder, L.S., Day, D.: The relationship of language and symbolic play in children with hearing loss. Volta Rev. **100**(3), 135–64 (1999)
777. Zanelli, P.: Uno sfondo per integrare: esperienze di programmazione di situazioni educative. Cappelli, Bologna, IT (1987)
778. Zanobini, M., Usai, M.C.: Psicologia della disabilità e dei disturbi dello sviluppo. Elementi di riabilitazione e di intervento, FrancoAngeli, Milano, IT (2011)
779. Zihl, J., Dutton, G.N.: Cerebral Visual Impairment in Children. Springer, Berlin, DE (2016)
780. Zimpel, A.F.: Trisomy 21: What we can learn from people with Down syndrome. Vandenhoeck & Ruprecht, Göttingen, DE (2016)
781. Ziviani, J., Rodger, S., Peters, S.: The play behaviour of children with and without autistic disorder in a clinical environment. N. Z. J. Occupat. Therapy **52**(2), 22–30 (2005)
782. Zlatev, J.: The epigenesis of meaning in human beings, and possibly in robots. Mind. Mach. **11**(2), 155–195 (2001)

Index

A. Bonarini and S. Besio, *Robot Play for All*, Research for Development,
https://doi.org/10.1007/978-3-031-05042-8